Lumbar Intervertebral Disk Degeneration

Guest Editors

DINO SAMARTZIS, DSc
KENNETH M.C. CHEUNG, MD, FRCS

ORTHOPEDIC CLINICS OF NORTH AMERICA

www.orthopedic.theclinics.com

October 2011 • Volume 42 • Number 4

SAUNDERS an imprint of ELSEVIER, Inc.

W.B. SAUNDERS COMPANY
A Division of Elsevier Inc.

1600 John F. Kennedy Blvd. • Suite 1800 • Philadelphia, PA 19103-2899.

http://www.orthopedic.theclinics.com

ORTHOPEDIC CLINICS OF NORTH AMERICA Volume 42, Number 4
October 2011 ISSN 0030-5898, ISBN-13: 978-1-4557-1113-0

Editor: David Parsons
Developmental Editor: Donald Mumford

Orthopedic Clinics of North America (ISSN 0030-5898) is published quarterly by Elsevier Inc., 360 Park Avenue South, New York, NY 10010-1710. Months of issue are January, April, July, and October. Business and Editorial Offices: 1600 John F. Kennedy Blvd., Suite 1800, Philadelphia, PA 19103-2899. Customer Service Office: 3251 Riverport Lane, Maryland Heights, MO 63043. Periodicals postage paid at New York, NY and additional mailing offices. Subscription prices are $269.00 per year for (US individuals), $513.00 per year for (US institutions), $318.00 per year (Canadian individuals), $615.00 per year (Canadian institutions), $392.00 per year (international individuals), $615.00 per year (international institutions), $132.00 per year (US students), $191.00 per year (Canadian and international students). Foreign air speed delivery is included in all *Clinics* subscription prices. All prices are subject to change without notice. **POSTMASTER:** Send change of address to *Orthopedic Clinics of North America*, **Elsevier Health Sciences Division, Subscription Customer Service, 3251 Riverport Lane, Maryland Heights, MO 63043. Customer Service (orders, claims, online, change of address): Elsevier Health Sciences Division, Subscription Customer Service, 3251 Riverport Lane, Maryland Heights, MO 63043. Tel: 1-800-654-2452 (U.S. and Canada); 314-447-8871 (outside U.S. and Canada). Fax: 314-447-8029. E-mail: journalscustomerservice-usa@elsevier. com (for print support); journalsonlinesupport-usa@elsevier.com (for online support).**

Reprints. For copies of 100 or more, of articles in this publication, please contact the Commercial Reprints Department, Elsevier Inc., 360 Park Avenue South, New York, NY 10010-1710. Tel.: 212-633-3812; Fax: 212-462-1935; E-mail: reprints@elsevier. com.

Orthopedic Clinics of North America is covered in *MEDLINE/PubMed* (*Index Medicus*), *Cinahl, Excerpta Medica, and Cumulative Index to Nursing and Allied Health Literature.*

Printed and bound by CPI Group (UK) Ltd, Croydon, CR0 4YY

Transferred to Digital Print 2011

Contributors

GUEST EDITORS

DINO SAMARTZIS, DSc, PhD (C), MSc, MACE, Dip EBHC, FRIPH
Research Assistant Professor and Honorary Assistant Professor, Department of Orthopaedics and Traumatology, Division of Spine Surgery, Li Ka Shing Faculty of Medicine, The University of Hong Kong, Pokfulam, Hong Kong SAR, China

KENNETH M.C. CHEUNG, MBBS(UK), MD (HK), FRCS, FHKCOS, FHKAM(Orth)
Clinical Professor, Department of Orthopaedics and Traumatology, Division of Spine Surgery, La Ka Shing Faculty of Medicine, The University of Hong Kong, Pokfulam, Hong Kong SAR, China

AUTHORS

GUNNAR B.J. ANDERSSON, MD, PhD
Department of Orthopaedic Surgery, Rush University Medical Center, Chicago, Illinois

WON C. BAE, PhD
Assistant Professor, Department of Radiology, University of California, San Diego, San Diego, California

BARBARA P. CHAN, PhD
Tissue Engineering Laboratory, Department of Mechanical Engineering, The University of Hong Kong, Hong Kong SAR, China

DANNY CHAN, PhD
Associate Professor, Department of Biochemistry, Li Ka Shing Faculty of Medicine, The University of Hong Kong, Hong Kong SAR, China

WILSON C.W. CHAN, PhD
Department of Biochemistry, The University of Hong Kong, Li Ka Shing Faculty of Medicine, Hong Kong SAR, China

KENNETH M.C. CHEUNG, MBBS(UK), MD (HK), FRCS, FHKCOS, FHKAM(Orth)
Clinical Professor, Department of Orthopaedics and Traumatology, Division of Spine Surgery, La Ka Shing Faculty of Medicine, The University of Hong Kong, Pokfulam, Hong Kong SAR, China

JEREMY C.T. FAIRBANK, MA, MD, FRCS
Nuffield Department of Orthopaedics, Rheumatology and Musculoskeletal Sciences, Oxford University, Oxford, United Kingdom

THIJS GRUNHAGEN, DPhil
Formerly, Department of Physiology, Anatomy and Genetics, Oxford University, Oxford, United Kingdom; Currently, Philips Research, Eindhoven, The Netherlands

SERENA HU, MD
Department of Orthopedic Surgery, University of California, San Francisco, San Francisco, California

NOZOMU INOUE, MD, PhD
Professor and Director, Spine Biomechanics Laboratory, Department of Orthopedic Surgery, Rush University Medical Center, Chicago, Illinois

JAMES D. KANG, MD
Co-Director, The Ferguson Laboratory for Orthopaedic and Spine Research; Executive Vice Chairman; Professor, Department of Orthopaedic Surgery, University of Pittsburgh Medical Center, Pittsburgh, Pennsylvania

PATRICK YU-PING KAO, PhD
Department of Biochemistry, Li Ka Shing Faculty of Medicine, The University of Hong Kong, Pokfulam, Hong Kong SAR, China

JARO KARPPINEN, MD, PhD
Institute of Clinical Sciences, Department of Physical and Rehabilitation Medicine, University of Oulu, Oulu, Finland

JOHN KURHANEWICZ, PhD
Department of Radiology and Biomedical Imaging, University of California, San Francisco, San Francisco, California

VICTOR Y.L. LEUNG, PhD
Department of Orthopaedics and Traumatology, The University of Hong Kong, Hong Kong SAR, China

THOMAS M. LINK, MD
Department of Radiology and Biomedical Imaging, University of California, San Francisco, San Francisco, California

KEITH D.K. LUK, MCh(Orth), FRCSE, FRCSG, FRACS, FHKAM(Orth)
Department of Orthopaedics and Traumatology, The University of Hong Kong, Pokfulam, Hong Kong SAR, China

TEIJA LUND, MD, PhD
Consultant Spine Surgeon, ORTON Orthopaedic Hospital, Tenholantie, Helsinki, Finland

SHARMILA MAJUMDAR, PhD
Departments of Radiology and Biomedical Imaging and Orthopedic Surgery, University of California, San Francisco, San Francisco, California

KOICHI MASUDA, MD
Professor, Department of Orthopaedic Surgery, University of California, San Diego, La Jolla, California

H. MICHAEL MAYER, MD, PhD
Professor of Neurosurgery, Paracelsus Medical School, Salzburg, Austria; Medical Director, Spine Center, Schön Klinik Muenchen-Harlaching, Munich, Germany

ALEJANDRO A. ESPINOZA ORÍAS, PhD
Instructor and Assistant Director, Spine Biomechanics Laboratory, Department of Orthopedic Surgery, Rush University Medical Center, Chicago, Illinois

THOMAS R. OXLAND, PhD
Professor, Departments of Orthopaedics and Mechanical Engineering, University of British Columbia, Vancouver, British Columbia, Canada

DAISUKE SAKAI, MD, PhD
Department of Orthopaedic Surgery, Surgical Science, and Research Center for Regenerative Medicine, Tokai University School of Medicine, Isehara, Kanagawa, Japan

DINO SAMARTZIS, DSc, PhD (C), MSc, MACE, Dip EBHC, FRIPH
Research Assistant Professor and Honorary Assistant Professor, Department of Orthopaedics and Traumatology, Division of Spine Surgery, Li Ka Shing Faculty of Medicine, The University of Hong Kong, Pokfulam, Hong Kong SAR, China

PAK CHUNG SHAM, BM BCh, PhD
Chair Professor, Department of Psychiatry, Li Ka Shing Faculty of Medicine, The University of Hong Kong, Hong Kong SAR, China

FRANCIS H. SHEN, MD
Department of Orthopaedic Surgery, University of Virginia, Charlottesville, Virginia

ABOULFAZL SHIRAZI-ADL, PhD
Génie mécanique, École Polytechnique, Montréal, Québec, Canada

CHRISTOPH J. SIEPE, MD, PhD
Associate Professor of Orthopaedic Surgery, Paracelsus Medical School, Salzburg, Austria; Spine Center, Schön Klinik Muenchen-Harlaching, Munich, Germany

YOU-QIANG SONG, PhD
Assistant Professor, Department of Biochemistry, Li Ka Shing Faculty of Medicine, The University of Hong Kong, Pokfulam, Hong Kong SAR, China

GWENDOLYN SOWA, MD, PhD
Co-Director, The Ferguson Laboratory for Orthopaedic and Spine Research; Assistant Professor, Department of Physical Medicine and Rehabilitation, University of Pittsburgh Medical Center, Pittsburgh, Pennsylvania

LYNNE S. STEINBACH, MD
Department of Radiology and Biomedical Imaging, University of California, San Francisco, San Francisco, California

KIT LING SZE, PhD
Department of Biochemistry, The University of Hong Kong, Li Ka Shing Faculty of Medicine, Hong Kong SAR, China

VIVIAN TAM, PhD
Department of Orthopaedics and Traumatology, The University of Hong Kong, Hong Kong SAR, China

JILL P.G. URBAN, PhD
Department of Physiology, Anatomy and Genetics, Oxford University, Oxford, United Kingdom

NAM VO, PhD
The Ferguson Laboratory for Orthopaedic and Spine Research; Department of Orthopaedic Surgery, University of Pittsburgh Medical Center, Pittsburgh, Pennsylvania

BARRETT I. WOODS, MD
Resident Physician, The Ferguson Laboratory for Orthopaedic and Spine Research; Department of Orthopaedic Surgery, University of Pittsburgh Medical Center, Pittsburgh, Pennsylvania

Contents

Preface: Lumbar Intervertebral Disk Degeneration xi

Dino Samartzis and Kenneth M.C. Cheung

Structure and Biology of the Intervertebral Disk in Health and Disease 447

Wilson C.W. Chan, Kit Ling Sze, Dino Samartzis, Victor Y.L. Leung, and Danny Chan

The intervertebral disks along the spine provide motion and protection against mechanical loading. The 3 structural components, nucleus pulposus, annulus fibrosus, and cartilage endplate, function as a synergistic unit, though each has its own role. The cells within each of these components have distinct origins in development and morphology, producing specific extracellular matrix proteins that are organized into unique architectures fit for intervertebral disk function. This article focuses on various aspects of intervertebral disk biology and disruptions that could lead to diseases such as intervertebral disk degeneration.

Intervertebral Disk Nutrition: A Review of Factors Influencing Concentrations of Nutrients and Metabolites 465

Thijs Grunhagen, Aboulfazl Shirazi-Adl, Jeremy C.T. Fairbank, and Jill P.G. Urban

The biomechanical behavior of the intervertebral disk ultimately depends on the viability and activity of a small population of resident cells that make and maintain the disk's extracellular matrix. Nutrients that support these cells are supplied by the blood vessels at the disks' margins and diffuse through the matrix of the avascular disk to the cells. This article reviews pathways of nutrient supply to these cells; examines factors that may interrupt these pathways, and discusses consequences for disk cell survival, disk degeneration, and disk repair.

Genetics of Lumbar Disk Degeneration: Technology, Study Designs, and Risk Factors 479

Patrick Yu-Ping Kao, Danny Chan, Dino Samartzis, Pak Chung Sham, and You-Qiang Song

Lumbar disk degeneration (LDD) is a common musculoskeletal condition. Genetic risk factors have been suggested to play a major role in its cause. This article reviews the main research strategies that have been used to study the genetics of LDD, and the genes that thus far have been identified to influence susceptibility to LDD. With the rapid progress in genomic technologies, further advances in the genetics of LDD are expected in the next few years.

Biomechanics of Intervertebral Disk Degeneration 487

Nozomu Inoue and Alejandro A. Espinoza Orías

Degenerative changes in the material properties of nucleus pulposus and anulus fibrosus promote changes in viscoelastic properties of the whole disk. Volume, pressure and hydration loss in the nucleus pulposus, disk height decreases and fissures in the anulus fibrosus, are some of the signs of the degenerative cascade that advances with age and affect, among others, spinal function and its stability. Much remains to be learned about how these changes affect the function of the motion segment and relate to symptoms such as low back pain and altered spinal biomechanics.

Diagnostic Tools and Imaging Methods in Intervertebral Disk Degeneration

501

Sharmila Majumdar, Thomas M. Link, Lynne S. Steinbach, Serena Hu, and John Kurhanewicz

Low back pain has a negative impact on the economy and society. Intervertebral disk degeneration is linked to the occurrence of low back pain. MRI provides three-dimensional morphologic and biochemical information regarding the status of the disk. This article reviews new and evolving MRI disk-imaging techniques, including grading, relaxation-time measurements, diffusion, and contrast perfusion. In addition, high-resolution magic-angle spinning methods to correlate in vitro disk degeneration (with pain, etc) and in vivo spectroscopic results are discussed. With the potential for morphologic and biochemical characterization of the intervertebral disk, MRI shows promise as a tool to quantitatively assess disk health.

Management of Degenerative Disk Disease and Chronic Low Back Pain

513

Jaro Karppinen, Francis H. Shen, Keith D.K. Luk, Gunnar B.J. Andersson, Kenneth M.C. Cheung, and Dino Samartzis

Degenerative disk disease is a strong etiologic risk factor of chronic low back pain (LBP). A multidisciplinary approach to treatment is often warranted. Patient education, medication, and cognitive behavioral therapies are essential in the treatment of chronic LBP sufferers. Surgical intervention with a rehabilitation regime is sometimes advocated. Prognostic factors related to the outcome of different treatments include maladaptive pain coping and genetics. The identification of pain genes may assist in determining individuals susceptible to pain and in patient selection for appropriate therapy. Biologic therapies show promise, but clinical trials are needed before advocating their use in humans.

Adjacent Level Disk Disease—Is it Really a Fusion Disease?

529

Teija Lund and Thomas R. Oxland

Adjacent segment degeneration (ASD) is a relatively common phenomenon after spinal fusion surgery. Whether ASD is a consequence of the previous fusion or an individual's predisposition to continued degeneration remains unsolved to date. This article summarizes the existing biomechanical and clinical literature on the causes and clinical impact of ASD, as well as possible risk factors. Further, the theoretical advantage of motion-preserving technologies that aim to preserve the adjacent segment is discussed.

Prosthetic Total Disk Replacement—Can We Learn from Total Hip Replacement?

543

H. Michael Mayer and Christoph J. Siepe

Total lumbar disk replacement has become a routine procedure in many countries. However, discussions regarding its use are ongoing. Issues focus on patient selection, technical limitations, and avoidance or management of complications or long-term outcomes. A review of the development of this technology, since the development of the first successful implantation of a total lumbar disk prosthesis in 1984, shows an amazing analogy to the history of total hip replacement. This article is a one-to-one comparison of the evolution of total hip and total lumbar disk replacement from "skunk works" to scientific evidence.

Stem Cell Regeneration of the Intervertebral Disk

555

Daisuke Sakai

The use of stem cell applications has been explored and aimed at regenerating the intervertebral disk. The microenvironment in which cells of the intervertebral disk reside is harsh; however, researchers have reported on many applications for stem cells, including research aimed at defining and stimulating endogenous stem cell populations, methods to induce stem cell differentiation toward intervertebral disk cell phenotype in vivo, and direct transplantation of stem cells into damaged intervertebral disk to promote transplanted site-dependant differentiation. Successful results have been reported, although limitations remain. This article reviews the current status of stem cell research as applied to the intervertebral disk.

Gene Therapy for Intervertebral Disk Degeneration

563

Barrett I. Woods, Nam Vo, Gwendolyn Sowa, and James D. Kang

Intervertebral disk degeneration is a common and potentially debilitating disease process affecting millions of Americans and other populations each year. Current treatments address resultant symptoms and not the underlying pathophysiology of disease. This has spawned the development of biologic treatments, such as gene therapy, which attempt to correct the imbalance between catabolism and anabolism within degenerating disk cells. The identification of therapeutic genes and development of successful delivery systems have resulted in significant advances in this novel treatment. Continued investigation of the pathophysiology of disk degeneration, however, and safety mechanisms for the application of gene therapy are required for clinical translation.

Tissue Engineering for Intervertebral Disk Degeneration

575

Victor Y.L. Leung, Vivian Tam, Danny Chan, Barbara P. Chan, and Kenneth M.C. Cheung

Many challenges confront intervertebral disk engineering owing to complexity and the presence of extraordinary stresses. Rebuilding a disk of native function could be useful for removal of the symptoms and correction of altered spine kinematics. Improvement in understanding of disk properties and techniques for disk engineering brings promise to the fabrication of a functional motion segment for the treatment of disk degeneration. Increasing sophistication of techniques available in biomedical sciences will bring its application into clinics. This review provides an account of current progress and challenges of intervertebral disk bioengineering and discusses means to move forward and toward bedside translation.

Emerging Technologies for Molecular Therapy for Intervertebral Disk Degeneration

585

Won C. Bae and Koichi Masuda

Intervertebral disks are biologically regulated by the maintenance of a balance between the anabolic and catabolic activities of disk cells. Therapeutic agents, initially evaluated using in vitro studies on disk cells and explants, have been used as intradiscal injections in preclinical settings to test in vivo efficacy. These include anabolic growth factors, other biostimulatory agents, and antagonistic agents against matrix-degrading enzymes and cytokines. Additional work is needed to identify patient populations, using methods such as MRI, and to better understand the mechanism of healing. Clinical trials are underway for a few of these agents and other promising candidates are on the horizon.

Index

603

Orthopedic Clinics of North America

FORTHCOMING ISSUES

January 2012

Complex Cervical Spine Disorders
Frank M. Phillips, MD, and
Safdar N. Khan, MD,
Guest Editors

April 2012

Cartilage Injuries in the Pediatric Knee
Harpal K. Gahunia, PhD, and
Paul Sheppard Babyn, MD, *Guest Editors*

July 2012

Lifetime Management of Hip Dysplasia
George Haidukewych, MD, and
Ernest Sink, MD, *Guest Editors*

October 2012

Emerging Concepts in Upper Extremity Trauma
Michael P. Leslie, DO, and
Seth D. Dodds, MD, *Guest Editors*

RECENT ISSUES

July 2011

Legg-Calvé-Perthes Disease
Charles T. Price, MD, and
Benjamin Joseph, MS Orth, MCh Orth,
Guest Editors

April 2011

**Current Status of Metal-on-Metal
Hip Resurfacing**
Harlan C. Amstutz, MD,
Joshua J. Jacobs, MD, and
Edward Ebramzadeh, PhD, *Guest Editors*

January 2011

Obesity in Orthopedics
George V. Russell, MD, *Guest Editor*

THE CLINICS ARE NOW AVAILABLE ONLINE!

Access your subscription at:
www.theclinics.com

Preface
Lumbar Intervertebral Disk Degeneration

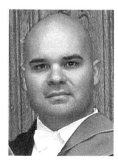

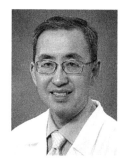

Dino Samartzis, DSc

Kenneth M.C. Cheung, MBBS(UK),
MD (HK), FRCS, FHKCOS, FHKAM(Orth)

Guest Editors

It has been our immense honor to serve as guest editors for this focus issue addressing lumbar intervertebral disk degeneration for the *Orthopedic Clinics of North America*. Throughout the years, we have come to appreciate and understand that disk degeneration is a complex, multifactorial condition that intrigues as well as perplexes. As such, disk degeneration continues to captivate the imagination and creativity of many physicians and researchers alike striving to understand its etiology and function, its role in the development of pain, and various treatment modalities. It is due to such devotion by many throughout the years that we are at an age where unique and novel therapies, such as artificial disk replacement, tissue engineering, molecular and genetic interventions, and stem cell use, have been developed to treat disk degeneration. Therefore, we hope that this focus issue will raise awareness of such developments and new technologies in the horizon.

This focus issue is not a product of one man or woman but a collaborative effort by many. We are fortunate to have contributions from worldwide leaders in the field of spine surgery, radiology, rehabilitation, epidemiology, and basic science that have come together to offer their insights toward a very complex topic. There is an old Chinese proverb that states, "In a dark world, do

not try to bring light to everything but try to light at least one candle." In line with this thinking, disk degeneration is regarded by many as the last frontier of spine conditions and disorders that at times its understanding is in our grasp and at other times it continues to elude us. Attempting to illuminate upon the complexities of this field is a daunting task. However, trying to bring to the forefront some of the more pressing issues will hopefully shed some light. We hope that each of these articles lights a "candle," stirring discussion and motivating action.

We would like to extend our sincerest gratitude to the journal's previous managing editor, Deb Dellapena, for her support of this focus issue. Furthermore, we are in tremendous appreciation of the current managing editor, David Parsons, and his entire staff for all of their countless hours and patience devoted to this initiative. We also extend our heartfelt gratitude to our families, friends, and colleagues for their support. In particular, we remain indebted to all of the authors of this focus issue and their wonderful contributions. Such collective contributions further stress the need for a multidisciplinary and collaborative approach toward advances in understanding and treating disk degeneration. In closing, we hope that this focus issue addressing lumbar intervertebral disk degeneration is

Orthop Clin N Am 42 (2011) xi–xii
doi:10.1016/j.ocl.2011.08.001

informative and insightful. However, more importantly, we hope this journal issue will inspire the physician and researcher to further broaden the understanding of this condition by striving to advance medical knowledge to ultimately improve patient care, outcomes, and quality of life.

Sincerely,

Dino Samartzis, DSc
Kenneth M.C. Cheung, MBBS(UK), MD (HK), FRCS, FHKCOS, FHKAM(Orth)

Department of Orthopaedics and Traumatology
Division of Spine Surgery
Li Ka Shing Faculty of Medicine
The University of Hong Kong
Professorial Block, 5th Floor
102 Pokfulam Road
Pokfulam, Hong Kong SAR, China

E-mail addresses:
dsamartzis@msn.com (D. Samartzis)
cheungmc@hku.hk (K.M.C. Cheung)

Structure and Biology of the Intervertebral Disk in Health and Disease

Wilson C.W. Chan, PhD[a], Kit Ling Sze, PhD[a],
Dino Samartzis, DSc[b], Victor Y.L. Leung, PhD[c],
Danny Chan, PhD[a],*

KEYWORDS

- Intervertebral disk • Degeneration • Extracellular matrix
- Development • Biology

Low back pain is a leading debilitating condition that affects every population worldwide,[1] and can lead to diminished physical function, loss of wages, decreased quality of life, and psychological distress.[1–4] In fact, chronic low back pain may also lead to brain tissue destruction.[5–8] As a consequence, low back pain is one of the most common conditions for which to seek medical consultation and one of those preeminent for analgesic use in the United States.[3,4] Furthermore, the management of patients with low back pain can be a challenge, often requiring a multidisciplinary approach to treatment (see the article by Karppinen and colleagues elsewhere in this issue).[9–13]

Although low back pain is a multifactorial condition (eg, biopsychological, muscular, socioeconomic), intervertebral disk (IVD) degeneration has been indicated to be a strong etiologic factor (Fig. 1).[14–24] Intervertebral disk degeneration occurs in every population worldwide, mainly involving the lower lumbar segments (L4 to S1) where disk height narrowing also commonly occurs and generally affects almost all individuals by the sixth and seventh decade of life.[24,25] However, the development or, rather, severity of IVD degeneration is not linearly based on age; degenerative changes can be noted in young children and not yet be manifested in other adults.[19,24] Overall, the true prevalence of IVD degeneration in populations has yet to be determined, due to improper surveillance methods (ie, patient-based versus population-based), sampling issues, heterogeneity in the operational definition and imaging modalities in assessing the phenotype of disk changes, and an incomplete understanding of the risk-factor profile and its interaction effects that may affect degenerative changes and their manifestation in different age, gender, and ethnic groups.[14,15,26] Along these lines, the incidence rates of annular tears, disk bulging, and endplate defects/abnormalities are also not conclusive, and vary between studies.

The development of IVD degeneration is a complex, multifaceted condition. Various studies have suggested that, age, male gender, abnormal physical loading, trauma, infection, hormonal, overweight and obesity, altered metabolism, Schmorl's

This work was supported by an Area of Excellence grant from the University Grants Committee of Hong Kong (AoE/M-04/04).

[a] Department of Biochemistry, The University of Hong Kong, LKS Faculty of Medicine, Laboratory Block, 3rd Floor, 21 Sassoon Road, Pokfulam, Hong Kong SAR, China

[b] Department of Orthopaedics and Traumatology, Division of Spine Surgery, Li Ka Shing Faculty of Medicine, The University of Hong Kong, Professorial Block, 5th Floor, 102 Pokfulam Road, Pokfulam, Hong Kong SAR, China

[c] Department of Orthopaedics & Traumatology, The University of Hong Kong, Professorial Block, 5th Floor, 102 Pokfulam Road, Pokfulam, Hong Kong SAR, China

* Corresponding author.
E-mail address: chand@hku.hk

Orthop Clin N Am 42 (2011) 447–464
doi:10.1016/j.ocl.2011.07.012

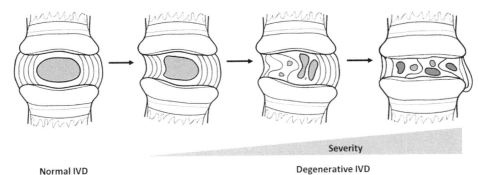

Severity

Normal IVD   Degenerative IVD

Fig. 1. Illustration of the different stages of intervertebral disk degeneration. Note the normal disk on the left and the progression of degenerative changes from left to right, which are characterized as chemical and structural changes of the disk (eg, dehydration of the nucleus pulposus, disruption of the annulus fibrosus, decreased disk height, and endplate changes). IVD, intervertebral disk.

nodes, cigarette smoking, and occupation are risk factors related to the development of IVD degeneration.[20,27–41] Several investigators have also noted that systemic conditions, such as atherosclerosis, may contribute to IVD degeneration, due to the "vascular insufficiency" provided to the vertebral body that may affect diffusion of metabolites and nutrients into the disk necessary to maintain a healthy environment.[42–46] Furthermore, it has been strongly suggested that IVD degeneration may be attributed to genetic factors. Familial aggregation studies have indicated that individuals with severe forms of IVD degeneration that are often symptomatic have family members with a history of disk-related problems, often seeking medical attention themselves.[47–51] Twin studies have also noted that more than 70% of variability of IVD degeneration may be attributed to genetics.[52–55] Moreover, observational cohort studies have identified specific genes that may play a role in the development of IVD degeneration, some of which may have a synergistic effect with environmental exposures and perhaps be age dependent (see the article by Kao and colleagues elsewhere in this issue).[56–59] As such, understanding the genetic epidemiology of IVD degeneration is imperative in comprehending the scope of the degenerative condition, why degenerative changes occur in certain individuals rather than others, and in developing a better understanding of the use of biological therapies for the prevention or regeneration of the disease process (see the articles by Sakai, Woods and colleagues, Leung and colleagues, and Bae and Masuda elsewhere in this issue). However, at a more basic level, understanding the structure and biology of the IVD in health and disease, in particular the developmental process, cellular origin, changes in the extracellular matrix (ECM) components, and maintenance in adult life, is essential.

INTERVERTEBRAL DISK

The IVD is a functional unit connecting the vertebral bodies of the spine. In humans there are 25 IVDs interposed from the axis to the sacrum. Each IVD consists of 3 structural components: a soft gelatinous nucleus pulposus (NP) in the center surrounded by a tough peripheral lamellar annulus fibrosus (AF), sandwiched between 2 cartilaginous endplates (EP) (**Fig. 2**). The components of the disk act synergistically, facilitating motions of the spine and acting as shock absorbers between vertebral bodies.[60–62]

Traditional concepts on the function of the disk relate to specific ECM proteins that assemble and interact to form the 3 distinct structures. While one can describe the NP, AF, and EP separately with distinct functions, the homeostasis of the IVD as a unit must have optimal function from all 3 structures. The impairment of one or more of these structures can lead to dire consequences with IVD degeneration. The ECM is produced and maintained by resident cells, and there are feedback mechanisms for cells to sense the ECM, while the ECM regulates extrinsic signals to cells for disk homeostasis.

DEVELOPMENT OF THE INTERVERTEBRAL DISK

The notochord is central to the development of IVD. The notochord is a rod-shaped midline structure of mesodermal origin found in chordate embryos during gastrulation, and represents a primitive axial skeleton.[63,64] As a structure that is recognized in all vertebrate embryos, its development has been well studied and described since the nineteenth century.[65] It is composed of cells derived from the organizer tissue at different stages of development.

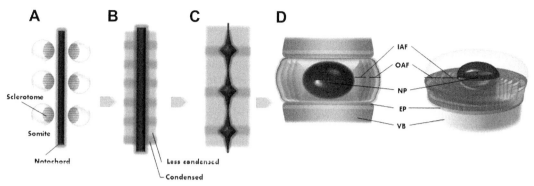

Fig. 2. Development of the intervertebral disk. (*A*) In early development, the notochord is localized adjacent to pairs of paraxial somites containing sclerotome cells. (*B*) Sclerotome cells migrate and condense around the notochord forming the perinotochordal sheath, with a metameric pattern of condensed and uncondensed regions (*C*) The notochord contracts within the developing vertebral bodies and expands within the future nucleus pulposus regions of the intervertebral disk. (*D*) Establishment of the basic structure of the intervertebral disk with formation of the cartilage endplate and the lamellar structures of the annulus fibrosus. EP, endplate; IAF, inner annulus fibrosus; NP, nucleus pulposus; OAF, outer annulus fibrosus; VB, vertebral body.

The contribution of the organizer to different regions of the notochord along the anterior-posterior axis is complex, but has been studied using cell-mapping tools and live time-lapse imaging.[66,67] In principle, the anterior notochord is formed by direct convergence of the anterior dispersed cells, the trunk notochord is formed by convergent extension of the node-derived cells, and the tail notochord is formed by posterior migration of the node-derived progenitors. The notochord is important not only as a signaling center but also as a structure that gives rise to the future NP.

In early gestation stages (30 days in human, 12 days in mouse), the notochord is located adjacent to the paraxial somites (see **Fig. 2**A) and can induce the differentiation of the ventral somatic derivatives into the sclerotome.[68] Sclerotome cells migrate and condense around the notochord, forming the perinotochordal sheath (see **Fig. 2**B). The cells form the unsegmented perichordal mesenchyme with a metameric pattern of condensed and uncondensed regions.[69] The condensed mesenchyme will give rise to the AF of the disk, whereas the uncondensed mesenchyme will form the future vertebral body, developed first as a continuous cartilaginous column forming around the notochord. As development progresses, the notochord is thought to be compressed or squeezed away from the cartilage anlagen regions of the vertebral bodies and expanded in the IVD anlagen regions (see **Fig. 2**C), giving rise to the future NP. In some instances remnants of the notochord can be detected within vertebral bodies, and are thought to be a possible origin of chordomas[69–71]; this would support the idea that notochordal cells may have progenitor properties.

Although this notion remains controversial, cell-tracking analysis of notochordal cells in the mouse suggests this may be the case, with perhaps subsequent differentiation to mature NP cells.[70]

To date, no cell-tracking data are available to confirm the origin of the AF cells, but it is thought to originate from the somites. Little is known regarding the origin of the cells in the EP and its formation. It was first postulated that the NP is not derived from the side of the vertebral body but from undifferentiated cells, which accumulate in early development and develop into an organized structure under mechanical influences. This hypothesis was later refined to suggest induction from mechanical stimulus due to actions of compressive forces, torsion, and shear stresses occurring in the IVD, similar to the mechanical stresses that induce thickening and delamination of connective tissues (see the article by Inoue and Espinoza Orias elsewhere in this issue). Thus, the hyaline cartilage EP represents the interface between the vertebral body and the disk, and the annular epiphysis of the vertebral body develops in the marginal part of the EP. These descriptions of IVD development are derived from previous detailed anatomic analyses that need to be revisited using modern tools in molecular genetics, such as those available in the mouse.

STRUCTURAL ORGANIZATION OF THE INTERVERTEBRAL DISK

The AF is made up of concentric angle-ply layers that cross one another obliquely in space (see **Fig. 2**D). The AF is divided into inner and outer regions, which have distinct biochemical and cellular composition as well as biomechanical properties. The outer AF is composed of fibroblastic cells, which produce type I collagen. The collagen fibrils form fibers, which run parallel within each lamella, organized into a ligamentous structure that inserts into the adjacent vertebral bodies.[72,73] Bundles of microfibrils are distributed within the interterritorial matrix and are colocalized with elastin fibers.[74] Cells in the inner AF are more chondrocyte-like, producing mainly type II collagen, and proteoglycans such as aggrecan. These changes give rise to a less fibrous and less organized structure compared with the outer AF.[75]

The vertebral EP is composed of two layers: an inner bony layer and an outer cartilaginous layer. The latter is a thin horizontal layer of articular cartilaginous structure, which interfaces the vertebral bodies and the IVDs. IVDs have limited nerve and blood vessel supply,[76,77] and the EPs act as the source and regulator of nutrient and oxygen diffusion from the vertebral bodies (see the article by Grunhagen and colleagues elsewhere in this issue).[78] The NP is an aggrecan-rich jellylike structure confined within the EP and AF. It is composed of chondrocyte-like cells producing polysaccharide/mucoprotein molecules, such as chondroitin sulfate, collagen, and elastin fibers. Aggrecan, with high anionic glycosaminoglycan content, is the major type of proteoglycan in the IVDs, providing the osmotic properties for compressive loading.[79] The specific matrix composition in each structural compartment supports the different mechanical role and cell signaling function of the disk cells.

The NP represents the center of the IVD. This region of the disk has attracted much attention, as it is thought to be where degeneration occurs with changes in cell morphology and ECM components, leading to reduced water content and narrowed disk height. In humans, studies have suggested that notochordal cells disappear after the establishment of the spinal column, and the cell population is gradually replaced by chondrocyte-like NP cells, whereas in mouse and other species notochordal cells are maintained in the NP.[80,81] There is also an apparent correlation between this maintenance of notochordal characteristics of cells in the NP and susceptibility to disk degeneration in the different species studied, including mouse, rat, rabbit, dog, sheep, and human. However, this is an area of controversy, as the "absence" of notochordal cells is based on morphologic and histologic studies.[82,83] Furthermore, notochordal-related molecular markers, such as cytokeratin types CK-8, CK-18, CK-19, and galectin-3, can be detected in adult human NP cells.[84–87] Thus, the precise fate of notochordal cells remains to be resolved.[70,87–91]

EXTRACELLULAR MATRIX AND IVD FUNCTION

The ECM in the IVD is a dynamic network of structural proteins that contributes to disk function, resisting mechanical loading and tensile force. While a key function of ECM is structural, one must also consider that the ECM provides the environment for cell maintenance and survival. In addition, the array of ECM components and the functionalities that they carry provide diverse interactions with soluble factors, such as growth factors, cytokines, morphogens, chemokines, and enzymes, modulating their interaction with or presentation to cells. The ECM is not an inert substance but continues to be produced and degraded in remodeling and repair processes. Throughout life, there are significant changes in the molecular composition and organization of the ECM network as part of development, growth, and aging.[92,93] Accelerated imbalance between anabolic and catabolic events within the IVD will affect the integrity of the matrix and disk function, leading to early IVD degeneration.[94–96]

In general, the major ECM components consist of collagens organized into various fibrillar networks providing the tensile strength required for specific tissue function.[97–99] The presence of elastin gives added elasticity to tissues.[100] Proteoglycans contain a small core protein, but have many highly negatively charged glycosaminoglycan (GAG) side chains, providing opportunities for interactions with other matrix molecules and soluble factors.[101,102] These GAG elements also attract cations with water retention properties, contributing to tissue hydration. Lastly, there is a huge array of structural glycoproteins, such as fibronectin,[103,104] laminins,[105] and tenasins.[106] These structural glycoproteins help to fine-tune tissue functionality as well as assist in the assembling and organization of the matrix. The ECM components and their role in IVD function are discussed here in relation to the specific IVD structures.

Annulus Fibrosus

The AF is a highly structured lamellar tissue, and can be subdivided into the outer annulus and inner annulus. In a healthy adult human disk, the outer annulus is made up of a series of 15 to 25 concentric lamellae with highly ordered collagen fibers oriented in sheets parallel with each lamella.[72,73] The outer annulus is composed of mainly type I collagen attributing to approximately 90% of the collagens in the IVD, together with smaller amounts of collagen types III, V, and VI.[107] Type III and V collagens can form heterotypic fibrils with type I collagen, providing diversity to fibril properties, whereas type VI collagen molecules assemble into beaded filaments.[108] These collagen fibrils network with adjacent lamellae, working cooperatively with each other during dynamic loading.

Elastic fibers, which make up only 2% of the AF dry weight, is another organized ECM network that aligns parallel with the lamellae. The outer annulus consists of a higher elastin density and has a greater elastin colocalization with mircofibrils in comparison with the inner annulus.[74] Elastin is concentrated between the lamellae and is thought to function in protecting the disk from delamination, as well as help with the recovery of the lamellar structure after deformation under radial loads.[74]

Of interest, a translamellar bridging network (TLBN) has been identified within the AF,[109] where there is a network consisting of translamellar bridging fibers within the inter bundle space of an individual lamella, connecting fibers of the adjacent lamellae. The structural alignment of TLBN is suggested to enhance resistance toward radial, lifting, and torsional forces, and prevents the disjunction of lamellae under torsional force.[109]

Toward the inner AF, there is a transition to a type II collagen-enriched structure, with higher content of proteoglycans such as aggrecan, biglycans, and lumican, which results in a less organized fibrous structure.[75] The reason for this transition is not clear; perhaps there is a need for a progressive change of AF to establish a functional link between inner AF and the type II collagen–enriched NP. Postnatally, the boundary between the outer and the inner AF become less distinct, as does the interface between the inner AF and the NP with aging.

Nucleus Pulposus

As the NP enlarges with growth, it is filled with a soft cartilaginous-like matrix, but consists of very high levels of proteoglycans entrapped in a randomly orientated type II collagen fibrous network (**Fig. 3**). Like cartilage, there are also small amounts of type XI and IX collagens. Type XI collagens associate with type II collagens to form heterotypic collagen fibrils, whereas type IX collagen is a fibril-associated collagen that coats the surface of these cartilage-like collagen fibrils. There are unique interruptions within the triple helix of type IX collagen molecules, allowing bending of the triple helical molecules. The arrangement of type IX collagen on the fibril surface is such that some domains are projected away from the fibril for interaction with other matrix molecules, acting as a bridge between collagen fibrils and other matrix components. A role for type IX collagen in IVD integrity is implicated, as two of the type IX collagen genes (COL9A2 and COL9A3) are associated with IVD degeneration.[110,111] It is significant that IVDs from patients with the risk Trp2 allele in the COL9A2 gene are mechanically impaired, with

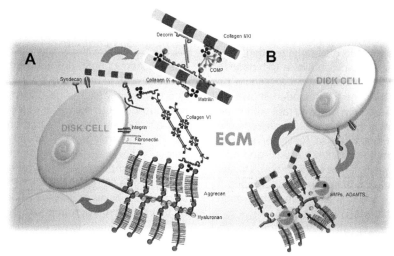

Fig. 3. Extracellular matrix components and environment in healthy and degenerated intervertebral disks. (*A*) Healthy disk cells producing the appropriate extracellular matrix (ECM) components for intervertebral disk function and interacting with the matrix components via specific receptors, such as integrin, responding to signals from the environment for tissue homeostasis. (*B*) Alteration in the disk cell environment with degrading extracellular matrix components altering the signals to disk cells, disrupting normal cell function and cell phenotype, with a negative impact on intervertebral disk function. ADAMTS, A Disintegrin And Metalloproteinase with Thrombospondin MotifS; COMP, Cartilage Oligomeric Matrix Protein; MMPs, matrix metalloproteins.

reduced water-retention property and resistance to compression.[56,57]

Chondroitin sulfate (CS) proteoglycan on the cell surface or ECM play important roles in the development and biological function of the IVD.[112] Similar to cartilage, the major CS proteoglycan in the ECM is aggrecan. Aggrecan has a relatively large core protein of about 2000 amino acids with distinct structural and functional regions. There are 3 globular domains (G1, G2, and G3). The first 2, G1 and G2, are localized toward the N-terminal region separated by a short interglobular domain (IGD). The third, the G3 domain, is localized near the C-terminal region of the core protein. Between the G2 and G3 domains are sites for the attachment of about 100 CS glycosaminoglycan side chains distributed along the CS1 and CS2 domains.[113] Nearer to the G2 domain are attachment sites for approximately 30 keratan sulfate (KS) glycosaminoglycan side chains that are short (22–30 disaccharide units) but highly variable.

The G1 domain mediates the interaction of aggrecan with hyaluronic acid (HA), and the interaction is stabilized by a small link protein that has properties similar to the G1 domain.[114,115] Up to 100 aggrecan molecules can be found on a single HA, resulting in a huge and highly charged aggregate with HA and other matrix molecules.[116]

The highly charged GAG chains attract and retain water in the NP, and produce a swelling pressure allowing resistance to compression from axial loading.[117] In human, the CS1 domain possesses a variable number of tandem repeats, and results in a variation of the length of the aggrecan core protein in different individuals.[118] It is suggested that individuals with a lower CS content are more susceptible to disk degeneration.[119,120] The G3 globular domain contains a C-type lectin motif, but no distinct carbohydrate binding has been identified. Recently, it has been shown that aggrecan via this domain can interact with matrix proteins containing EGF repeats, such as fibulins and tenasins. Fibulins are a family of secreted glycoproteins that interact with elastin and many other matrix proteins.[121] As such, the organization and assembly of the ECM can be established by the networking of aggrecan with other matrix proteins in the tissues.

Small leucine repeat proteins/proteoglycans (SLRP) are also present in the NP. The SLRPs include the small cartilage proteoglycans, such as fibromodulin, decorin, and lumican. These molecules have a central portion consisting of 10 or 11 repeats of approximately 25 amino acids with leucine residues at conserved sites. These SLRPs contain 1 or 2 keratan sulfate chains attached to the repeating units. The polysaccharides can directly interact with collagen and can serve to cross-bridge and cross-link collagen fibers, and regulate collagen fibril assembly. Decorin, via its core protein, can also bind to beaded filaments of type VI collagen at the N-terminal part of this collagen,[122] again acting as bridging molecules in the ECM. SLRPs can also bind growth factors, in particular transforming growth factor (TGF)-β, to regulate tissue homeostasis.[123]

Other SLRPs such as asporin and chondroadherin do not contain GAG side chains. Asporin also binds collagen via its leucine-rich repeat domain.[124] This molecule contains an N-terminal extension with a variable number of aspartic acid residues, and is a polymorphic region of the gene in the human population, ranging from 8 to 19 continuous aspartic acid (D) residues. It has been shown in Asian populations that individuals with the 14-repeat (D14) allele have a higher incidence of osteoarthritis and IVD degeneration, and is upregulated in cartilage of osteoarthritic patients and in patients with IVD degeneration.[125] Asporin also binds TGF-β, and the D14 variant was shown to bind TGF-β with a higher affinity than the common allele (D13) with 13 repeats.[126] A hypothesis is that asporin could regulate the availability of TGF-β and thus modulate the synthesis of matrix molecules. Chondroadherin does not have the N-terminal extension; however, like other SLRPs it interacts with collagen but also interacts with α2β1 integrin, a cell surface receptor by which cells sense their environment, and this interaction is thought to enhance matrix production.[127]

Cartilaginous Endplate

The biochemical composition of the cartilaginous EP is similar to the articular cartilage of joints. The ECM components described for the NP are also applicable to the EP. It must be emphasized that although many of the components found in the NP are cartilage ECM proteins, their relative amounts are very different, and thus differ in form and function. As in hyaline cartilage, this thin cartilage NP layer is composed of a network of randomly oriented collagen fibers within a gel of hydrated proteoglycans. At the junction with the inner annulus fibrosus the collagen network is more organized, oriented more horizontal and parallel to the vertebral bodies, with the collagen fibers running continually into the inner annulus. In cartilaginous endplate, the major proteoglycan is also aggrecan, but the relative level is lower than in the NP.[93,128] In cartilage, the length of the CS side chains appears to be longer and is higher in proportion relative to the KS side chains.

As a thin horizontal layer lying at the interface between the disk and the adjacent vertebral bodies, the NP acts as a selectively permeable barrier in which small and uncharged solutes can diffuse across readily, whereas the movement of anions or larger solutes is restricted.[78] However, permeability studies suggest that diffusion mainly occurs between the subchondral space and the central zone of the disk.[129] Type X collagen is normally found in hypertrophic cartilage undergoing mineralization. Its function in the ECM is not clear, but it is thought to have a role in cartilage mineralization.[130] Type X collagen is found in the central region of the cartilaginous endplate with aging,[131–133] and could be related to hypertrophic differentiation of chondrocytes and calcification within the endplate, impairing diffusion and thus nutritional supply to disk cells (see the article by Grunhagen and colleagues elsewhere in this issue).[41,134]

ECM HOMEOSTASIS AND DEGENERATIVE STATES

The ECM in the IVD undergoes extensive remodeling throughout development, growth, and aging. The balance between the process of matrix degradation, synthesis, and deposition determines the matrix composition in the IVD. This balance not only is critical for the quality and integrity of the matrix but also determines biological changes of disk cells in the control of differentiation, maintenance of cell phenotype, cell proliferation, and cell death. Conversely, maintenance of cell function and activity dictates the tolerance to physiologic stresses before a pathologic condition arises. A progressive imbalance and accumulative stress in cell function would manifest a degenerative phenomenon. The observation of loss of cellularity and altered disk cell activity or phenotype in the degenerated IVD is consistent with such a notion.

What causes disk degeneration is still not clear, but from the analysis of magnetic resonance imaging (MRI) studies, there are several structural abnormalities that can be considered. It is generally accepted that dehydration of the nucleus pulposus, as analyzed by MRI, is an indication of degeneration that progressively worsens, and can be associated with "tears" within the AF (high-intensity zones) or the cartilage endplate (ie, Schmorl's nodes). In some instances, the NP can herniate through a disrupted AF. These MRI changes are thought to be caused by failure of the tissue structures from alterations of the ECM. For example, the NP can lose its hydration property from a reduced proteoglycan content. The tears within the AF may occur via disruption of the organized collagen and/or elastin networks within the lamellae, or mineralization of the cartilaginous endplate affecting nutrition supply to the disk, causing early cellular senescence or cell death and impairing the capacity for tissue maintenance and repair.

Because of the similarity of the matrix components of the IVD to that of the cartilage in a joint, the lessons learnt from cartilage biology and pathology are frequently applied to the disk, bearing in mind the similarities and differences. Destruction of cartilage in osteoarthritis is used as a model system to look for similar occurrences in the disk.

Cytokines, Matrix Metalloproteinase, and Disk Degeneration

Cytokines are important in the biology and pathology of the IVD because of their potential role in regulating the integrity of connective tissues; they influence the synthesis and degradation of the ECM, ingrowth of nerves and blood vessels, and accumulation of macrophages that are characteristic of disk degeneration. These cytokines include tumor necrosis factor (TNF), TWEAK (TNF-like weak inducer of apoptosis), interleukin (IL)-1, IL-10, platelet-derived growth factor, vascular endothelial growth factor, insulin-like growth factor, TGF-β, endothelial growth factor (EGF), and fibroblast growth factor.[135–137] Whereas anabolic cytokines such as TGF-β can promote the synthesis of collagens and proteoglycans,[138,139] catabolic cytokines, such as TNF-α and IL-1, have received considerable attention because of their involvement in cartilage homeostasis and their ability to switch chondrocytes from an anabolic to a catabolic state.[140–142] TNF-α and IL-1 and their respective receptors are elevated in human degenerative IVD.[143,144] These proinflammatory cytokines can increase production of matrix-degradative enzymes, and enhance the breakdown of collagens and proteoglycans.[145,146] Thus, the expression or activity of a range of matrix metalloproteinases (MMPs) such as MMP-1, -3, -7, -9, -10 and -13,[146,147] as well as ADAMTS (A Disintegrin And Metalloproteinase with Thrombospondin MotifS)-4 and -5,[145,148] are increased in disk cells with age and degeneration. Significantly, the levels of some of these enzymes and their activities appear to correlate with the degree of degeneration.[144,149] ADAMTS-4 and -5 have high specificity for the cleavage of aggrecan and are also known as aggrecanase-1 and -2, respectively.

Degradation of type II collagen is initiated by cleavage of the triple helix at a specific MMP cleavage site,[150] whereas numerous MMPs and ADAMTSs may be involved in the degradation of aggrecan in response to cytokine stimulation.[151–153]

Given dehydration of the NP is a key feature of IVD degeneration, the degradation of aggrecan is a prime-candidate biological process in the initiation of degenerative changes. The enzymes and their kinetics for the cleavage of aggrecan have been intensively studied because of their involvement in osteoarthritis; however, their role in the degenerative process and how they cooperate are still largely unclear.

Studies have shown that MMPs in general have a lower efficiency for cleaving aggrecan within the IGD and CS2 regions compared with ADAMTS-4 and ADAMTS-5.[153,154] In vivo, activities of MMPs are regulated by the presence of tissue inhibitors of metalloproteinase (TIMP). In degenerated IVD, expression of the general MMP inhibitors, TIMP-1 and TIMP-2, are upregulated, whereas TIMP-3, a specific inhibitor for ADAMTS, remains relatively unchanged compared with the enhanced ADAMTS-4 and -5 expressions, suggesting ADAMTS enzyme activity may be an important factor in IVD degeneration. A recent study using a rabbit annular puncture model of IVD degeneration showed that suppressing ADAMTS-5 activity by siRNA injection reduces degradation within the NP, and improves MRI and histologic scores for IVD degeneration.[155] This result would be consistent with the finding that mice with genetic inactivation of the *Adamts-5* gene are more resistant to surgically induced osteoarthritis of knee joints.[156] A clear understanding of the degradative processes within the disk would be beneficial for the development of specific therapeutic targets.

As MMPs cleave matrix proteins at very specific sites, it is possible to follow the cleavage occurrences with neo-epitope antibodies that can recognize newly exposed N- or C-termini. This method was successfully applied to studies of aggrecan degradation from specific cleavage within the core protein.[157,158] Again, lessons from cartilage degradation suggest that cytokines that trigger the secretion of proteolytic enzymes may initially degrade aggrecan, followed by the release of other molecules such as COMP (Cartilage Oligomeric Matrix Protein) and fibromodulin, and progressively to the release of collagen fragments as the major type II collagen–containing fibrillar network is eroded away.[159] The MMP cleavage site for type II collagen is clearly defined, and neo-epitope antibodies are available for the specific detection and localization of these cleavage fragments.[92,160]

Extracellular Matrix Protein Changes in Disk Degeneration

In early stages of degeneration there are several changes in the pattern of matrix protein synthesis, reflecting an altered homeostasis. For instance, more type I collagen is found within the NP, whereas more type II collagen is detected in the outer annulus but less so in the endplates.[161] Although both type I and II collagens are fibrillar collagens, they assemble and organize into distinct fibrils of different size and supramolecular aggregates, and are not redundant in function. In fact, it could be detrimental for tissue function if these collagens are expressed ectopically.

The synthesis of proteoglycans is also altered with decreased aggrecan, increased versican, and other small leucine-rich repeat protein/proteoglycans, such as asporin, biglycan, and decorin, in human disk samples.[162–164] The relative proportion of GAGs also changes, from a chondroitin sulfate–enriched matrix to that of keratan sulfate, thus reducing the hydration property of the tissue.[165,166] This change is related to the higher content of sulfate of chondroitin sulfate GAGs being more negatively charged, able to attract more cations and contribute to the water-binding capacity. While the hydroxyl groups on disaccharide units of chondroitin sulfate GAG are differentially sulfated, contributing to structural heterogeneity, specific sulfation motif epitopes can be recognized by a variety of monoclonal antibodies, and have been used to study their pattern in development and postnatal growth[167] as well as degeneration of the IVD.[166,168] The findings are supportive of a significant role for chondroitin sulfate in IVD development and maintenance. In degeneration, an involvement in cellular reparatory processes was proposed.

With degeneration the cellular microenvironment becomes more hostile, with a high level of cytokines and a low level of oxygen and nutritional contents. Of interest, studies have demonstrated that cells in NP have the potential to repair the degenerated disk by generating more matrix molecules. For example, it was shown that the NP cells in degenerated IVD retain the ability to synthesize large aggrecan molecules with intact HA-binding regions.[169] It is also thought that in the early stages of IVD degeneration, disk cells attempt to restore normal function by synthesizing more water-attracting matrix proteins. However, it would be important to consider a reparatory process using more stringent criteria, perhaps from high-throughput global proteomic studies comparing proteins produced by IVD cells at different stages of development and degeneration.

As degeneration progresses the less hydrated and more fibrous NP fails to withstand the compressive loading, resulting in uneven distribution of forces to the surrounding AF. Additional stress is imposed on the AF, which will lead to the formation of radial tears or bulge, or tears to the cartilaginous endplates.[170,171] This line of thinking is very much centered on dehydration of the NP. However, it is also possible that IVD degeneration could be initiated from the surrounding AF or the cartilaginous endplate. Indeed, there is evidence for changes in the endplate that alter nutritional supply to the nucleus, or changes in cell phenotype in the AF prior to dehydration of the NP. This predicament will only be resolved when researchers have good animal models for IVD degeneration, allowing detailed analysis of the sequence of molecular and cellular events.

DISK CELLS INTERACTING WITH THE ENVIRONMENT

In addition to structural support for tissue function, the ECM also provides information cues to inform cellular response. Disk cells are embedded in a sea of ECM. Cells sense their environment via cell surface receptors that directly interact with specific motifs or domains present within the matrix components. There are many cell surface receptors that can mediate cell-matrix interactions, of which integrins is a major class. Integrins function as heterodimers, consisting of one α and one β subunit, which combine to form 24 distinct integrin receptors.[172] Specific heterodimer combinations present cells with defined binding properties. On binding, specific downstream cellular effects are transduced, affecting cell fate, proliferation, and migration. Functions of integrins have been studied in many systems including cartilaginous tissues. For example, inactivation of the $\beta1$ integrin gene in chondrocytes affects the columnar structure of proliferating chondrocytes in the cartilage growth plate, critical for the linear growth of long bones.[173]

In human IVD, integrin subunits involved in the binding of collagens ($\alpha1$, $\beta1$) and fibronectins ($\alpha5$, αv, $\beta1$, $\beta3$, $\beta5$) have been detected in both the AF and NP.[174] The precise function of integrins in IVDs in not clear. However, an involvement in mechanotransduction has been suggested for a class of integrins that bind to the RGD (arginine-glycine-aspartic acid) sequence motif of the ligand.[175] This proposal would be consistent with the variations in expression profiles between the AF and NP[174]; tissues within the IVD with different mechanical properties. Of interest, cells from nondegenerated and degenerated IVD behaved differently in response to hydrostatic loading, suggesting altered mechanotransduction pathways.[175,176] This possibility would be consistent with the notion that cell-matrix interaction is impaired in degeneration, perhaps arising from

an alteration in the ECM composition with a feedback loop that has a negative impact on cell function and phenotype.

CELL MAINTENANCE AND DISEASE STATES

Degenerative disease of the IVD is a disruption of homeostasis, contributed by deregulation of function or metabolism of cells in the system. Conversely, maintenance of cell function and activity dictates the tolerance to physiologic stresses before a pathologic condition arises. A progressive imbalance and accumulative stress would manifest a degenerative phenomenon. The observation of loss of cellularity and an altered disk cell phenotype in degenerated disk is consistent with such a notion.

Whereas IVD has few pain receptors except in the periphery of the disk [177,178] and may not be irritated until inflammation becomes moderate to severe, IVD degeneration may render the motion segments unstable under load, which results in tension and strain (see the article by Inoue and Espinoza Orias elsewhere in this issue).[179] The NP appears to be the first place of degeneration with observable changes, although it may not correspond to the primary site of defect. One working hypothesis points to the reduction of nutritional exchange through the ossification of endplate (see the article by Grunhagen and colleagues elsewhere in this issue). Additional theories include disk overload due to obesity or altered metabolism and/or introduction of low-grade inflammation brought on by fat cells and weight gain.[20,180] Insights from transgenic models imply that hyperactivity of muscles may also induce the degeneration.[181,182]

Association studies suggest that most cases of degeneration may be related to age-related processes together with multiple intrinsic and extrinsic components that accelerate the process; these include genetic factors and environmental stresses. Individuals who are genetically compromised in disk cell function may have abnormal adaptive response to stress and subsequently be more susceptible to IVD degeneration. Through studying disk microenvironments, it is becoming clear that disk cells have an extraordinary capacity to adapt to adverse microenvironments, including mechanical shear, tension in oxygen supply, nutrition and waste exchange, and osmotic pressure.

Intervertebral disks, especially on the lumbar levels, are subjected to high compressive load, which place excessive stress on disk cells.[183] Although disk cells may benefit from mechanical stimulation, excess load in the long term is thought to be detrimental. Symptomatic subjects suffering from IVD degeneration may show signs of pain relief and disk height restoration after nonsurgical distraction,[184] and distraction devices may induce IVD regeneration in animal models, suggesting that mechanical stress may contribute to degeneration. However, disk cells have been shown to exhibit higher matrix anabolism and viability under a regime of dynamic and cyclic loading that mimics the loading in humans, implying that disk cells are in fact designed to adapt to physiologic mechanical stress.[185,186]

The IVD, especially the NP, suffers from hypoxia because of limited vascularization. However, like other cells in minimally vascularized tissues such as cartilage, disk cells are able to withstand low oxygen tension, in part by activating hypoxia-inducible factors (HIFs) to adjust their metabolic activities and protect from apoptosis. Reports show that low oxygen content appears not to impair disk cell metabolism or functionality in vitro,[187] indicating its limited effects on disk homeostasis. Nonetheless, recent study has shown that notochordal NP cells are more susceptible to oxygen deprivation than chondrocyte-like NP cells,[91] suggesting that loss of notochordal cells and hence IVD degeneration may indeed be linked to oxygen stress. HIF-1α regulates chondrocyte survival and production of aggrecan and collagen II.[188,189] In vitro studies have reported a similar function of HIF in NP cells,[190,191] suggesting disk cells are normally adapted to hypoxic conditions.

Albeit with low metabolic activity, disk cells also encounter low energy supply and high waste accumulation, again due to a lack of blood supply. This scenario includes low glucose and high lactic acid, and other metabolites.[192] How disk cells can cope with these aspects is still largely unclear, other than through the general exchange via surrounding vasculature and NP diffusion. A balanced waste production and removal is vital to maintain a minimal baseline level of stress for cells.[193] Inefficient waste removal and presence of cell corpses could induce inflammation, leading to a cascade of destructive events. It is thought that because of disk motion, exercise may prevent IVD degeneration through increased solute transport, reducing waste accumulation and boosting nutrient supply.[194]

Disk cells also live under a microenvironment of high osmotic pressure, established by the high hydrophilicity of the GAG chains in the aggrecan-rich matrix in the extracellular space. Thus, gradient of osmotic pressure will drive water into the disk cells. It is thought that disk cells may modulate the osmotic potential through the action of aquaporin-2 (a tonicity-sensitive water channel), TonEBP (Tonicity-responsive Enhancer Binding Protein), and acid-sensing ion channel 3 present on the membranes, regulating intracellular tonicity.[195,196] It has also been proposed that the vacuoles of NP contain ionic pumps, which have a function in regulating the cytoplasm tonicity under hypotonic stress.[197] It is not clear whether a deregulation in the antiosmotic pressure system may cause degeneration, but reports have shown that osmotic pressure has an impact on the disk cell proliferation, matrix production, and cellular response to cytokines.[198,199]

Disk cell apoptosis[200,201] has been associated with IVD degeneration. However, recent reports suggest that IVD degeneration is attributed to a loss of disk cell function rather than a loss of disk cells[202] owing to cell senescence.[203–205] Whether these cellular changes are related to the cause or consequence of IVD degeneration is not clear but is likely to be a combination of both, leading to a detrimental outcome. In degenerative disks, cells within the NP appear as clusters more characteristic of chondrocytes than NP cells. The origin and exact phenotype of these cell clusters is not clear. It is possible that their presence may reflect a compensation strategy of the disk to mount a self-repair process, albeit limited. These changes in disk cell activities, irrespective to how they are initiated, can result in presentation of factors associated with IVD degeneration. Cartilage matrix cannot replace the function of NP matrix. Proteoglycan to collagen ratio is a major parameter that differentiates NP from hyaline cartilage.[206] It is noteworthy that there is a gradual change in proteoglycan/collagen content in degenerative disks associated with a transformation from a gelatinous to cartilaginous structure in humans and various animal models.

The authors' previous population-based MRI study showed that 80% of the population by the age of 50 years will have lumbar IVD degeneration.[24] Such significant presentation implies that the degeneration is an inevitable age-related process. Strikingly, disk degeneration is also present in a large proportion of younger individuals between the age of 20 and 40 years.[24] Conversely, there are aged individuals who have no disk degeneration. Therefore, while there are risk factors that may contribute to early disk degeneration, there are also protective factors that prevent disk degeneration. Genetics have been shown to be a significant contributing factor, which is likely to be translated to cellular function to maintain disk homeostasis.

One important area that needs to be addressed is whether the disk has the ability for self repair, and how this endogenous repair mechanism can be harnessed for therapeutic strategies; in the absence of such a repair mechanism, exogenous biological stimulus may be considered, for which cells and growth factors can be introduced to mount a repair (see the articles by Sakai, Woods and colleagues, Leung and colleagues, and Bae and Masuda elsewhere in this issue). Thus, the finding of a potential endogenous pool of progenitor cells in the IVD is exciting in that it may facilitate maintenance of homeostasis.[207,208] Better understanding of these progenitor cells, their source, and their maintenance would be of paramount importance. This understanding, together with a clearer understanding of the control of disk cell differentiation from progenitors as well as their applications in tissue engineering and cell therapy strategies, may hold the future for the management of IVD degeneration.

REFERENCES

1. Andersson GB. Epidemiological features of chronic low-back pain. Lancet 1999;354:581–5.
2. Deyo RA, Mirza SK, Martin BI, et al. Trends, major medical complications, and charges associated with surgery for lumbar spinal stenosis in older adults. JAMA 2010;303:1259–65.
3. Deyo RA, Tsui-Wu YJ. Descriptive epidemiology of low-back pain and its related medical care in the United States. Spine 1987;12:264–8.
4. Hart LG, Deyo RA, Cherkin DC. Physician office visits for low back pain. Frequency, clinical evaluation, and treatment patterns from a U.S. national survey. Spine 1995;20:11–9.
5. Apkarian AV. Functional magnetic resonance imaging of pain consciousness: cortical networks of pain critically depend on what is implied by "pain." Curr Rev Pain 1999;3:308–15.
6. Apkarian AV, Krauss BR, Fredrickson BE, et al. Imaging the pain of low back pain: functional magnetic resonance imaging in combination with monitoring subjective pain perception allows the study of clinical pain states. Neurosci Lett 2001; 299:57–60.
7. Apkarian AV, Sosa Y, Krauss BR, et al. Chronic pain patients are impaired on an emotional decision-making task. Pain 2004;108:129–36.
8. Apkarian AV, Sosa Y, Sonty S, et al. Chronic back pain is associated with decreased prefrontal and thalamic gray matter density. J Neurosci 2004;24: 10410–5.
9. Danon-Hersch N, Samartzis D, Wietlisbach V, et al. Appropriateness criteria for surgery improve clinical outcomes in patients with low back pain and/or sciatica. Spine (Phila Pa 1976) 2010. [Epub ahead of print].
10. Shen FH, Samartzis D, Andersson GB. Nonsurgical management of acute and chronic low back pain. J Am Acad Orthop Surg 2006;14:477–87.
11. van Middelkoop M, Rubinstein SM, Kuijpers T, et al. A systematic review on the effectiveness of physical and rehabilitation interventions for chronic non-specific low back pain. Eur Spine J 2011;20: 19–39.
12. Ravenek MJ, Hughes ID, Ivanovich N, et al. A systematic review of multidisciplinary outcomes in the management of chronic low back pain. Work 2010;35:349–67.
13. Negrini S, Minozzi S, Taricco M, et al. A systematic review of physical and rehabilitation medicine topics as developed by the Cochrane Collaboration. Eura Medicophys 2007;43:381–90.
14. Chou R, Qaseem A, Owens DK, et al. Diagnostic imaging for low back pain: advice for high-value health care from the American College of Physicians. Ann Intern Med 2011;154:181–9.
15. Fourney DR, Andersson GBJ, Arnold PM, et al. Chronic low back pain: a heterogeneous condition with challenges for an evidence-based approach. Spine, in press.
16. Kjaer P, Leboeuf-Yde C, Korsholm L, et al. Magnetic resonance imaging and low back pain in adults: a diagnostic imaging study of 40-year-old men and women. Spine (Phila Pa 1976) 2005;30:1173–80.
17. Kjaer P, Leboeuf-Yde C, Sorensen JS, et al. An epidemiologic study of MRI and low back pain in 13-year-old children. Spine (Phila Pa 1976) 2005; 30:798–806.
18. Luoma K, Riihimaki H, Luukkonen R, et al. Low back pain in relation to lumbar disc degeneration. Spine (Phila Pa 1976) 2000;25:487–92.
19. Samartzis D, Karppinen J, Chan D, et al. The association of disc degeneration based on magnetic resonance imaging and the presence of low back pain. Presented at: World Forum for Spine Research: Intervertebral Disc. Montreal (Canada), July 5–8, 2010.
20. Samartzis D, Karppinen J, Mok F, et al. A population-based study of juvenile disc degeneration and its association with overweight and obesity, low back pain, and diminished functional status. J Bone Joint Surg Am 2011;93:662–70.
21. Savage RA, Whitehouse GH, Roberts N. The relationship between the magnetic resonance imaging appearance of the lumbar spine and low back pain, age and occupation in males. Eur Spine J 1997;6:106–14.
22. Visuri T, Ulaska J, Eskelin M, et al. Narrowing of lumbar spinal canal predicts chronic low back pain more accurately than intervertebral disc degeneration: a magnetic resonance imaging study in young Finnish male conscripts. Mil Med 2005;170:926–30.

23. Takatalo J, Karppinen J, Niinimäki J, et al. Does lumbar disc degeneration on MRI associate with low back symptom severity in young Finnish adults? Spine (Phila Pa 1976) 2011. [Epub ahead of print].

24. Cheung KM, Karppinen J, Chan D, et al. Prevalence and pattern of lumbar magnetic resonance imaging changes in a population study of one thousand forty-three individuals. Spine 2009;34:934–40.

25. Battie MC, Videman T, Parent E. Lumbar disc degeneration: epidemiology and genetic influences. Spine 2004;29:2679–90.

26. Battie MC, Videman T. Lumbar disk degeneration: epidemiology and genetics. J Bone Joint Surg Am 2006;88(Suppl 2):3–9.

27. Mok FP, Samartzis D, Karppinen J, et al. ISSLS prize winner: Prevalence, determinants, and association of Schmorl nodes of the lumbar spine with disc degeneration: a population-based study of 2449 individuals. Spine 2010;35:1944–52.

28. Cheung KM, Samartzis D, Karppinen J, et al. Intervertebral disc degeneration: new insights based on "skipped" level disc pathology. Arthritis Rheum 2010;62:2392–400.

29. Adams MA, Freeman BJ, Morrison HP, et al. Mechanical initiation of intervertebral disc degeneration. Spine 2000;25:1625–36.

30. Roberts S, Menage J, Urban JP. Biochemical and structural properties of the cartilage end-plate and its relation to the intervertebral disc. Spine 1989;14:166–74.

31. Battie MC, Videman T, Gill K, et al. 1991 Volvo Award in clinical sciences. Smoking and lumbar intervertebral disc degeneration: an MRI study of identical twins. Spine 1991;16:1015–21.

32. Jhawar BS, Fuchs CS, Colditz GA, et al. Cardiovascular risk factors for physician-diagnosed lumbar disc herniation. Spine J 2006;6:684–91.

33. Leino-Arjas P, Kaila-Kangas L, Solovieva S, et al. Serum lipids and low back pain: an association? A follow-up study of a working population sample. Spine (Phila Pa 1976) 2006;31:1032–7.

34. Leino-Arjas P, Kauppila L, Kaila-Kangas L, et al. Serum lipids in relation to sciatica among Finns. Atherosclerosis 2008;197:43–9.

35. Bibby RL, Webster-Brown JG. Characterisation of urban catchment suspended particulate matter (Auckland region, New Zealand); a comparison with non-urban SPM. Sci Total Environ 2005;343: 177–97.

36. Bibby SR, Fairbank JC, Urban MR, et al. Cell viability in scoliotic discs in relation to disc deformity and nutrient levels. Spine (Phila Pa 1976) 2002;27:2220–8 [discussion: 2227–8].

37. Ohshima H, Urban JP. The effect of lactate and pH on proteoglycan and protein synthesis rates in the intervertebral disc. Spine (Phila Pa 1976) 1992;17: 1079–82.

38. Urban JP, McMullin JF. Swelling pressure of the lumbar intervertebral discs: influence of age, spinal level, composition, and degeneration. Spine 1988; 13:179–87.

39. Samartzis D, Karppinen J, Luk KD, et al. Body mass index and its association with lumbar disc degeneration in adults. Global Spine Congress. San Francisco (CA); 2009.

40. Rajasekaran S, Vidyadhara S, Subbiah M, et al. ISSLS prize winner: A study of effects of in vivo mechanical forces on human lumbar discs with scoliotic disc as a biological model: results from serial postcontrast diffusion studies, histopathology and biochemical analysis of twenty-one human lumbar scoliotic discs. Spine 2010;35:1930–43.

41. Rajasekaran S, Babu JN, Arun R, et al. ISSLS prize winner: a study of diffusion in human lumbar discs: a serial magnetic resonance imaging study documenting the influence of the endplate on diffusion in normal and degenerate discs. Spine 2004;29:2654–67.

42. Kauppila LI. Prevalence of stenotic changes in arteries supplying the lumbar spine. A postmortem angiographic study on 140 subjects. Ann Rheum Dis 1997;56:591–5.

43. Kauppila LI. Atherosclerosis and disc degeneration/ low-back pain—a systematic review. Eur J Vasc Endovasc Surg 2009;37:661–70.

44. Kauppila LI, McAlindon T, Evans S, et al. Disc degeneration/back pain and calcification of the abdominal aorta. A 25-year follow-up study in Framingham. Spine (Phila Pa 1976) 1997;22:1642–7 [discussion: 1648–9].

45. Kurunlahti M, Tervonen O, Vanharanta H, et al. Association of atherosclerosis with low back pain and the degree of disc degeneration. Spine (Phila Pa 1976) 1999;24:2080–4.

46. Shiri R, Karppinen J, Leino-Arjas P, et al. Cardiovascular and lifestyle risk factors in lumbar radicular pain or clinically defined sciatica: a systematic review. Eur Spine J 2007;16:2043–54.

47. Frino J, McCarthy RE, Sparks CY, et al. Trends in adolescent lumbar disk herniation. J Pediatr Orthop 2006;26:579–81.

48. Matsui H, Kanamori M, Ishihara H, et al. Familial predisposition for lumbar degenerative disc disease. A case-control study. Spine (Phila Pa 1976) 1998;23:1029–34.

49. Postacchini F, Lami R, Pugliese O. Familial predisposition to discogenic low-back pain. An epidemiologic and immunogenetic study. Spine (Phila Pa 1976) 1988;13:1403–6.

50. Simmons ED Jr, Guntupalli M, Kowalski JM, et al. Familial predisposition for degenerative disc disease. A case-control study. Spine (Phila Pa 1976) 1996;21:1527–9.

51. Varlotta GP, Brown MD, Kelsey JL, et al. Familial predisposition for herniation of a lumbar disc in

patients who are less than twenty-one years old. J Bone Joint Surg Am 1991;73:124–8.

52. Battie MC, Haynor DR, Fisher LD, et al. Similarities in degenerative findings on magnetic resonance images of the lumbar spines of identical twins. J Bone Joint Surg Am 1995;77:1662–70.

53. Battie MC, Videman T, Gibbons LE, et al. 1995 Volvo Award in clinical sciences. Determinants of lumbar disc degeneration. A study relating lifetime exposures and magnetic resonance imaging findings in identical twins. Spine (Phila Pa 1976) 1995;20: 2601–12.

54. Battie MC, Videman T, Levalahti E, et al. Heritability of low back pain and the role of disc degeneration. Pain 2007;131:272–80.

55. Sambrook PN, MacGregor AJ, Spector TD. Genetic influences on cervical and lumbar disc degeneration: a magnetic resonance imaging study in twins. Arthritis Rheum 1999;42:366–72.

56. Aladin DM, Cheung KM, Chan D, et al. Expression of the Trp2 allele of COL9A2 is associated with alterations in the mechanical properties of human intervertebral discs. Spine 2007;32:2820–6.

57. Jim JJ, Noponen-Hietala N, Cheung KM, et al. The TRP2 allele of COL9A2 is an age-dependent risk factor for the development and severity of intervertebral disc degeneration. Spine 2005;30:2735–42.

58. Song YQ, Cheung KM, Ho DW, et al. Association of the asporin D14 allele with lumbar-disc degeneration in Asians. Am J Hum Genet 2008;82:744–7.

59. Cheung KM, Chan D, Karppinen J, et al. Association of the Taq I allele in vitamin D receptor with degenerative disc disease and disc bulge in a Chinese population. Spine 2006;31:1143–8.

60. Guerin HL, Elliott DM. Quantifying the contributions of structure to annulus fibrosus mechanical function using a nonlinear, anisotropic, hyperelastic model. J Orthop Res 2007;25:508–16.

61. Heuer F, Schmidt H, Wilke HJ. The relation between intervertebral disc bulging and annular fiber associated strains for simple and complex loading. J Biomech 2008;41:1086–94.

62. Schmidt H, Kettler A, Heuer F, et al. Intradiscal pressure, shear strain, and fiber strain in the intervertebral disc under combined loading. Spine 2007;32:748–55.

63. Adams DS, Keller R, Koehl MA. The mechanics of notochord elongation, straightening and stiffening in the embryo of *Xenopus laevis*. Development 1990;110:115–30.

64. Hogan BL, Thaller C, Eichele G. Evidence that Hensen's node is a site of retinoic acid synthesis. Nature 1992;359:237–41.

65. Jurand A. Some aspects of the development of the notochord in mouse embryos. J Embryol Exp Morphol 1974;32:1–33.

66. Kinder SJ, Tsang TE, Wakamiya M, et al. The organizer of the mouse gastrula is composed of a dynamic population of progenitor cells for the axial mesoderm. Development 2001;128: 3623–34.

67. Yamanaka Y, Tamplin OJ, Beckers A, et al. Live imaging and genetic analysis of mouse notochord formation reveals regional morphogenetic mechanisms. Dev Cell 2007;13:884–96.

68. Pourquie O, Coltey M, Teillet MA, et al. Control of dorsoventral patterning of somitic derivatives by notochord and floor plate. Proc Natl Acad Sci U S A 1993;90:5242–6.

69. Aszodi A, Chan D, Hunziker E, et al. Collagen II is essential for the removal of the notochord and the formation of intervertebral discs. J Cell Biol 1998; 143:1399–412.

70. Choi KS, Cohn MJ, Harfe BD. Identification of nucleus pulposus precursor cells and notochordal remnants in the mouse: implications for disk degeneration and chordoma formation. Dev Dyn 2008;237:3953–8.

71. Grotmol S, Kryvi H, Nordvik K, et al. Notochord segmentation may lay down the pathway for the development of the vertebral bodies in the Atlantic salmon. Anat Embryol 2003;207:263–72.

72. Cassidy JJ, Hiltner A, Baer E. Hierarchical structure of the intervertebral disc. Connect Tissue Res 1989;23:75–88.

73. Marchand F, Ahmed AM. Investigation of the laminate structure of lumbar disc annulus fibrosus. Spine 1990;15:402–10.

74. Yu J, Tirlapur U, Fairbank J, et al. Microfibrils, elastin fibres and collagen fibres in the human intervertebral disc and bovine tail disc. J Anat 2007;210:460–71.

75. Humzah MD, Soames RW. Human intervertebral disc: structure and function. Anat Rec 1988;220:337–56.

76. Roberts S, Eisenstein SM, Menage J, et al. Mechanoreceptors in intervertebral discs. Morphology, distribution, and neuropeptides. Spine 1995;20: 2645–51.

77. Crock HV, Goldwasser M. Anatomic studies of the circulation in the region of the vertebral end-plate in adult Greyhound dogs. Spine 1984;9:702–6.

78. Urban JP, Smith S, Fairbank JC. Nutrition of the intervertebral disc. Spine 2004;29:2700–9.

79. Watanabe H, Yamada Y, Kimata K. Roles of aggrecan, a large chondroitin sulfate proteoglycan, in cartilage structure and function. J Biochem 1998; 124:687–93.

80. Butler WF. Comparative anatomy and development of the mammalian disc. CRC Press; 1989.

81. Hunter CJ, Matyas JR, Duncan NA. The functional significance of cell clusters in the notochordal nucleus pulposus: survival and signaling in the canine intervertebral disc. Spine 2004;29:1099–104.

82. Peacock A. Observations on the prenatal development of the intervertebral disc in man. J Anat 1951; 85:260–74.

83. Peacock A. Observations on the postnatal structure of the intervertebral disc in man. J Anat 1952;86:162–79.

84. Gotz W, Kasper M, Fischer G, et al. Intermediate filament typing of the human embryonic and fetal notochord. Cell Tissue Res 1995;280:455–62.

85. Gotz W, Kasper M, Miosge N, et al. Detection and distribution of the carbohydrate binding protein galectin-3 in human notochord, intervertebral disc and chordoma. Differentiation 1997;62: 149–57.

86. Naka T, Iwamoto Y, Shinohara N, et al. Cytokeratin subtyping in chordomas and the fetal notochord: an immunohistochemical analysis of aberrant expression. Mod Pathol 1997;10:545–51.

87. Weiler C, Nerlich AG, Schaaf R, et al. Immunohistochemical identification of notochordal markers in cells in the aging human lumbar intervertebral disc. Eur Spine J 2010;19:1761–70.

88. Salisbury JR. The pathology of the human notochord. J Pathol 1993;171:253–5.

89. Pazzaglia UE, Salisbury JR, Byers PD. Development and involution of the notochord in the human spine. J R Soc Med 1989;82:413–5.

90. Rastogi A, Thakore P, Leung A, et al. Environmental regulation of notochordal gene expression in nucleus pulposus cells. J Cell Physiol 2009;220: 698–705.

91. Guehring T, Wilde G, Sumner M, et al. Notochordal intervertebral disc cells: sensitivity to nutrient deprivation. Arthritis Rheum 2009;60:1026–34.

92. Antoniou J, Steffen T, Nelson F, et al. The human lumbar intervertebral disc: evidence for changes in the biosynthesis and denaturation of the extracellular matrix with growth, maturation, ageing, and degeneration. J Clin Invest 1996;98:996–1003.

93. Antoniou J, Goudsouzian NM, Heathfield TF, et al. The human lumbar endplate. Evidence of changes in biosynthesis and denaturation of the extracellular matrix with growth, maturation, aging, and degeneration. Spine 1996;21:1153–61.

94. Buckwalter JA. Aging and degeneration of the human intervertebral disc. Spine 1995;20:1307–14.

95. Singh K, Masuda K, Thonar EJ, et al. Age-related changes in the extracellular matrix of nucleus pulposus and annulus fibrosus of human intervertebral disc. Spine 2009;34:10–6.

96. Roughley PJ. Biology of intervertebral disc aging and degeneration: involvement of the extracellular matrix. Spine 2004;29:2691–9.

97. Yang CL, Rui H, Mosler S, et al. Collagen II from articular cartilage and annulus fibrosus. Structural and functional implication of tissue specific posttranslational modifications of collagen molecules. Eur J Biochem 1993;213:1297–302.

98. Wu JJ, Eyre DR. Intervertebral disc collagen. Usage of the short form of the alpha1(IX) chain in bovine nucleus pulposus. J Biol Chem 2003;278:24521–5.

99. Duance VC, Crean JK, Sims TJ, et al. Changes in collagen cross-linking in degenerative disc disease and scoliosis. Spine 1998;23:2545–51.

100. Yu J. Elastic tissues of the intervertebral disc. Biochem Soc Trans 2002;30:848–52.

101. Bushell GR, Ghosh P, Taylor TF, et al. Proteoglycan chemistry of the intervertebral disks. Clin Orthop Relat Res 1977;(129):115–23.

102. Roughley PJ, Alini M, Antoniou J. The role of proteoglycans in aging, degeneration and repair of the intervertebral disc. Biochem Soc Trans 2002;30:869–74.

103. Oegema TR Jr, Johnson SL, Aguiar DJ, et al. Fibronectin and its fragments increase with degeneration in the human intervertebral disc. Spine 2000; 25:2742–7.

104. Greg Anderson D, Li X, Tannoury T, et al. A fibronectin fragment stimulates intervertebral disc degeneration in vivo. Spine 2003;28:2338–45.

105. Chen J, Jing L, Gilchrist CL, et al. Expression of laminin isoforms, receptors, and binding proteins unique to nucleus pulposus cells of immature intervertebral disc. Connect Tissue Res 2009;50:294–306.

106. Gruber HE, Ingram JA, Hanley EN Jr. Tenascin in the human intervertebral disc: alterations with aging and disc degeneration. Biotech Histochem 2002;77:37–41.

107. Eyre DR, Muir H. Quantitative analysis of types I and II collagens in human intervertebral discs at various ages. Biochim Biophys Acta 1977;492:29–42.

108. Engvall E, Hessle H, Klier G. Molecular assembly, secretion, and matrix deposition of type VI collagen. J Cell Biol 1986;102:703–10.

109. Schollum ML, Robertson PA, Broom ND. A microstructural investigation of intervertebral disc lamellar connectivity: detailed analysis of the translamellar bridges. J Anat 2009;214:805–16.

110. Annunen S, Paassilta P, Lohiniva J, et al. An allele of COL9A2 associated with intervertebral disc disease. Science 1999;285:409–12.

111. Paassilta P, Lohiniva J, Goring HH, et al. Identification of a novel common genetic risk factor for lumbar disk disease. JAMA 2001;285:1843–9.

112. Hayes AJ, Benjamin M, Ralphs JR. Extracellular matrix in development of the intervertebral disc. Matrix Biol 2001;20:107–21.

113. Doege KJ, Sasaki M, Kimura T, et al. Complete coding sequence and deduced primary structure of the human cartilage large aggregating proteoglycan, aggrecan. Human-specific repeats, and additional alternatively spliced forms. J Biol Chem 1991;266:894–902.

114. Watanabe H, Cheung SC, Itano N, et al. Identification of hyaluronan-binding domains of aggrecan. J Biol Chem 1997;272:28057–65.

115. Morgelin M, Paulsson M, Hardingham TE, et al. Cartilage proteoglycans. Assembly with hyaluronate and link protein as studied by electron microscopy. Biochem J 1988;253:175–85.

116. Heinegard D, Hascall VC. Characterization of chondroitin sulfate isolated from trypsin-chymotrypsin digests of cartilage proteoglycans. Arch Biochem Biophys 1974;165:427–41.

117. Taylor JR, Scott JE, Cribb AM, et al. Human intervertebral disc acid glycosaminoglycans. J Anat 1992;180(Pt 1):137–41.

118. Doege KJ, Coulter SN, Meek LM, et al. A human-specific polymorphism in the coding region of the aggrecan gene. Variable number of tandem repeats produce a range of core protein sizes in the general population. J Biol Chem 1997;272:13974–9.

119. Kawaguchi Y, Osada R, Kanamori M, et al. Association between an aggrecan gene polymorphism and lumbar disc degeneration. Spine 1999;24:2456–60.

120. Kim NK, Shin DA, Han IB, et al. The association of aggrecan gene polymorphism with the risk of intervertebral disc degeneration. Acta Neurochir 2011;153:129–33.

121. Roark EF, Keene DR, Haudenschild CC, et al. The association of human fibulin-1 with elastic fibers: an immunohistological, ultrastructural, and RNA study. J Histochem Cytochem 1995;43:401–11.

122. Wiberg C, Hedbom E, Khairullina A, et al. Biglycan and decorin bind close to the n-terminal region of the collagen VI triple helix. J Biol Chem 2001;276:18947–52.

123. Hildebrand A, Romaris M, Rasmussen LM, et al. Interaction of the small interstitial proteoglycans biglycan, decorin and fibromodulin with transforming growth factor beta. Biochem J 1994;302(Pt 2):527–34.

124. Kalamajski S, Aspberg A, Lindblom K, et al. Asporin competes with decorin for collagen binding, binds calcium and promotes osteoblast collagen mineralization. Biochem J 2009;423:53–9.

125. Nakamura T, Shi D, Tzetis M, et al. Meta-analysis of association between the ASPN D-repeat and osteoarthritis. Hum Mol Genet 2007;16:1676–81.

126. Kizawa H, Kou I, Iida A, et al. An aspartic acid repeat polymorphism in asporin inhibits chondrogenesis and increases susceptibility to osteoarthritis. Nat Genet 2005;37:138–44.

127. Camper L, Heinegard D, Lundgren-Akerlund E. Integrin alpha2beta1 is a receptor for the cartilage matrix protein chondroadherin. J Cell Biol 1997;138:1159–67.

128. Inkinen RI, Lammi MJ, Agren U, et al. Hyaluronan distribution in the human and canine intervertebral disc and cartilage endplate. Histochem J 1999;31:579–87.

129. Nachemson A, Lewin T, Maroudas A, et al. In vitro diffusion of dye through the end-plates and the annulus fibrosus of human lumbar inter-vertebral discs. Acta Orthop Scand 1970;41:589–607.

130. Kwan KM, Pang MK, Zhou S, et al. Abnormal compartmentalization of cartilage matrix components in mice lacking collagen X: implications for function. J Cell Biol 1997;136:459–71.

131. Boos N, Norlich AG, Wiest I, et al. Immunolocalization of type X collagen in human lumbar intervertebral discs during ageing and degeneration. Histochem Cell Biol 1997;108:471–80.

132. Itoh H, Asou Y, Hara Y, et al. Enhanced type X collagen expression in the extruded nucleus pulposus of the chondrodystrophoid dog. J Vet Med Sci 2008;70:37–42.

133. Aigner T, Gresk-otter KR, Fairbank JC, et al. Variation with age in the pattern of type X collagen expression in normal and scoliotic human intervertebral discs. Calcif Tissue Int 1998;63:263–8.

134. Rutges JP, Duit RA, Kummer JA, et al. Hypertrophic differentiation and calcification during intervertebral disc degeneration. Osteoarthritis Cartilage 2010;18:1487–95.

135. Kang JD, Georgescu HI, McIntyre-Larkin L, et al. Herniated lumbar intervertebral discs spontaneously produce matrix metalloproteinases, nitric oxide, interleukin-6, and prostaglandin E2. Spine 1996;21:271–7.

136. Tolonen J, Gronblad M, Virri J, et al. Platelet-derived growth factor and vascular endothelial growth factor expression in disc herniation tissue: and immunohistochemical study. Eur Spine J 1997;6:63–9.

137. Igarashi T, Kikuchi S, Shubayev V, et al. 2000 Volvo Award winner in basic science studies: Exogenous tumor necrosis factor-alpha mimics nucleus pulposus-induced neuropathology. Molecular, histologic, and behavioral comparisons in rats. Spine 2000;25:2975–80.

138. Arend WP, Dayer JM. Inhibition of the production and effects of interleukin-1 and tumor necrosis factor alpha in rheumatoid arthritis. Arthritis Rheum 1995;38:151–60.

139. Chikanza IC, Roux-Lombard P, Dayer JM, et al. Dysregulation of the in vivo production of interleukin-1 receptor antagonist in patients with rheumatoid arthritis. Pathogenetic implications. Arthritis Rheum 1995;38:642–8.

140. Grimaud E, Heymann D, Redini F. Recent advances in TGF-beta effects on chondrocyte metabolism. Potential therapeutic roles of TGF-beta in cartilage disorders. Cytokine Growth Factor Rev 2002;13:241–57.

141. Shikhman AR, Brinson DC, Lotz MK. Distinct pathways regulate facilitated glucose transport in

human articular chondrocytes during anabolic and catabolic responses. Am J Physiol Endocrinol Metab 2004;286:E980–5.

142. Fernandes JC, Martel-Pelletier J, Pelletier JP. The role of cytokines in osteoarthritis pathophysiology. Biorheology 2002;39:237–46.

143. Bachmeier BE, Nerlich AG, Weiler C, et al. Analysis of tissue distribution of TNF-alpha, TNF-alpha-receptors, and the activating TNF-alpha-converting enzyme suggests activation of the TNF-alpha system in the aging intervertebral disc. Ann N Y Acad Sci 2007;1096:44–54.

144. Richardson SM, Doyle P, Minogue BM, et al. Increased expression of matrix metalloproteinase-10, nerve growth factor and substance P in the painful degenerate intervertebral disc. Arthritis Res Ther 2009;11:R126.

145. Le Maitre CL, Freemont AJ, Hoyland JA. Localization of degradative enzymes and their inhibitors in the degenerate human intervertebral disc. J Pathol 2004;204:47–54.

146. Le Maitre CL, Pockert A, Buttle DJ, et al. Matrix synthesis and degradation in human intervertebral disc degeneration. Biochem Soc Trans 2007;35:652–5.

147. Goupille P, Jayson MI, Valat JP, et al. Matrix metalloproteinases: the clue to intervertebral disc degeneration? Spine 1998;23:1612–26.

148. Hatano E, Fujita T, Ueda Y, et al. Expression of ADAMTS-4 (aggrecanase-1) and possible involvement in regression of lumbar disc herniation. Spine 2006;31:1426–32.

149. Pockert AJ, Richardson SM, Le Maitre CL, et al. Modified expression of the ADAMTS enzymes and tissue inhibitor of metalloproteinases 3 during human intervertebral disc degeneration. Arthritis Rheum 2009;60:482–91.

150. Fukui N, McAlinden A, Zhu Y, et al. Processing of type II procollagen amino propeptide by matrix metalloproteinases. J Biol Chem 2002;277:2193–201.

151. Sztrolovics R, Alini M, Roughley PJ, et al. Aggrecan degradation in human intervertebral disc and articular cartilage. Biochem J 1997;326(Pt 1):235–41.

152. Durigova M, Roughley PJ, Mort JS. Mechanism of proteoglycan aggregate degradation in cartilage stimulated with oncostatin M. Osteoarthritis Cartilage 2008;16:98–104.

153. Durigova M, Troeberg L, Nagase H, et al. Involvement of ADAMTS5 and hyaluronidase in aggrecan degradation and release from OSM-stimulated cartilage. Eur Cell Mater 2011;21:31–45.

154. Durigova M, Nagase H, Mort JS, et al. MMPs are less efficient than ADAMTS5 in cleaving aggrecan core protein. Matrix Biol 2011;30:145–53.

155. Seki S, Asanuma-Abe Y, Masuda K, et al. Effect of small interference RNA (siRNA) for ADAMTS5 on intervertebral disc degeneration in the rabbit annular needle-puncture model. Arthritis Res Ther 2009;11:R166.

156. Botter SM, Glasson SS, Hopkins B, et al. ADAMTS5-/- mice have less subchondral bone changes after induction of osteoarthritis through surgical instability: implications for a link between cartilage and subchondral bone changes. Osteoarthritis Cartilage 2009;17:636–45.

157. Rogerson FM, Stanton H, East CJ, et al. Evidence of a novel aggrecan-degrading activity in cartilage: Studies of mice deficient in both ADAMTS-4 and ADAMTS-5. Arthritis Rheumatism 2008;58:1664–73.

158. East CJ, Stanton H, Golub SB, et al. ADAMTS-5 deficiency does not block aggrecanolysis at preferred cleavage sites in the chondroitin sulfate-rich region of aggrecan. J Biol Chem 2007;282:8632–40.

159. Heathfield TF, Onnerfjord P, Dahlberg L, et al. Cleavage of fibromodulin in cartilage explants involves removal of the N-terminal tyrosine sulfate-rich region by proteolysis at a site that is sensitive to matrix metalloproteinase-13. J Biol Chem 2004;279:6286–95.

160. Lee ER, Lamplugh L, Kluczyk B, et al. Neoepitopes reveal the features of type II collagen cleavage and the identity of a collagenase involved in the transformation of the epiphyses anlagen in development. Dev Dyn 2009;238:1547–63.

161. Takaishi H, Nemoto O, Shiota M, et al. Type-II collagen gene expression is transiently upregulated in experimentally induced degeneration of rabbit intervertebral disc. J Orthop Res 1997;15:528–38.

162. Gruber HE, Ingram JA, Hoelscher GL, et al. Asporin, a susceptibility gene in osteoarthritis, is expressed at higher levels in the more degenerate human intervertebral disc. Arthritis Res Ther 2009;11:R47.

163. Inkinen RI, Lammi MJ, Lehmonen S, et al. Relative increase of biglycan and decorin and altered chondroitin sulfate epitopes in the degenerating human intervertebral disc. J Rheumatol 1998;25:506–14.

164. Cs-Szabo G, Ragasa-San Juan D, Turumella V, et al. Changes in mRNA and protein levels of proteoglycans of the annulus fibrosus and nucleus pulposus during intervertebral disc degeneration. Spine 2002;27:2212–9.

165. Pearce RH, Grimmer BJ, Adams ME. Degeneration and the chemical composition of the human lumbar intervertebral disc. J Orthop Res 1987;5:198–205.

166. Roberts S, Caterson B, Evans H, et al. Proteoglycan components of the intervertebral disc and cartilage endplate: an immunolocalization study of animal and human tissues. Histochem J 1994;26:402–11.

167. Hayes AJ, Hughes CE, Ralphs JR, et al. Chondroitin sulphate sulphation motif expression in the

ontogeny of the intervertebral disc. Eur Cell Mater 2011;21:1–14.

168. Johnson WE, Eisenstein SM, Roberts S. Cell cluster formation in degenerate lumbar intervertebral discs is associated with increased disc cell proliferation. Connect Tissue Res 2001;42:197–207.

169. Johnstone B, Bayliss MT. The large proteoglycans of the human intervertebral disc. Changes in their biosynthesis and structure with age, topography, and pathology. Spine 1995;20:674–84.

170. Adams MA, McNally DS, Dolan P. 'Stress' distributions inside intervertebral discs. The effects of age and degeneration. J Bone Joint Surg Br 1996;78:965–72.

171. Vernon-Roberts B, Moore RJ, Fraser RD. The natural history of age-related disc degeneration: the pathology and sequelae of tears. Spine (Phila Pa 1976) 2007;32:2797–804.

172. Legate KR, Wickstrom SA, Fassler R. Genetic and cell biological analysis of integrin outside-in signaling. Genes Dev 2009;23:397–418.

173. Aszodi A, Hunziker EB, Brakebusch C, et al. Beta1 integrins regulate chondrocyte rotation, G1 progression, and cytokinesis. Genes Dev 2003;17:2465–79.

174. Nettles DL, Richardson WJ, Setton LA. Integrin expression in cells of the intervertebral disc. J Anat 2004;204:515–20.

175. Le Maitre CL, Frain J, Millward-Sadler J, et al. Altered integrin mechanotransduction in human nucleus pulposus cells derived from degenerated discs. Arthritis Rheumatism 2009;60:460–9.

176. Gilchrist CL, Chen J, Richardson WJ, et al. Functional integrin subunits regulating cell-matrix interactions in the intervertebral disk. J Orthop Res 2007;25:829–40.

177. Fagan A, Moore R, Vernon Roberts B, et al. ISSLS prize winner: The innervation of the intervertebral disc : a quantitative analysis. Spine 2003;28:2570–6.

178. Freemont AJ, Peacock TE, Goupille P, et al. Nerve ingrowth into diseased intervertebral disc in chronic back pain. Lancet 1997;350:178–81.

179. Farfan HF, Gracovetsky S. The nature of instability. Spine 1984;9:714–9.

180. Liuke M, Solovieva S, Lamminen A, et al. Disc degeneration of the lumbar spine in relation to overweight. Int J Obes 2005;29:903–8.

181. Hamrick MW, Pennington C, Byron CD. Bone architecture and disc degeneration in the lumbar spine of mice lacking GDF-8 (myostatin). J Orthop Res 2003;21:1025–32.

182. Panjabi MM. A hypothesis of chronic back pain: ligament subfailure injuries lead to muscle control dysfunction. Eur Spine J 2006;15:668–76.

183. Setton LA, Chen J. Mechanobiology of the intervertebral disc and relevance to disc degeneration. J Bone Joint Surg Am 2006;88(Suppl 2):52–7.

184. Apfel CC, Cakmakkaya OS, Martin W, et al. Restoration of disk height through non-surgical spinal

decompression is associated with decreased discogenic low back pain: a retrospective cohort study. BMC Musculoskelet Disord 2010;11:155.

185. Illien-Junger S, Gantenbein-Ritter B, Grad S, et al. The combined effects of limited nutrition and high-frequency loading on intervertebral discs with endplates. Spine 2010;35:1744–52.

186. Gantenbein B, Grunhagen T, Lee CR, et al. An in vitro organ culturing system for intervertebral disc explants with vertebral endplates: a feasibility study with ovine caudal discs. Spine 2006;31:2665–73.

187. Mwale F, Ciobanu I, Giannitsios D, et al. Effect of oxygen levels on proteoglycan synthesis by intervertebral disc cells. Spine 2011;36:E131–8.

188. Schipani E, Ryan HE, Didrickson S, et al. Hypoxia in cartilage: HIF-1alpha is essential for chondrocyte growth arrest and survival. Genes Dev 2001; 15:2865–76.

189. Duval E, Leclercq S, Elissalde JM, et al. Hypoxia-inducible factor 1alpha inhibits the fibroblast-like markers type I and type III collagen during hypoxia-induced chondrocyte redifferentiation: hypoxia not only induces type II collagen and aggrecan, but it also inhibits type I and type III collagen in the hypoxia-inducible factor 1alpha-dependent redifferentiation of chondrocytes. Arthritis Rheumatism 2009;60:3038–48.

190. Zeng Y, Danielson KG, Albert TJ, et al. HIF-1 alpha is a regulator of galectin-3 expression in the intervertebral disc. J Bone Miner Res 2007;22:1851–61.

191. Agrawal A, Guttapalli A, Narayan S, et al. Normoxic stabilization of HIF-1alpha drives glycolytic metabolism and regulates aggrecan gene expression in nucleus pulposus cells of the rat intervertebral disc. Am J Physiol Cell Physiol 2007;293: C621–31.

192. Grunhagen T, Wilde G, Soukane DM, et al. Nutrient supply and intervertebral disc metabolism. J Bone Joint Surg Am 2006;88(Suppl 2):30 6.

193. Bibby SR, Jones DA, Ripley RM, et al. Metabolism of the intervertebral disc: effects of low levels of oxygen, glucose, and pH on rates of energy metabolism of bovine nucleus pulposus cells. Spine 2005;30:487–96.

194. Arun R, Freeman BJ, Scammell BE, et al. 2009 ISSLS Prize Winner: What influence does sustained mechanical load have on diffusion in the human intervertebral disc? an in vivo study using serial postcontrast magnetic resonance imaging. Spine 2009;34:2324–37.

195. Gajghate S, Hiyama A, Shah M, et al. Osmolarity and intracellular calcium regulate aquaporin2 expression through TonEBP in nucleus pulposus cells of the intervertebral disc. J Bone Miner Res 2009;24:992–1001.

196. Uchiyama Y, Cheng CC, Danielson KG, et al. Expression of acid-sensing ion channel 3 (ASIC3)

in nucleus pulposus cells of the intervertebral disc is regulated by p75NTR and ERK signaling. J Bone Miner Res 2007;22:1996–2006.

197. Hunter CJ, Bianchi S, Cheng P, et al. Osmoregulatory function of large vacuoles found in notochordal cells of the intervertebral disc running title: an osmoregulatory vacuole. Mol Cell Biomech 2007; 4:227–37.

198. Mavrogonatou E, Kletsas D. Effect of varying osmotic conditions on the response of bovine nucleus pulposus cells to growth factors and the activation of the ERK and Akt pathways. J Orthop Res 2010;28:1276–82.

199. Wuertz K, Urban JP, Klasen J, et al. Influence of extracellular osmolarity and mechanical stimulation on gene expression of intervertebral disc cells. J Orthop Res 2007;25:1513–22.

200. Wang HQ, Yu XD, Liu ZH, et al. Deregulated miR-155 promotes Fas-mediated apoptosis in human intervertebral disc degeneration by targeting FADD and caspase-3. J Pathol 2011. DOI:10.1002/path.2931. [Epub ahead of print].

201. Zhang L, Niu T, Yang SY, et al. The occurrence and regional distribution of DR4 on herniated disc cells: a potential apoptosis pathway in lumbar intervertebral disc. Spine 2008;33:422–7.

202. Liebscher T, Haefeli M, Wuertz K, et al. Age-related variation in cell density of human lumbar intervertebral disc. Spine 2011;36:153–9.

203. Gruber HE, Ingram JA, Norton HJ, et al. Senescence in cells of the aging and degenerating intervertebral disc: immunolocalization of senescence-associated beta-galactosidase in human and sand rat discs. Spine 2007;32:321–7.

204. Le Maitre CL, Freemont AJ, Hoyland JA. Accelerated cellular senescence in degenerate intervertebral discs: a possible role in the pathogenesis of intervertebral disc degeneration. Arthritis Res Ther 2007;9:R45.

205. Roberts S, Evans EH, Kletsas D, et al. Senescence in human intervertebral discs. Eur Spine J 2006; 15(Suppl 3):S312–6.

206. Mwale F, Roughley P, Antoniou J. Distinction between the extracellular matrix of the nucleus pulposus and hyaline cartilage: a requisite for tissue engineering of intervertebral disc. Eur Cell Mater 2004;8:58–63 [discussion: 64].

207. Risbud MV, Guttapalli A, Tsai TT, et al. Evidence for skeletal progenitor cells in the degenerate human intervertebral disc. Spine 2007;32:2537–44.

208. Feng G, Yang X, Shang H, et al. Multipotential differentiation of human annulus fibrosus cells: an in vitro study. J Bone Joint Surg Am 2010;92:675–85.

Intervertebral Disk Nutrition: A Review of Factors Influencing Concentrations of Nutrients and Metabolites

Thijs Grunhagen, DPhil[a,b], Aboulfazl Shirazi-Adl, PhD[c],
Jeremy C.T. Fairbank, MA, MD, FRCS[d], Jill P.G. Urban, PhD[a,*]

KEYWORDS

- Oxygen • Glucose • Diffusion • pH • End plate
- Calcification • Intervertebral • Disk

The normal adult human disk is virtually avascular. Nutrients, principally glucose and oxygen, necessary for survival and activity of disk cells are transported from blood vessels at its margins to the cells deep within the disk matrix, mainly by diffusion; products of metabolism, principally lactic acid, are removed by the reverse route. Loss of adequate nutrient supply has long been associated with the development and progression of disk degeneration because it adversely affects activity and even the viability of disk cells. Although the disk has only a small number of cells, these cells play a vital role. Such cells are responsible for making and maintaining the macromolecules of the disk matrix and, hence, ultimately govern tho diok'o biomcchanical functioning.

Here the authors discuss some of the factors that determine the rate at which nutrients can reach the disk cells. The authors review how these change with degeneration and age. The authors also discuss how the balance between rate of nutrient supply and rate of demand influences the nutrient-metabolite milieu of disk cells and, hence, their activity and survival. Finally, the authors assess the role of nutrient supply in developing successful biologic treatments for disk degeneration.

FACTORS INFLUENCING RATE OF SUPPLY OF NUTRIENTS TO THE DISK CELLS
Blood Supply to the Disks

The adult human disk is virtually avascular apart from a small number of capillaries that penetrate only a few millimeters into the outermost annulus. The disk is, thus, nourished by blood vessels at its margins.[1,2] Those arising in the vertebral bodies feed most of the disk; only the outer annulus is nourished by blood vessels in the soft tissues at the annulus periphery.[3,4] The supply through the vertebral bodies is, thus, critical for disk health.[4] The blood supply to the vertebral column has

The authors thank the European Community's Seventh Framework Program (FP7, 2007–2013) under grant agreement HEALTH-F2-2008-201626 for support.
[a] Department of Physiology, Anatomy and Genetics, Oxford University, Le Gros Clark Building, South Parks Road, Oxford OX1 3QX, UK
[b] Philips Research, High Tech Campus 5, 5656 AE, Eindhoven, The Netherlands
[c] Génie mécanique, École Polytechnique, Montréal, Québec, Canada H3C 3A7
[d] Nuffield Department of Orthopaedics, Rheumatology and Musculoskeletal Sciences, Oxford University, Oxford, OX3 7LD, UK
* Corresponding author.
E-mail address: jill.urban@dpag.ox.ac.uk

Orthop Clin N Am 42 (2011) 465–477
doi:10.1016/j.ocl.2011.07.010

been mapped at different stages of development and aging by several angiographic studies.[5–9] In healthy young adults, the first through fourth lumbar vertebral bodies are supplied by pairs of arteries rising from the posterior wall of the abdominal aorta, whereas the fifth lumbar vertebral body is mainly supplied by arteries originating in the aortic bifurcation.[10] These arteries branch into a complex system of smaller vessels that give rise to the capillaries responsible for supplying nutrients to the disk (**Fig. 1**). These capillaries penetrate the marrow spaces of the subchondral plate of the vertebral body and terminate in loops at the interface between the vertebral body and cartilaginous end plate.[11–17] They contain muscarinic receptors[18] and, therefore, are not passive conduits[19] because flow through the capillary bed is regulated by drugs, such as acetyl choline and those in cigarette smoke,[19–21] and possibly other physiologic signals, such as vibration. In addition to causing the capillary bed to constrict, these stimuli can also lead it to remodel in the long-term.[22]

Transport of Nutrients from the Blood Vessels to the Disk Cells: Fluid Flow or Diffusion

The adult lumbar disks are large; the anterior height of the lower lumbar disks may be more than 20 mm and the mid-disk height more than 15 mm.[23,24] Nutrients, thus, have to move long distances (about 5–8 mm) from the capillaries at the end plate-disk interface through a dense matrix to reach cells in the disk center.

Potentially, nutrients could move by diffusion under gradients set up by the cells' metabolic demands. As is often suggested, nutrients could

also be transported to the disk cells by fluid pumped in and out of the disk during customary daily changes in load.[25] Although convective flow can enhance the transport of large molecules, several experimental and theoretical studies have shown that movement of small solutes, such as glucose and oxygen, through cartilage matrices is predominantly by diffusion rather than by convection.[26–28] Indeed, if convection rather than diffusion played a major role in delivery of nutrients to the disk cells, the nutrient supply would be compromised during any prolonged period of inactivity; moreover, the cells would, in general, have a lower nutrient supply during the day's activities when, as a result of the overall increased and sustained compression loading,[29,30] there is a considerable net movement of fluid out of the disk.[31]

The Cartilaginous End Plate

All nutrients supplied by the blood vessels arising in the vertebral body have to diffuse through the cartilaginous end plate, a thin layer of rigid hyaline cartilage lying between the vertebral body and the disk itself.[16,17,32] In young humans, in addition to the layer of hyaline cartilage, there is a zone of growth cartilage adjacent to the bone,[32] which is penetrated by cartilage canals[33] facilitating nutrient transport into this area of the disk during growth. With the increase in maturity, the cartilage canals vanish and the growth cartilage thins to disappear in late adolescence.[32,34] The disk then has to rely on nutrients supplied by small capillaries that penetrate the subchondral plate of the vertebral body and terminate in loops at the cartilage end plate[15,17] (see **Fig. 1**) and possibly from

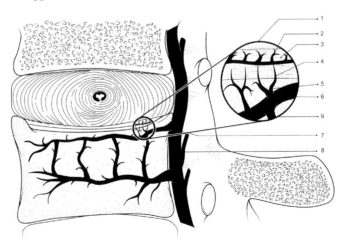

Fig. 1. The organization of the venous system in a human vertebral body. The inset shows an enlarged section of the disk-bone interface with the intervertebral disk (1), the capillary bed through which nutrients to the disk are provided (2–3), the venous system perforating the subchondral plate and the collecting vein (4–5), and the venous system of the vertebral body (6–9). (*From* Crock HV, Yoshizawa H, Kame SK. Observations on the venous drainage of the human vertebral body. J Bone Joint Surg Br 1973;55(3):528–33; with permission.)

transport via marrow spaces, which occupy around 20% of the cartilage/bone interface; these spaces seem directly related to permeability of the subchondral bone as measured in vitro.[17,25,32]

Because all nutrients supplied by the capillaries of the end-plate route must pass through the cartilaginous end plate, transport properties of the end plate regulate movement of solutes into and out of the disk.[35] As in other cartilages, penetration of solutes into the end plate depends on their charge, shape, and molecular weight; end-plate cartilage, thus, acts as a selective permeability barrier, allowing for easier passage of small solutes, such as glucose and oxygen, but severely impeding the transport of large solutes, such as growth factors and matrix macromolecules.[35,36] Calcification of this end plate severely restricts the transport of even small solutes through the cartilaginous end plate as discussed later.[35]

Diffusion Through the Disk Matrix

As in the cartilaginous end plate, movement of solutes through the disk itself is governed by factors that depend both on matrix composition and on solute properties.[35,37–41] Solute movement through the matrix is restricted by its dense proteoglycan network, which regulates the size of pores available to solutes; the higher the proteoglycan concentration, the smaller the average pore size. In general, only a small fraction of pores are accessible to large solutes, limiting their concentration in the tissue to low levels. However, small solutes, such as oxygen, can penetrate into most of the available pores. As the disk degenerates and proteoglycans are lost, pore size increases, allowing access to large molecules, such as growth factors or cytokines, which are virtually excluded from normal disks.

The rate of movement of solutes through the matrix is regulated by solute diffusivity, which again depends on water content and matrix properties, particularly proteoglycan concentration. For instance, loss of hydration during loading, which increases proteoglycan concentration, will decrease diffusivity.[42] Thus, for any solute, diffusivity varies with the position in the disk and depends on local proteoglycan concentration. In the annulus, diffusivity also depends on direction, differing radially from axially.[38,39] Solute diffusivity also varies with solute molecular weight and shape.[43] Diffusivities of small solutes, such as glucose and oxygen, are considerably greater than that of large proteins.

The amount diffusing into the disk is very sensitive to disk dimensions, particularly disk height (**Fig. 2**). Diffusion to the center of the disk will be

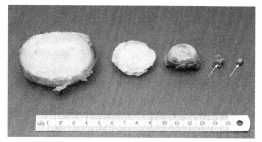

Fig. 2. Variation of dimensions of disks from different spinal levels and different animal species. From left to right, the figure shows human lumbar L4-L5, Bovine caudal C1-C2, sheep thoracic T11-T12, rat lumbar disk, rat tail disk (*arrows* demonstrate disk location). (*From* Alini M, Eisenstein SM, Ito K, et al. Are animal models useful for studying human disk disorders/degeneration? Eur Spine J 2008;17(1):2–19; with permission.)

much more rapid in a small animal disk than in a large human lumbar disk[44]; and, thus, potential nutritional problems may be missed in animal disk degeneration models. In human disks, diffusion will also be affected by the load-induced variations in disk height because the disk may lose and regain more than 20% of its height during the diurnal cycle.[31,45,46] Fluid loss increases proteoglycan content and, hence, decreases porosity, thus, leading to a decrease in solute diffusivity. It also, however, reduces disk height, potentially increasing the rate of transport to the disk center. Calculations and experiments show that these 2 opposing effects balance each other out for nutrients, such as oxygen and glucose, so that the diurnal loss and regain of fluid has little effect on nutrient concentration profiles, at least in normal disks.[42,47] However, for solutes even as small as 500 daltons, long-term static loading seems to significantly impede transport into the center of the disks[48]; but it is unclear whether it is through alterations in blood flow or in transport through the matrix.

FAILURE OF NUTRIENT TRANSPORT AND ASSOCIATION WITH DISK DEGENERATION
Disturbances of Nutrient Transport with Ageing and Pathology

Nutrients are supplied to the disk from capillaries, which are fed by blood flowing through the arteries of the vertebral bodies. Nutrients must then be able to pass from the capillaries through the cartilaginous endplate into the disk matrix. Several studies have shown that pathologic changes to any of these spinal structures can influence nutrient pathways and transport adversely and are associated with disk degeneration (see article by Chan and colleagues).

Although interest has focused on changes at the bone-disk junction, atherosclerosis of the lumbar arteries restricting blood flow to the lumbar spine has also been associated with disk degeneration and back pain. Kauppila[49] has recently reviewed the evidence for this. For instance, chronic back pain was significantly more common in those with occluded or narrowed lumbar arteries[50]; calcification and stenotic changes seen in the abdominal aorta were associated with disk degeneration,[51,52] as were high levels of cholesterol and triglycerides.[53,54] However, it should be noted that disk degeneration is evident in many people in the first and second decade of life,[55] well before atherosclerosis develops (see article by Chan and colleagues).

Disorders that affect the microcirculation, such as sickle-cell anemia, Gaucher disease, and Caisson disease, which all can restrict capillary flow, are also associated with disk degeneration.[56] The effects of environmental factors, such as smoking, which can also restrict blood flow through the capillaries feeding the disk,[20] are, however, controversial.[57–60] Moreover, although several mechanisms linking smoking to disk degeneration have been proposed,[20,21,61,62] there is no direct evidence to show that any association between smoking and disk degeneration is causal.

Pathologic changes that influence the pathway between blood supply and disk have long been shown to affect transport to the disk.[63] Sclerosis of the bony end plate and increase in bone mineral density decrease contact area with the cartilaginous end plate and, hence, reduce end-plate permeability and are associated with an increase in disk degeneration.[64–67] The cartilaginous end plate, a critical component in the transport pathway, shows early signs of degeneration with cracks, irregularities, protrusions of nucleus material through the end plate, and Schmorl nodes evident even by the second decade.[68] Moreover, the end plate calcifies, which can severely impede transport from the blood supply to the disk.[35] The degree of calcification of the end plate, as well as other irregularities, increases with ageing[32,68] and also with disk degeneration (**Fig. 3**).[69,70] The cartilage end plates of scoliotic disks are also often heavily calcified,[71] and here direct measurement has shown such calcification impedes transport from the blood supply into the disk.[72,73]

Direct Visualization of Transport of Solutes into the Disk

Over the past decade, the development of relatively noninvasive magnetic resonance imaging (MRI) techniques for following movement of contrast medium has provided insights into how pathologic changes affect transport into the disk.[74–76] In these studies, the enhancement of the signal in the disk following intravenous injection of a paramagnetic contrast agent is monitored over several hours (**Fig. 4**). Comparison of the precontrast and postcontrast enhancement gives a semiquantitative measure of the rate of transport of the agent into the disk.[77]

These studies have shown first of all that transport into disks is slow and in line with that expected from diffusion; the contrast agent moves forward as a diffusion front and only reaches the center of normal lumbar disks at around 6 hours.[77] They have also shown definitively that degeneration of the disk affects transport of solutes into it; even with mild degeneration, transport is both reduced in extent and delayed.[75,77] In degenerate disks, however, the pattern of enhancement is irregular and enhancement may be rapid with spikes within 10 minutes after injection,[77] possibly because of vascular ingrowth and the breaches of the end plate. Rajasekaran and colleagues[78] have devised an end-plate score, which relates to the extent of disk degeneration to patterns of postcontrast movement into the disk. This score could potentially be used as a diagnostic tool, but it needs further validation.

Because postcontrast serial MRI studies can be performed noninvasively and require only clinical MRI equipment, it is hoped that they increase our understanding of factors influencing nutrient transport and their relationship to disk failure. To date, postcontrast serial MRI has been used to study the effects of vasoactive drugs on nutrient transport.[78] The administration of nimodepine, a vasodilator, increased signal intensity in the disk by approximately 15%, indicating the importance of blood flow rate on the delivery of nutrients to the disk. It has also been used to examine the effect of mechanical loading, whereby 4.5 hours of sustained creep loading reduced solute diffusion into the disk[48] under static load. The reduction of transport into scoliotic disks, which undergo long-term sustained loading in vivo with consequent remodeling, was even more marked and was apparent before other MRI changes were visible.[73]

THE EXTRACELLULAR NUTRIENT-METABOLITE MILIEU REGULATES CELL VIABILITY AND ACTIVITY

As previously discussed, nutrients are transported to the disk cells from the arterial blood supply by a long and complex pathway that can be affected

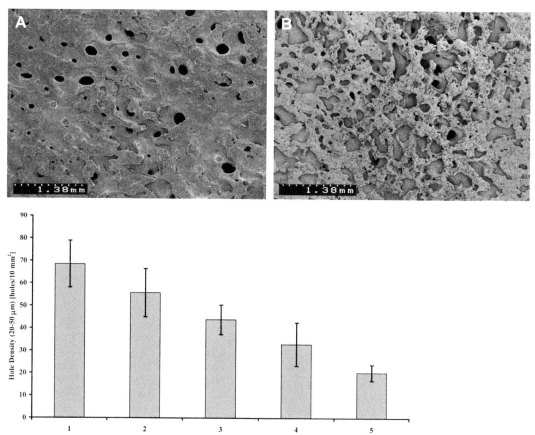

Fig. 3. Calcification of the endplate increases with age and degree of degeneration. (*A*) and (*B*) show a scanning electron micrograph of the disk-bone interface after soft tissue has been removed from human lumbar disks by enzyme digestion at 30 years (*A*) and 80 years (*B*). The graph shows the decrease in density of the open holes, 20 to 50 μm in diameter per 10-mm² area of nucleus pulposus endplate, with increase in disk degeneration (*solid lines*) are error bars (1 standard error of the mean). (*Adapted from* Benneker LM, Heini PF, Alini M, et al. 2004 Young Investigator Award Winner: vertebral endplate marrow contact channel occlusions and intervertebral disk degeneration. Spine 2005;30(2):167–73; with permission.)

adversely by aging and degeneration. However, the local nutrient-metabolite milieu does not only depend on transport of nutrients to the cells but also by rates of cellular activity. It is this local milieu that determines cell function and, if nutrients or pH decrease to critical levels, cell survival. Cellular activity, particularly the production of matrix macromolecules, is strongly dependent on maintenance of an appropriate level of nutrients and metabolites. A decrease in oxygen tension, glucose levels, or in pH leads to a marked reduction in matrix gene expression and production of sulfated glycosaminoglycans, for instance.[79–81] Furthermore, cells will not survive if glucose levels decrease less than approximately 0.5 mm or if lactic acid is not removed and consequently the extracellular pH decreases to less than approximately pH 6.7.[82,83]

Rates of Cell Metabolism Regulate the Local Nutrient-Metabolite Milieu

The rates at which these disk cells consume nutrients, such as glucose and oxygen, and produce metabolic by-products, such as lactic acid, are critical determinants of the nutrient concentrations throughout the disk. For example, all disk cells consume sulfate to produce the sulfated glycosaminoglycan side chains of proteoglycans. However, actual rates of sulfate incorporation are very low compared with the concentration of sulfate available, so that sulfate concentration is hardly affected by cellular activity and the gradient is almost flat.[84] For glucose, the situation is different, even though concentrations and diffusivities of sulfate and glucose are similar, disk cells consume glucose at rates that almost deplete it from the disk center.[85] The rates of energy

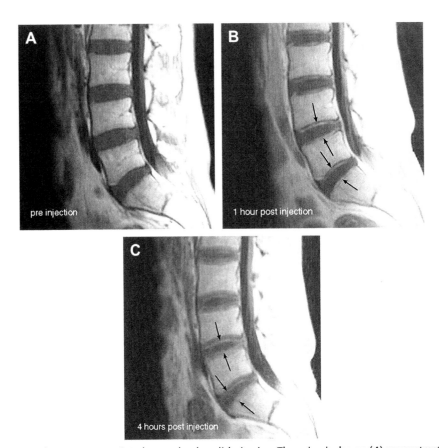

Fig. 4. Transport of contrast agent into human lumbar disks in vivo. The spine is shown (*A*) precontrast, (*B*) 1 hour after intravenous injection of contrast, and (*C*) 4 hours after contrast injection. The diffusion of contrast from the blood supply into the disk is visible and can be quantitated. Arrows show movement of contrast medium into the disk. (*Adapted from* Bydder GM. New approaches to magnetic resonance imaging of intervertebral disks, tendons, ligaments, and menisci. Spine 2002;27(12):1264–8; with permission.)

metabolism per cell vary with disk cell phenotype. Notochordal nucleus pulposus cells found in infant humans and in animals, such as rodents and pigs, consume oxygen and glucose at a much higher rate than the chondrocytelike nucleus cells seen in adult human disks. Moreover, other factors, such as the presence of cytokines and growth factors; mechanical stress; and levels of pH, oxygen, and glucose, also alter rates of nutrient consumption and lactic acid production. Thus, a disk that has an adequate nutrient supply under normal conditions, may be placed under nutrient stress by inflammatory signals or by inappropriate mechanical stresses.

Measured Nutrient-Metabolite Concentrations

There is little direct information on nutrient or metabolite concentrations in the disk because measurements of glucose, oxygen, lactate, and pH levels at the required sensitivity can now only be made invasively. Oxygen concentrations have

been measured by inserting needle microelectrodes into disk explants in vitro[38,42] and in vivo into disks of dogs[85] (**Fig. 5**A) and human surgical patients.[83,86] Intradiscal pH has also been measured in situ using electrodes.[61,87,88] Lactate and glucose have, however, only been measured biochemically in explants or in tissue segments taken at surgery.[73,83,85,86,89] All of these measurements confirm that there are concentration gradients of nutrients and metabolites in the disk, that these are consistent with those expected for transport of these solutes into and out of the disk by diffusion, and that pathologic changes can influence metabolite and nutrient concentrations considerably (see **Fig. 5**B) and lead to situations whereby disk cells can no longer function or even survive.

The Importance of Modeling Nutrient Concentrations

It is difficult, if not impossible, particularly in humans, to obtain more than a limited snapshot of local levels of nutrients in the disk by direct measurement. Thus,

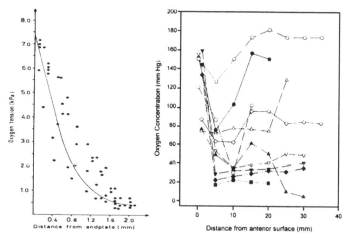

Fig. 5. Oxygen profiles measured in vivo using oxygen needle microelectrodes. The left hand sides shows concentrations measured from the endplate toward the nucleus center in animal disks. The right hand sides shows oxygen concentrations measured in lumbar disks of patients undergoing routine surgery for treatment of low-back pain via an anterior approach. Even though these profiles were measured in different directions, it is evident that oxygen tensions in the healthy animal disk fall continuously with distance from the blood supply in all animals tests, whereas the oxygen tension in patients' disks, although falling across the outer annulus in virtually all patients, follows a much more erratic course toward the inner annulus and nucleus, with very high oxygen tensions in some patients (vascular ingrowth or dead cells) and very low tensions in others, probably because patterns of pathologic changes and degree of degeneration varied from patient to patient. (*From* Holm S, Maroudas A, Urban JP, et al. Nutrition of the intervertebral disk: solute transport and metabolism. Connect Tissue Res 1981;8(2):101–19; with permission; and Bartels EM, Fairbank JC, Winlove CP, et al. Oxygen and lactate concentrations measured in vivo in the intervertebral disks of scoliotic and back pain patients. Spine 1998;231–8; with permission.)

measurement cannot provide an understanding of how ageing and pathologic changes or environmental factors, such as mechanical load, affect the extracellular nutrient-metabolite milieu. However, as previously discussed, nutrients are small molecules that move through the disk matrix almost entirely by diffusion under gradients set up by cellular metabolic activity.[26–28] Levels of nutrients can, thus, be calculated using standard diffusion equations. The validity of diffusive models has been demonstrated in animal experiments in vivo and in model systems in vitro. In these cases, changes in concentration across the disk could be measured experimentally, and measured profiles were in good agreement with those calculated from diffusion-reaction models.[42,84] Therefore, modeling is able to provide insight into nutrient-concentration profiles throughout the disk for situations whereby measurement is difficult, if not impossible.

The first models were analytical[44,90] and, hence, were limited in scope. Nevertheless, they demonstrated how nutrient-concentration profiles were governed by the balance between rates of transport of nutrients into the disk and rates of cellular metabolism; thereby, cell density and the rate of metabolism per cell were critical parameters. A significant advance was provided by the

incorporation of finite element methods,[91] allowing calculation of profiles resulting from diffusion from both the endplate and the annulus periphery. A further advance in modeling arose when data on the interrelationships of metabolic rates became available.[92] Metabolic profiles calculated using this information showed that profiles of nutrients and metabolites through the disk are interdependent[93]; hence, for example, in regions where oxygen tensions are low, glucose concentrations are necessarily also low and lactic acid concentrations high. Modeling has been further extended to examine diffusive profiles in a realistic 3-dimensional (3D) geometry.[94] As such, the results demonstrate the importance of considering a 3D geometry for understanding details of the local nutrient-metabolite milieu, particularly in areas distant from the nutrient supply (**Fig. 6**). A recent axisymmetric model that calculated effect of variations in end-plate permeability on nutrient and pH gradients used this information together with data on the critical nutrient concentrations necessary for cells to stay alive to calculate nutrient concentration levels, cell death, and viable cell densities in relation to end-plate properties.[95]

Although they are limited by availability of data, both as input into the models and for subsequent validation of predictions, parametric studies have

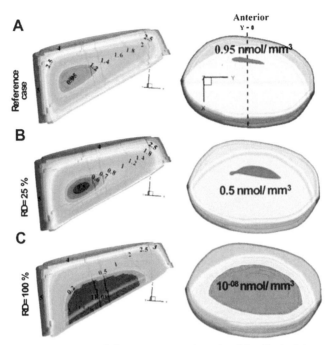

Fig. 6. Results of 3-dimentional modeling of glucose transport into the disk; effect of changes in relative diffusivity across the distal endplate on glucose concentration profiles. The left hand side figures shows a midsagittal view of the glucose concentration profiles (critical glucose concentrations shown in purple). The right hand sides figures shows a top view of the disk with critical region in gray. The results were calculated for distal endplate diffusivities of 100% (*A*), 25% (*B*), and 5% (*C*). The simulation shows how reduction in transport through the central region of the distal endplate alone can lead to large regions of the disk unable to support viable and active cells. (*From* Mokhbi SD, Shirazi-adl A, Urban JP. Investigation of solute concentrations in a 3D model of intervertebral disk. Eur Spine J 2009;18(2):254–62; with permission.)

shown the relative sensitivity of the nutrient-metabolite milieu to factors, such as changes in metabolic rates, diffusivity, hydration, or end-plate permeability. Such studies have investigated how the milieu is affected by mechanical loading, disk deformation, and disk degeneration.[47,93,94,96] These studies have considerably increased understanding of which factors are important regulators of nutrient concentrations and, hence, cellular activity in the disk. The models confirm the critical role of end-plate permeability in maintaining disk health. They have demonstrated that concentrations are governed not only by the adequacy of the supply but also by cellular demand. For instance, growth factors or inflammation by increasing glucose consumption rates can deplete nutrients from the center of the disk.[94] Importantly, they have shown that a decrease in end-plate permeability to less than threshold levels leads to cell death in central regions of the disk.[95] Models, thus, can increase the understanding of how nutrient supply and changes consequent on degeneration regulate the density of viable cells that can be supported in a disk.

NUTRITION AND BIOLOGIC THERAPIES

There is considerable interest in the possibility of using biologic therapies to repair or regenerate the disk matrix and restore disk biomechanical function[97–99] (see articles by Sakai, Woods and colleagues, Leung and colleagues, and Bae and Masuda). Until recently, most emphasis has been expended on repairing the nucleus pulposus that involves strategies for implanting new active cells or tissues into a degenerate disk or stimulating resident cells to produce matrix or suppress production of degradative factors by the injection of bioactive compounds or by gene therapy.[100–103] These therapies have shown promise when tested in degenerate disks of animals, such as rabbits and dogs.[104–106] It should be noted, however, that these tests are almost invariably performed in young animals whereby disk degeneration has been induced acutely[107] and, thus, the remodeling of the disk and other spinal structures seen in human disk degeneration does not occur. Moreover, the nucleus of rabbits and rodents is populated by notochordal cells rather than the chondrocytelike cells found in the human nucleus pulposus. These animal models, thus, may not reflect all changes in the disk and other spinal structures seen in humans with degenerate disks.[107]

Despite the promise shown in animal studies, there are several severe technical limitations that have to be overcome before these biologic therapies can be applied successfully in humans.[98,108] Among these limitations, and probably the most difficult to deal with, is nutrient supply. As previously discussed, solute transport to and from disk cells is impeded even in mildly degenerate disks,[76] with adverse effects on cellular activity and viability. If nutrient supply is not adequate to maintain the function of the resident population of cells, implanted cells will also not function. Moreover, injections of growth factors that stimulate energy demand of the resident cells can place increasing demand on an already restricted nutrient supply; therefore, the net effect may not be beneficial. Thus, unless the nutrient supply can support the implanted cells or stimulated resident cells, biologic therapies are unlikely to repair or regenerate a damaged disk.

Nevertheless, as a result of the success in animals, cell therapies have been used clinically to treat patients. Cells isolated from surgical waste tissue obtained during routine operations to relieve sciatic pain have been expanded in culture and reintroduced into the surgical site[109] and are claimed to have a good outcome; but only limited results have been reported to date, and there is no adequate control group for comparison. A clinical trial for treating early disk degeneration by intradiscal injection of rhGDF-5 is underway,[110] but no results are yet available.

Biologic therapies may have a role to play in some patients. However, identifying patients who might benefit from such treatments will be demanding and has received relatively little attention. Moreover, as previously discussed, biologic treatments will only succeed where the nutrient supply to the disks is adequate; some validated method of assessing this seems essential before such therapies are introduced into the clinic. Also, despite the great advances in imaging, identification of painful disks is clinically challenging. Discography is widely used for this purpose; but its use is controversial, primarily because it seems to be a poor predictor of outcomes to fusion,[111] and long-term adverse effects have been noted in disks subjected to discography.[112] This finding means that designing entry criteria for clinical trials of biologic and other interventions will be difficult.

REFERENCES

1. Beadle OA. The intervertebral discs. Observations on their normal and morbid anatomy in relation to certain spinal deformities. London: His Majesty's Stationery Office; 1931.
2. Nerlich AG, Schaaf R, Walchli B, et al. Temporospatial distribution of blood vessels in human lumbar intervertebral discs. Eur Spine J 2007; 16(4):547–55.
3. Brodin H. Paths of nutrition in articular cartilage and intervertebral discs. Acta Orthop Scand 1955;24:177–83.
4. Ogata K, Whiteside LA. 1980 Volvo award winner in basic science. Nutritional pathways of the intervertebral disc. An experimental study using hydrogen washout technique. Spine 1981;6:211–6.
5. Ratcliffe JF. The arterial anatomy of the developing human dorsal and lumbar vertebral body. A microarteriographic study. J Anat 1981;133(Pt 4):625–38.
6. Hassler O. The human intervertebral disc. A microangiographical study of its vascular supply at various ages. Acta Orthop Scand 1970;40:765–72.
7. Crock HV, Yoshizawa H, Kame SK. Observations on the venous drainage of the human vertebral body. J Bone Joint Surg Br 1973;55(3):528–33.
8. Crock HV, Yoshizawa H. The blood supply of the vertebral column. Clin Orthop Relat Res 1976; 115:6–21.
9. Ratcliffe JF. The arterial anatomy of the adult human lumbar vertebral body: a microarteriographic study. J Anat 1980;131(1):57–79.
10. Ratcliffe JF. The anatomy of the fourth and fifth lumbar arteries in humans: an arteriographic study in one hundred live subjects. J Anat 1982; 135:753–61.
11. Crock HV, Goldwasser M. Anatomic studies of the circulation in the region of the vertebral end-plate in adult greyhound dogs. Spine 1984;9:702–6.
12. Crock HV, Goldwasser M, Yoshizawa H. Vascular anatomy related to the intervertebral disc. In: Ghosh P, editor. Biology of the intervertebral disc. Boca Raton (FL): CRC Press; 1991. p. 109–33.
13. Chandraraj S, Briggs CA, Opeskin K. Disc herniations in the young and end-plate vascularity. Clin Anat 1998;11(3):171–6.
14. Kobayashi S, Baba H, Takeno K, et al. Fine structure of cartilage canal and vascular buds in the rabbit vertebral endplate. Laboratory investigation. J Neurosurg Spine 2008;9(1):96–103.
15. Oki S, Matsuda Y, Itoh T, et al. Scanning electron microscopic observations of the vascular structure of vertebral end-plates in rabbits. J Orthop Res 1994;12(3):447–9.
16. Moore RJ. The vertebral end-plate: what do we know? Eur Spine J 2000;9(2):92–6.

17. Roberts S, Menage J, Urban JP. Biochemical and structural properties of the cartilage end-plate and its relation to the intervertebral disc. Spine 1989;14:166–74.

18. Brown MF, Hukkanen MV, McCarthy ID, et al. Sensory and sympathetic innervation of the vertebral endplate in patients with degenerative disc disease. J Bone Joint Surg Br 1997;79(1): 147–53.

19. Wallace AL, Wyatt BC, McCarthy ID, et al. Humoral regulation of blood flow in the vertebral endplate. Spine 1994;19(12):1324–8.

20. Holm S, Nachemson A. Nutrition of the intervertebral disc: acute effects of cigarette smoking. An experimental animal study. Ups J Med Sci 1988; 93(1):91–9.

21. Uematsu Y, Matuzaki H, Iwahashi M. Effects of nicotine on the intervertebral disc: an experimental study in rabbits. J Orthop Sci 2001;6(2): 177–82.

22. Iwahashi M, Matsuzaki H, Tokuhashi Y, et al. Mechanism of intervertebral disc degeneration caused by nicotine in rabbits to explicate intervertebral disc disorders caused by smoking. Spine 2002; 27(13):1396–401.

23. Amonoo-Kuofi HS. Morphometric changes in the heights and anteroposterior diameters of the lumbar intervertebral discs with age. J Anat 1991; 175:159–68.

24. Aydinlioglu A, Diyarbakirli S, Keles P. Heights of the lumbar intervertebral discs related to age in Turkish individuals. Tohoku J Exp Med 1999; 188(1):11–22.

25. Laffosse JM, Accadbled F, Molinier F, et al. Correlations between effective permeability and marrow contact channels surface of vertebral endplates. J Orthop Res 2010;28(9):1229–34.

26. Urban JP, Holm S, Maroudas A, et al. Nutrition of the intervertebral disc: effect of fluid flow on solute transport. Clin Orthop 1982;170:296–302.

27. Katz MM, Hargens AR, Garfin SR. Intervertebral disc nutrition. Diffusion versus convection. Clin Orthop 1986;(210):243–5.

28. Ferguson SJ, Ito K, Nolte LP. Fluid flow and convective transport of solutes within the intervertebral disc. J Biomech 2004;37(2):213–21.

29. Nachemson A, Elfstrom G. Intravital dynamic pressure measurements in lumbar discs. A study of common movements, maneuvers and exercises. Scand J Rehabil Med 1970;2(Suppl 1):1–40.

30. Wilke HJ, Neef P, Caimi M, et al. New in vivo measurements of pressures in the intervertebral disc in daily life. Spine 1999;24(8):755–62.

31. Boos N, Wallin A, Gbedegbegnon T, et al. Quantitative MR imaging of lumbar intervertebral discs and vertebral bodies: influence of diurnal water content variations. Radiology 1993;188:351–4.

32. Bernick S, Cailliet R. Vertebral end-plate changes with aging of human vertebrae. Spine 1982;7(2): 97–102.

33. Whalen JL, Parke WW, Mazur JM, et al. The intrinsic vasculature of developing vertebral end plates and its nutritive significance to the intervertebral discs. J Pediatr Orthop 1985;5(4): 403–10.

34. Rudert M, Tillmann B. Detection of lymph and blood vessels in the human intervertebral disc by histochemical and immunohistochemical methods. Anat Anz 1993;175(3):237–42.

35. Roberts S, Urban JPG, Evans H, et al. Transport properties of the human cartilage endplate in relation to its composition and calcification. Spine 1996;21:415–20.

36. Shibuya K. Experimental and clinical studies on metabolism with the intervertebral disc. Nihon Seikeigeka Gakkai Zasshi 1970;44:1–24.

37. Travascio F, Jackson AR, Brown MD, et al. Relationship between solute transport properties and tissue morphology in human annulus fibrosus. J Orthop Res 2009;27(12):1625–30.

38. O'Hare D, Winlove CP, Parker KH. Electrochemical method for direct measurement of oxygen concentration and diffusivity in the intervertebral disc: electrochemical characterization and tissue-sensor interactions. J Biomed Eng 1991;13(4): 304–12.

39. Jackson A, Gu W. Transport properties of cartilaginous tissues. Curr Rheumatol Rev 2009;5(1):40–50.

40. Bartels E, Fairbank JC, Winlove CP, et al. Measurement of hydrogen and oxygen in isolated intervertebral discs. J Physiol 1995;483:126.

41. Maroudas A. Transport of solutes through cartilage: permeability to large molecules. J Anat 1976; 122(2):335–47.

42. Grunhagen T. Nutrient transport into intervertebral discs; modelling and electrochemical measurements [thesis/dissertation]. Oxford (UK): University of Oxford; 2010.

43. Maroudas A. Biophysical chemistry of cartilaginous tissues with special reference to solute and fluid transport. Biorheology 1975;12(3–4):233–48.

44. Stairmand JW, Holm S, Urban JP. Factors influencing oxygen concentration gradients in the intervertebral disc. A theoretical analysis. Spine (Phila Pa 1976) 1991;16(4):444–9.

45. de Puky P. The physiological oscillation of the length of the body. Acta Orthop Scand 1935;6:338–47.

46. Tyrrell AR, Reilly T, Troup JD. Circadian variation in stature and the effects of spinal loading. Spine 1985;10:161–4.

47. Soukane DM, Shirazi-adl A, Urban JP. Computation of coupled diffusion of oxygen, glucose and lactic acid in an intervertebral disc. J Biomech 2007; 40(12):2645–54.

48. Arun R, Freeman BJ, Scammell BE, et al. 2009 ISSLS Prize Winner: What influence does sustained mechanical load have on diffusion in the human intervertebral disc? an in vivo study using serial postcontrast magnetic resonance imaging. Spine (Phila Pa 1976) 2009;34(21):2324–37.

49. Kauppila LI. Atherosclerosis and disc degeneration/low-back pain–a systematic review. Eur J Vasc Endovasc Surg 2009;37(6):661–70.

50. Kauppila LI. Prevalence of stenotic changes in arteries supplying the lumbar spine. A postmortem angiographic study on 140 subjects. Ann Rheum Dis 1997;56(10):591–5.

51. Kauppila LI, McAlindon T, Evans S, et al. Disc degeneration/back pain and calcification of the abdominal aorta. A 25-year follow-up study in Framingham. Spine 1997;22(14):1642–7.

52. Kurunlahti M, Tervonen O, Vanharanta H, et al. Association of atherosclerosis with low back pain and the degree of disc degeneration. Spine 1999; 24(20):2080–4.

53. Hangai M, Kaneoka K, Kuno S, et al. Factors associated with lumbar intervertebral disc degeneration in the elderly. Spine J 2008;8(5):732–40.

54. Leino-Arjas P, Kaila-Kangas L, Solovieva S, et al. Serum lipids and low back pain: an association? A follow-up study of a working population sample. Spine (Phila Pa 1976) 2006;31(9):1032–7.

55. Miller J, Schmatz C, Schultz A. Lumbar disc degeneration: correlation with age, sex, and spine level in 600 autopsy specimens. Spine 1988;13:173–8.

56. Jones JP Jr, Engleman EP. Osseous avascular necrosis associated with systemic abnormalities. Arthritis Rheum 1966;9(5):728–36.

57. Leboeuf-yde C. Smoking and low back pain. A systematic literature review of 41 journal articles reporting 47 epidemiologic studies. Spine (Phila Pa 1976) 1999;24(14):1463–70.

58. Goldberg MS, Scott SC, Mayo NE. A review of the association between cigarette smoking and the development of nonspecific back pain and related outcomes. Spine (Phila Pa 1976) 2000;25(8): 995–1014.

59. Hassett G, Hart DJ, Manek NJ, et al. Risk factors for progression of lumbar spine disc degeneration: the Chingford Study. Arthritis Rheum 2003;48(11): 3112–7.

60. Battie MC, Videman T, Gill K, et al. 1991 Volvo Award in clinical sciences. Smoking and lumbar intervertebral disc degeneration: an MRI study of identical twins. Spine 1991;16(9):1015–21.

61. Hambly MF, Mooney V. Effect of smoking and pulsed electromagnetic fields on intradiscal pH in rabbits. Spine 1992;17(Suppl 6):S83–5.

62. Fogelholm RR, Alho AV. Smoking and intervertebral disc degeneration. Med Hypotheses 2001;56(4): 537–9.

63. Nachemson A, Lewin T, Maroudas A, et al. In vitro diffusion of dye through the end-plates and annulus fibrosus of human lumbar intervertebral discs. Acta Orthop Scand 1970;41:589–607.

64. Pye SR, Reid DM, Lunt M, et al. Lumbar disc degeneration: association between osteophytes, end-plate sclerosis and disc space narrowing. Ann Rheum Dis 2007;66(3):330–3.

65. Muraki S, Yamamoto S, Ishibashi H, et al. Impact of degenerative spinal diseases on bone mineral density of the lumbar spine in elderly women. Osteoporos Int 2004;15(9):724–8.

66. Rutges JP, Jagt van der OP, Oner FC, et al. Micro-CT quantification of subchondral endplate changes in intervertebral disc degeneration. Osteoarthritis Cartilage 2011;19(1):89–95.

67. Laffosse JM, Kinkpe C, Gomez-Brouchet A, et al. Micro-computed tomography study of the subchondral bone of the vertebral endplates in a porcine model: correlations with histomorphometric parameters. Surg Radiol Anat 2010;32(4):335–41.

68. Weiler C, Nerlich AG, Zipperer J, et al. 2002 SSE Award Competition in Basic Science: expression of major matrix metalloproteinases is associated with intervertebral disc degradation and resorption. Eur Spine J 2002;11(4):308–20.

69. Benneker LM, Heini PF, Alini M, et al. 2004 Young Investigator Award Winner: vertebral endplate marrow contact channel occlusions and intervertebral disc degeneration. Spine 2005;30(2):167–73.

70. Vernon-Roberts B. Disc pathology and disease states. In: Ghosh P, editor. The biology of the intervertebral disc. Boca Raton (FL): CRC press; 1988. p. 73–119.

71. Roberts S, Menage J, Eisenstein SM. The cartilage end-plate and intervertebral disc in scoliosis: calcification and other sequelae. J Orthop Res 1993; 11(5):747–57.

72. Urban MR, Fairbank JC, Etherington PJ, et al. Electrochemical measurement of transport into scoliotic intervertebral discs in vivo using nitrous oxide as a tracer. Spine 2001;26(8):984–90.

73. Rajasekaran S, Vidyadhara S, Subbiah M, et al. ISSLS prize winner: a study of effects of in vivo mechanical forces on human lumbar discs with scoliotic disc as a biological model: results from serial postcontrast diffusion studies, histopathology and biochemical analysis of twenty-one human lumbar scoliotic discs. Spine (Phila Pa 1976) 2010;35(21):1930–43.

74. Bydder GM. New approaches to magnetic resonance imaging of intervertebral discs, tendons, ligaments, and menisci. Spine 2002;27(12):1264–8.

75. Nguyenminh C, Riley L, Ho KC, et al. Effect of degeneration of the intervertebral disk on the process of diffusion. AJNR Am J Neuroradiol 1997;18(3):435–42.

76. Rajasekaran S, Naresh-Babu J, Murugan S. Review of postcontrast MRI studies on diffusion of human

lumbar discs. J Magn Reson Imaging 2007;25(2): 410–8.

77. Rajasekaran S, Babu JN, Arun R, et al. ISSLS prize winner: a study of diffusion in human lumbar discs: a serial magnetic resonance imaging study documenting the influence of the endplate on diffusion in normal and degenerate discs. Spine 2004; 29(23):2654–67.

78. Rajasekaran S, Venkatadass K, Naresh BJ, et al. Pharmacological enhancement of disc diffusion and differentiation of healthy, ageing and degenerated discs: results from in-vivo serial post-contrast MRI studies in 365 human lumbar discs. Eur Spine J 2008;17(5):626–43.

79. Razaq S, Wilkins RJ, Urban JP. The effect of extracellular pH on matrix turnover by cells of the bovine nucleus pulposus. Eur Spine J 2003;12(4):341–9.

80. Ishihara H, Urban JP. Effects of low oxygen concentrations and metabolic inhibitors on proteoglycan and protein synthesis rates in the intervertebral disc. J Orthop Res 1999;17(6):829–35.

81. Rinkler C, Heuer F, Pedro MT, et al. Influence of low glucose supply on the regulation of gene expression by nucleus pulposus cells and their responsiveness to mechanical loading. J Neurosurg Spine 2010;13(4):535–42.

82. Bibby SR, Urban JP. Effect of nutrient deprivation on the viability of intervertebral disc cells. Eur Spine J 2004;13(8):695–701.

83. Bibby SR, Fairbank JC, Urban MR, et al. Cell viability in scoliotic discs in relation to disc deformity and nutrient levels. Spine 2002;27(20):2220–8.

84. Urban JP, Holm S, Maroudas A. Diffusion of small solutes into the intervertebral disc: as in vivo study. Biorheology 1978;15(3–4):203–21.

85. Holm S, Maroudas A, Urban JP, et al. Nutrition of the intervertebral disc: solute transport and metabolism. Connect Tissue Res 1981;8(2):101–19.

86. Bartels EM, Fairbank JCT, Winlove CP, et al. Oxygen and lactate concentrations measured in vivo in the intervertebral discs of scoliotic and back pain patients. Spine 1998;23:1–7.

87. Nachemson A. Intradiscal measurements of pH in patients with lumbar rhizopathies. Acta Orthop Scand 1969;40:23–42.

88. Kitano T, Zerwekh JE, Usui Y, et al. Biochemical changes associated with the symptomatic human intervertebral disc. Clin Orthop 1993;(293):372–7.

89. Holm S, Selstam G, Nachemson A. Carbohydrate metabolism and concentration profiles of solutes in the canine lumbar intervertebral disc. Acta Physiol Scand 1982;115(1):147–56.

90. Maroudas A, Stockwell RA, Nachemson A, et al. Factors involved in the nutrition of the human lumbar intervertebral disc: cellularity and diffusion of glucose in vitro. J Anat 1975;120(1):113–30.

91. Selard E, Shirazi-adl A, Urban JP. Finite element study of nutrient diffusion in the human intervertebral disc. Spine 2003;28(17):1945–53.

92. Bibby SR, Jones DA, Ripley RM, et al. Metabolism of the intervertebral disc: effects of low levels of oxygen, glucose, and pH on rates of energy metabolism of bovine nucleus pulposus cells. Spine 2005;30(5):487–96.

93. Soukane DM, Shirazi-adl A, Urban JP. Analysis of nonlinear coupled diffusion of oxygen and lactic acid in intervertebral discs. J Biomech Eng 2005; 127(7):1121–6.

94. Soukane DM, Shirazi-adl A, Urban JP. Investigation of solute concentrations in a 3D model of intervertebral disc. Eur Spine J 2009;18(2):254–62.

95. Shirazi-adl A, Taheri M, Urban JP. Analysis of cell viability in intervertebral disc: effect of endplate permeability on cell population. J Biomech 2010; 43(7):1330–6.

96. Magnier C, Boiron O, Wendling-Mansuy S, et al. Nutrient distribution and metabolism in the intervertebral disc in the unloaded state: a parametric study. J Biomech 2009;42(2):100–8.

97. Bron JL, Helder MN, Meisel HJ, et al. Repair, regenerative and supportive therapies of the annulus fibrosus: achievements and challenges. Eur Spine J 2009;18(3):301–13.

98. Kandel R, Roberts S, Urban JP. Tissue engineering and the intervertebral disc: the challenges. Eur Spine J 2008;17(Suppl 4):480–91.

99. Kalson NS, Richardson S, Hoyland JA. Strategies for regeneration of the intervertebral disc. Regen Med 2008;3(5):717–29.

100. Masuda K. Biological repair of the degenerated intervertebral disc by the injection of growth factors. Eur Spine J 2008;17(Suppl 4):441–51.

101. Hubert MG, Vadala G, Sowa G, et al. Gene therapy for the treatment of degenerative disc disease. J Am Acad Orthop Surg 2008;16(6):312–9.

102. Le Maitre CL, Hoyland JA, Freemont AJ. Interleukin-1 receptor antagonist delivered directly and by gene therapy inhibits matrix degradation in the intact degenerate human intervertebral disc: an in situ zymographic and gene therapy study. Arthritis Res Ther 2007;9(4):R83.

103. Sakai D. Future perspectives of cell-based therapy for intervertebral disc disease. Eur Spine J 2008; 17(Suppl 4):452–8.

104. Serigano K, Sakai D, Hiyama A, et al. Effect of cell number on mesenchymal stem cell transplantation in a canine disc degeneration model. J Orthop Res 2010;28(10):1267–75.

105. Miyamoto K, Masuda K, Kim JG, et al. Intradiscal injections of osteogenic protein-1 restore the viscoelastic properties of degenerated intervertebral discs. Spine J 2006;6(6):692–703.

106. Ganey T, Hutton WC, Moseley T, et al. Intervertebral disc repair using adipose tissue-derived stem and regenerative cells: experiments in a canine model. Spine (Phila Pa 1976) 2009;34(21): 2297–304.

107. Alini M, Eisenstein SM, Ito K, et al. Are animal models useful for studying human disc disorders/ degeneration? Eur Spine J 2008;17(1):2–19.

108. Paesold G, Nerlich AG, Boos N. Biological treatment strategies for disc degeneration: potentials and shortcomings. Eur Spine J 2007;16(4): 447–68.

109. Hohaus C, Ganey TM, Minkus Y, et al. Cell transplantation in lumbar spine disc degeneration disease. Eur Spine J 2008;17(Suppl 4):492–503.

110. A clinical trial to evaluate the safety, tolerability and preliminary effectiveness of single administration intradiscal rhGDF-5 for the treatment of early stage lumbar disc degeneration. Available at: http://clinicaltrials.gov/ct2/show/NCT01158924. 2011. Accessed August 17, 2011.

111. Carragee EJ, Tanner CM, Khurana S, et al. The rates of false-positive lumbar discography in select patients without low back symptoms. Spine (Phila Pa 1976) 2000;25(11):1373–80.

112. Carragee EJ, Don AS, Hurwitz EL, et al. 2009 ISSLS Prize Winner: Does discography cause accelerated progression of degeneration changes in the lumbar disc: a ten-year matched cohort study. Spine (Phila Pa 1976) 2009;34(21):2338–45.

Genetics of Lumbar Disk Degeneration: Technology, Study Designs, and Risk Factors

Patrick Yu-Ping Kao, PhD[d], Danny Chan, PhD[a],
Dino Samartzis, DSc[b], Pak Chung Sham, BM BCh, PhD[c],
You-Qiang Song, PhD[a],*

KEYWORDS

- Genetics • Lumbar disk degeneration • Association study
- Twin studies • Familial aggregation

Low-back pain (LBP) is a common musculoskeletal disorder and a global burden. Approximately 70% to 80% of people have experienced LBP at some point in their life.[1] The annual prevalence of LBP ranges from 15% to 45%, but is largely dependent on the population being studied and surveillance methods.[1,2] Low-back pain can lead to diminished function, loss of productivity, loss of work, psychological distress, and increased health care costs. As such, LBP poses considerable financial burden to nations through the direct cost of LBP treatments and the indirect cost due to loss of working productivity.[3,4] In the United States, one of the most frequent reasons for medical consultation is LBP.[1,3,4] Therefore, the impact of LBP on society is substantial, and understanding its development is imperative (see article by Karppinen and colleagues elsewhere in this issue).

Although LBP is a prevailing disorder, the factors that contribute to LBP are still not fully understood. A variety of factors, such as occupation, biopsychological factors, cardiovascular disorders, smoking, and obesity, have been suggested to be associated with LBP.[5–9] Conversely, British twin studies showed that there is excessive concordance of LBP for monozygotic (MZ) twins compared with dizygotic (DZ) twins, resulting in heritabilities ranging from 52% to 68% for various lumbar disk degeneration (LDD) phenotypes.[10] In addition, in a study by Battie and colleagues[11] of Finnish twins, heritability estimates ranged from 30% to 39% for various definitions of back pain problems during the prior year. Apparently, genetic factors play a vital role in the cause of LBP.

Intervertebral disk (IVD) degeneration is one proxy by which genetic risk factors act to influence LBP,[10,11] as revealed by studies that found IVD degeneration to be associated with LBP.[11–20] Although LBP is a multifactorial condition, discogenic origin can be mediated by such mechanisms as nerve ingrowth in degenerated disks, nerve root compression from herniated disks, and inflammatory responses of surrounding tissues in response to disk pathology.[11,21] Because of the close relationship

This work was supported by an Area of Excellence grant from the University Grants Committee of Hong Kong (AoE/M-04/04), as well as a grant from the Genomics Strategic Research Theme, the University of Hong Kong.
[a] Department of Biochemistry, Li Ka Shing Faculty of Medicine, University of Hong Kong, 3/F. Laboratory Block, 21 Sassoon Road, Pokfulam, Hong Kong SAR, China
[b] Department of Orthopaedics and Traumatology, Division of Spine Surgery, Li Ka Shing Faculty of Medicine, The University of Hong Kong, Professorial Block, 5th Floor, 102 Pokfulam Road, Pokfulam, Hong Kong SAR, China
[c] Department of Psychiatry, Li Ka Shing Faculty of Medicine, University of Hong Kong, Queen Mary Hospital, 102 Pokfulam Road, Hong Kong SAR, China
* Corresponding author.
E-mail address: songy@hku.hk

between LBP and LDD, and because both LDD and LBP have a large genetic component in their cause, it is worthwhile to investigate the genetics of LDD to unveil the mechanism by which LDD, and thus LBP, develop. Thus, this article discusses and raises awareness of genetic factors related to LDD. Furthermore, this article also addresses the genetic-based technologies, methodologies, and study designs that have been developed to assess LDD.

GENETIC COMPONENT OF LDD

The first step in studying the genetics of a condition is to ask whether there is a genetic component for a disease or its symptoms. The initial step in approaching this issue is to determine whether there is familial aggregation, that is, whether a higher number of occurrences of diseased individuals exist among family members than nondiseased individuals. On that basis, various studies were performed to decipher whether familial aggregation is present in LDD. Varlotta and colleagues[22] found that, in adolescent patients with disk herniation, a larger proportion of individuals had a positive family history of disk herniation than in control subjects. This finding was subsequently further supported by other investigators, such as Frino and colleagues[23] and Matsui and colleagues.[24] According to a study by Postacchini and colleagues[25] consisting of patients with discogenic LBP, the investigators noted a large proportion of first relatives who had experienced discogenic LBP and who had undergone disk surgery. Moreover, based on a study by Simmons and colleagues,[26] patients who had undergone spine surgery had a greater frequency of relatives who had experienced LBP and sciatica. Other reports have also noted a positive family history of LBP[27] and disk degeneration[28,29] in patients who had had spine surgery. These reports and others have indicated the presence of familial aggregation for LDD and, as such, the possibility of the influence of a genetic component on LDD.

Although studies have shown an association between familial aggregation and LDD, they only suggest a possibility of a genetic component, because it is still necessary to differentiate between familial aggregation that is caused by social-behavioral factors from that attributed to genetic factors. This differentiation can be achieved through twin studies that assess differences in disease concordance rates between MZ twins and DZ twins. If there is a strong genetic background for a disease, MZ twins should have a greater concordance rate in disease status than DZ twins. From the twin studies, heritability, defined as the proportion of a population's phenotypic differences caused by genetic

variation, can be estimated. In 1995, based on 155 identical male twins of the Finnish Twin Spine Study, Battie and colleagues[30] found that genetic risk factors play a major role in the development of LDD as noted on magnetic resonance imaging (MRI), explaining 77% of the variability. In 1999, and based on the UK Twin Study, Sambrook and colleagues[31] assessed LDD based on MRI of 172 MZ twins and 154 DZ twins, and noted a 74% heritability rate of LDD. The findings from these seminal studies based on Finnish and UK twins greatly substantiated the role of genetics as a causal risk factor in the development of LDD.

Although the importance of genetics can be established, there are 2 interesting points to note. First, there is no single gene that is responsible for causing LDD. Based on a study by Livshits and colleagues[32] assessing an Arabic pedigree, the investigators reported that a family history was found to be a risk factor for the development of LDD. A simple monogenic mendelian pattern of inheritance was rejected, suggesting that there could be a more complex mode of inheritance for LDD involving multiple genes. Second, genetic factors may interact with environmental factors in the causal framework of LDD. For example, based on early reports of the Finnish Twin Study, cigarette smoking status was found to greatly increase the ability to predict LDD.[33] Therefore, because gene-environment interaction effects may be present and often may be complex to disseminate, this presents a challenge to the identification of the disease mechanism of LDD.

DEFINING THE PHENOTYPE OF DISK DEGENERATION

Throughout the years, the integrity of the intervertebral disks has been assessed by various imaging modalities, such as plain radiographs, discography, computed tomography (CT), and MRI.[14,34–37] Standing plain radiographs are commonly used to assess disk space height and sclerosis of the end plate as well as other spinal and alignment abnormalities; however, this imaging lacks the ability to assess the soft tissue of the disk. Discography entails injection of provocative material directly into the disk to identify the discogenic origin of the pain source. This methodology is often uncomfortable to the individual and may accelerate LDD because of the direct disk injury that may be induced by the needle puncture.[38] CT is a method widely used for chest and abdominal imaging. However, it is less useful for examining soft tissues of the disk and is associated with excessively high levels of ionizing radiation exposure. Because the hallmark of disk degeneration entails the loss of water and proteoglycan content in the nucleus pulposus with structural changes of the disk and adjacent end plate (see article by Chan and colleagues elsewhere in this issue), this process entails various stages of degeneration that are best assessed with imaging that is sensitive to such alterations. MRI is a noninvasive method of imaging that allows direct evaluation of the soft tissues of the disk and, as such, is a desirable method, or rather a more sensitive method than the alternative imaging modalities for intervertebral disk imaging in assessing the phenotype of LDD. Throughout the years, MRI technology has further been developed to assess the integrity of the disk in a more sensitive and quantitative manner (see article by Majumdar and colleagues elsewhere in this issue). Nonetheless, because of the variety of imaging modalities in existence and the presence of numerous classification schemes in assessing disk degeneration, this has posed a dilemma in adopting a universal methodology to assess the phenotype of LDD.[13,39] Therefore, heterogeneity exists in the imaging phenotype of LDD between various observational cohort and genetic studies.

INTEGRATION OF KNOWLEDGE OF THE HUMAN GENOME FOR GENETIC STUDIES

The study of genetics was pioneered by Gregor Mendel who developed Mendel's laws of genetics, which allowed differences in genetic material (ie, DNA) of organisms to be related to appearances or conditions that are observable (ie, phenotypes). Two major factors have advanced genetics even further: knowledge of all the variants present in our genome, and advancement in capturing these variations, or genotyping technologies.

Each unit of DNA consists of an alkaline structure, known as a base pair. Single-nucleotide polymorphisms (SNPs) are single base pair changes among individuals. Microsatellites are short, repeated DNA fragments. Copy number variations (CNVs) are longer (>1 kb, kilo base pair) DNA fragments that have a different number of copies compared with a reference genome. Before the first decade of the twenty-first century genetic studies mainly focused on microsatellite and SNP markers. Nowadays, considerable attention has been given to the importance of CNVs. Presently, in comparison with SNP and CNVs, microsatellites are seldom used for genetic studies.

GENOME PROJECTS FOR HUMAN GENETICS

Improvements in genotyping technologies have enriched the knowledge on the relationship between genetic sequence and disease. The large-scale study of this relationship was made possible by the Human Genome Project,[40] which provided the first reference human genome sequence. Later, the HapMap project was initiated, with the main goal of capturing the pattern of SNPs, the most common type of genetic variation among individuals, within the human genome.[41,42] The initial stages of the project included Yoruban individuals from Africa, white individuals from the United States, Chinese, and Japanese individuals. Around 3.1 million SNPs were successfully genotyped.[41] The success of the HapMap project was a big step forward in supporting genetic studies. It improved understanding of the linkage disequilibrium (LD) pattern within the human genome, making it possible to choose only 1 or a small number of tagging SNPs within a high-LD (low recombination rate) region to genotype to obtain almost complete common variant information on a particular genomic region. This process helps save a huge amount of resources for genetic studies. Recently, the 1000 Genome Consortium has completed its initial sequencing of 179 individuals,[43] signifying the next era of genetic studies, which consists of sequencing each base pair of DNA, known as deep resequencing, as opposed to genotyping, which captures only known varying regions of the genome. In terms of disease genetic study, sequencing information makes it possible to study rare and previously unknown sequence variants. The 1000 Genome Project data are also valuable in allowing the genotypes of SNPs not genotyped in the experiment to be predicted by a computational process known as imputation.[44] With the denser map, locations of disease-causing variants can be determined with more precision.

GENOTYPING TECHNOLOGIES

Modern genotyping technologies are divided into 2 main categories: (1) those that are suitable for genotyping a larger number of SNPs and are thus suitable for genome-wide association studies (GWAS), and (2) those that are optimal for large samples size and are thus suitable for replication studies.[45] The most popular GWAS genotyping platforms are Ilumina's Infinium BeadChip and Affymetrix GeneChip, whereas other assays such as Perlegen and Invader are also available.[45] Illumina BeadChip and Affymetrix GeneChip are now capable of genotyping more than 1 million SNPs and CNVs in the genome. Because of the design of the products, Illumina BeadChip has a higher genomic coverage, meaning that the SNPs of the product are more capable of capturing information about the genome.[46] However, both Affymetrix and Illumina can also be used for genotyping smaller, more confined genotypic regions.

Sequenom MassArray is a platform used for a larger sample number with a small number of SNPs. I-plex assays for MassArray are used for genotyping up to 40 SNPs. Alternatively, the Taqman assay (from Applied Biosystems) uses a real-time method based on the polymerase chain reaction for SNP detection. Different alleles have different fluorescent probes. Therefore, the detection of different alleles can be achieved from signals given by their corresponding probes. The accuracy of this assay can reach up to 99%.[45] Other genotyping assays, such as Pyrosequencing, are also available.[47]

MAIN GENETIC STUDY STRATEGIES
Linkage and Association Strategies of Genetic Studies

Genetic studies are divided into 2 main streams: (1) family linkage analysis, and (2) the case-control association approach. In family linkage analysis, the pattern of inheritance of a disease is compared with the pattern of disease markers. If a particular region of markers is observed to be inherited in the same way as the disease, then the disease-causing variant may lie within the region. Family data are required to perform linkage studies.

In the case-control association approach, unrelated individuals with extreme disease statuses, namely the case group (those with the phenotype) and the control (those without the phenotype) group, are recruited. The allele frequencies of the genetic variants between cases and controls are compared. Disease-causing variants are identified by searching for markers that show statistically significant differences in allele frequencies between the 2 groups.

Association within family trios can also be performed using the transmission disequilibrium test (TDT). This test is conducted by observing in heterozygous parents whether there is one allele with higher transmission frequency to the offspring than the other.[48] This design is better than the case-control design because it avoids false-positives caused by the differences in population composition between the case and control groups. However, the power of this test is lower than that of the case-control design because the 2 parents are approximately equivalent in information to only 1 unrelated control subject.[48]

Depending on the SNP selection strategy, the case-control association approach can be divided further into the candidate gene and genome-wide approaches. The candidate gene approach has the main advantage that it is more specific, because the selection of SNPs is based on prior knowledge on the biology of the disease. When a high-throughput genotyping platform is not so readily available, this approach has been shown to be successful in identifying several genetic risk variants for some complex diseases. Currently, because of the availability of whole-genome genotyping platforms, the genome-wide approach for association studies has been made possible. The main advantage of this approach is that regions of interest need not be confined in particular genomic regions, relying on investigators' knowledge. Therefore, novel genetic variants are more readily identified.

Strengths and Weaknesses of Linkage and Association Approaches

Linkage studies were attractive at the time when genetic marker maps and genotyping technologies allowed few markers to be studied (**Table 1**), because linkage can be detected at long distances

Table 1
Advantages (✓) and disadvantages (×) of various genetic study methodologies

	Association (Candidate Gene Approach)	Association (Genome-Wide Approach)	Linkage
No knowledge of gene functions required	×	✓	✓
Localization to small genomic region	✓	✓	×
Cost	✓	×	✓
Families not required	✓	✓	×
Not easily affected by population stratification	×	×	✓
Power to detect common alleles (MAFs>5%) of modest effect	✓	✓	×
Power to detect rare alleles (MAFs<1%)	×	×	✓

Abbreviation: MAF, minor allele frequency.

Modified from Hirschhorn JN, Daly MJ. Genome-wide association studies for common diseases and complex traits. Nat Rev Genet 2005;6:96; with permission.

from a disease susceptibility loci. Alternatively, an important disadvantage of linkage studies is that they are powerful only when the mutation has a high probability of causing disease (high penetrance). Association studies rely on LD between genetic markers and disease susceptibility loci, and this typically requires the 2 loci to be very close to each other. In consequence, association studies were for a long time confined to the study of specific candidate genes supported by a strong hypothesis, and a genome-wide screen using association was not feasible until the recent developments in genotyping technologies mentioned earlier. An important advantage of association rather than linkage is that association has greater power to detect a locus with small or modest effect size. However, linkage is more robust to allelic heterogeneity, which refers to the presence of multiple risk alleles at a locus. With modern sequencing technology, linkage and association are best considered to be 2 complementary ways of using genetic markers to study the genetic basis of simple and complex diseases.

FINDINGS ON THE GENETICS OF LDD
Candidate Gene Studies

Genetic risk factors of LDD have been extensively studied in light of the findings from family and twins studies, which show that LDD has a substantial genetic component. Several articles have reviewed these genetic risk factors.[49–52] Most of the genetic studies of LDD now adopt the candidate gene approach. Genetic studies on LDD have focused on the genes that code for the functioning molecules in the disk, including the components of collagen IX,[53–55] aggrecan,[56,57] degrading enzymes such as matrix metalloproteinase II[58] and III,[59,60] and inflammatory signaling molecules such as interleukin I (IL -1)[61–63] Other genes identified as being associated with LDD are susceptibility genes related to other diseases. For instance, asporin[64] was first identified in rheumatoid arthritis,[65] osteoarthritis (OA), and knee OA[64,66,67]; collagen I[68] and vitamin D receptor (VDR)[69–71] are related to osteoporosis (collagen I[72–74]; VDR[75,76]), and CILP[77] is found in cartilage.[78]

However, most of these studies need to be confirmed with a larger sample size or a meta-analysis. A linkage study is also being performed by our group (unpublished). The results show that both association and linkage approaches can identify genetic risk factors of LDD.

CURRENT AND FUTURE TRENDS

Because genetics is rapidly developing, genetic studies on LDD will become more comprehensive

and more powerful. This article discusses areas of advancement and future trends in genetics of LDD.

Marker Selection and Analysis

Genetic studies on LDD have previously concentrated on the candidate gene approach. Although this approach has fulfilled its mission successfully in the past, it is heavily dependent on what is known about the disease, making finding novel genes difficult. Therefore, our study group has initiated genome-wide linkage and association approaches to fill the knowledge gap and lead to the identification of novel genes in relation to LDD. In our linkage study, we recruited patients with early-onset LDD and their family members for whole-genome linkage scan. For our GWAS, we selected individuals with extreme disk degeneration status, after having corrected for age. The synergy of the 2 approaches can help locate genetic risk factors with different properties, thus making our knowledge base for the genetics of LDD more complete. In the future, the genomes and exomes of individuals are expected to be sequenced with next-generation sequencing methodologies, making it possible to look directly for rare variants in individuals and helping to decipher the genetic mechanism related to LDD.

Aside from genes that increase the risk of LDD, the focus can be placed on searching for protective genes. This broadening of the mindset will facilitate the discovery of gene sets that may influence LDD through other mechanisms.

In statistical methodologies, multivariate approaches are currently being developed. These statistical approaches can make use of information from several genetic variants and phenotypes. By combining information from different genes, it will be possible to consider variants within genes as whole or genetic information across different genes. The combined effects of different genes can then be considered simultaneously. Moreover, disk degeneration phenotypes can be combined similarly. This combination may help us identify whether certain combinations of genes or phenotypes are related and, therefore, share similar pathologic mechanisms. Considering the sets of phenotypes and genes can also reduce the number of statistical tests required and increase the statistical power.

Study Design

Most LDD genetic studies are cross-sectional, which means only disease condition at a certain time point is observed. As databases of volunteers develop, a longitudinal study approach can be adopted by recruiting the volunteers for a second imaging. The possibility of a dynamic assessment of the progression of LDD condition allows investigation of the influence of genetic risk factors to LDD and validation of hypotheses about their effects.

Increasing Sample Size by International Collaboration

In genetic studies, statistical power is one of the most important considerations for likely success. The most efficient and economical way (from each research center's point of view) to increase sample size is to combine study results from different research groups. Meta-analysis methodologies can directly combine the significance and effects from multiple studies. With this method, samples from different collaborators are virtually combined in a simple way. Currently, many of the GWAS are performed by meta-analysis across different populations. This trend is expected to continue for polygenic diseases like LDD, and is probably a good way to take advantage of improving technologies.

SUMMARY

Genetics has a role in the cause of LDD. However, it may either exert an effect by itself or with other environmental factors. Moreover, knowledge of the genetic risk factors of LDD is not complete. In future, together with knowledge and advancement in genotyping technologies, the study approach can be extended in the directions of finding novel genes that are related to LDD, and analyzing LDD causes with other behavioral and environmental factors.

REFERENCES

1. Andersson GB. Epidemiological features of chronic low-back pain. Lancet 1999;354:581–5.
2. Manchikanti L, Singh V, Datta S, et al. Comprehensive review of epidemiology, scope, and impact of spinal pain. Pain Physician 2009;12:E35–70.
3. Deyo RA, Tsui-Wu YJ. Descriptive epidemiology of low-back pain and its related medical care in the United States. Spine 1987;12:264–8.
4. Hart LG, Deyo RA, Cherkin DC. Physician office visits for low back pain. Frequency, clinical evaluation, and treatment patterns from a U.S. national survey. Spine 1995;20:11–9.
5. Samartzis D, Karppinen J, Mok F, et al. A population-based study of juvenile disc degeneration and its association with overweight and obesity, low back pain, and diminished functional status. J Bone Joint Surg Am 2011;93:662–70.
6. Shiri R, Karppinen J, Leino-Arjas P, et al. The association between obesity and low back pain: a meta-analysis. Am J Epidemiol 2010;171:135–54.
7. Shiri R, Solovieva S, Husgafvel-Pursiainen K, et al. The association between obesity and the prevalence of low back pain in young adults: the Cardiovascular Risk in Young Finns Study. Am J Epidemiol 2008; 167:1110–9.
8. van Tulder M, Koes B, Bombardier C. Low back pain. Best Pract Res Clin Rheumatol 2002;16:761–75.
9. Videman T, Nurminen M, Troup JD. 1990 Volvo Award in Clinical Sciences. Lumbar spinal pathology in cadaveric material in relation to history of back pain, occupation, and physical loading. Spine 1990;15:728–40.
10. MacGregor AJ, Andrew T, Sambrook PN, et al. Structural, psychological, and genetic influences on low back and neck pain: a study of adult female twins. Arthritis Rheum 2004;51:160–7.
11. Battie MC, Videman T, Levalahti E, et al. Heritability of low back pain and the role of disc degeneration. Pain 2007;131:272–80.
12. Luoma K, Riihimaki H, Luukkonen R, et al. Low back pain in relation to lumbar disc degeneration. Spine (Phila Pa 1976) 2000;25:487–92.
13. Chou R, Qaseem A, Owens DK, et al. Diagnostic imaging for low back pain: advice for high-value health care from the American College of Physicians. Ann Intern Med 2011;154:181–9.
14. de Schepper EI, Damen J, van Meurs JB, et al. The association between lumbar disc degeneration and low back pain: the influence of age, gender, and individual radiographic features. Spine (Phila Pa 1976) 2010;35:531–6.
15. Kjaer P, Leboeuf-Yde C, Korsholm L, et al. Magnetic resonance imaging and low back pain in adults: a diagnostic imaging study of 40-year-old men and women. Spine (Phila Pa 1976) 2005;30:1173–80.
16. Kjaer P, Leboeuf-Yde C, Sorensen JS, et al. An epidemiologic study of MRI and low back pain in 13-year-old children. Spine (Phila Pa 1976) 2005;30:798–806.
17. Samartzis D, Karppinen J, Chan D, et al. The association of disc degeneration based on magnetic resonance imaging and the presence of low back pain. Presented at the World Forum for Spine Research: Intervertebral Disc. Montreal (Canada), July 5–8, 2010.
18. Savage RA, Whitehouse GH, Roberts N. The relationship between the magnetic resonance imaging appearance of the lumbar spine and low back pain, age and occupation in males. Eur Spine J 1997;6:106–14.
19. Takatalo J, Karppinen J, Niinimäki J, et al. Does lumbar disc degeneration on MRI associate with low back symptom severity in young Finnish adults? Spine (Phila Pa 1976) 2011. [Epub ahead of print]. DOI:10.1097/BRS.0b013e3182077122.
20. Visuri T, Ulaska J, Eskelin M, et al. Narrowing of lumbar spinal canal predicts chronic low back pain more accurately than intervertebral disc degeneration: a magnetic resonance imaging study in young Finnish male conscripts. Mil Med 2005;170:926–30.

21. Freemont AJ, Peacock TE, Goupille P, et al. Nerve ingrowth into diseased intervertebral disc in chronic back pain. Lancet 1997;350:178–81.

22. Varlotta GP, Brown MD, Kelsey JL, et al. Familial predisposition for herniation of a lumbar disc in patients who are less than twenty-one years old. J Bone Joint Surg Am 1991;73:124–8.

23. Frino J, McCarthy RE, Sparks CY, et al. Trends in adolescent lumbar disc herniation. J Pediatr Orthop 2006;26:579–81.

24. Matsui H, Terahata N, Tsuji H, et al. Familial predisposition and clustering for juvenile lumbar disc herniation. Spine (Phila Pa 1976) 1992;17:1323–8.

25. Postacchini F, Lami R, Pugliese O. Familial predisposition to discogenic low-back pain. An epidemiologic and immunogenetic study. Spine (Phila Pa 1976) 1988;13:1403–6.

26. Simmons ED Jr, Guntupalli M, Kowalski JM, et al. Familial predisposition for degenerative disc disease. A case-control study. Spine (Phila Pa 1976) 1996;21:1527–9.

27. Saftic R, Grgic M, Ebling B, et al. Case-control study of risk factors for lumbar intervertebral disc herniation in Croatian island populations. Croat Med J 2006;47:593–600.

28. Richardson JK, Chung T, Schultz JS, et al. A familial predisposition toward lumbar disc injury. Spine (Phila Pa 1976) 1997;22:1487–92 [discussion: 93].

29. Matsui H, Kanamori M, Ishihara H, et al. Familial predisposition for lumbar degenerative disc disease. A case-control study. Spine (Phila Pa 1976) 1998;23:1029–34.

30. Battie MC, Videman T, Gibbons LE, et al. 1995 Volvo Award in Clinical Sciences. Determinants of lumbar disc degeneration. A study relating lifetime exposures and magnetic resonance imaging findings in identical twins. Spine (Phila Pa 1976) 1995;20:2601–12.

31. Sambrook PN, MacGregor AJ, Spector TD. Genetic influences on cervical and lumbar disc degeneration: a magnetic resonance imaging study in twins. Arthritis Rheum 1999;42:366–72.

32. Livshits G, Cohen Z, Higla O, et al. Familial history, age and smoking are important risk factors for disc degeneration disease in Arabic pedigrees. Eur J Epidemiol 2001;17:643–51.

33. Battie MC, Haynor DR, Fisher LD, et al. Similarities in degenerative findings on magnetic resonance images of the lumbar spines of identical twins. J Bone Joint Surg Am 1995;77:1662–70.

34. Molinari RW, Bridwell KH, Lenke LG, et al. Complications in the surgical treatment of pediatric high-grade, isthmic dysplastic spondylolisthesis. A comparison of three surgical approaches. Spine (Phila Pa 1976) 1999;24:1701–11.

35. Pfirrmann CW, Metzdorf A, Zanetti M, et al. Magnetic resonance classification of lumbar intervertebral disc degeneration. Spine 2001;26:1873–8.

36. Schneiderman G, Flannigan B, Kingston S, et al. Magnetic resonance imaging in the diagnosis of disc degeneration: correlation with discography. Spine 1987;12:276–81.

37. Tilson ER, Strickland GD, Gibson SD. An overview of radiography, computed tomography, and magnetic resonance imaging in the diagnosis of lumbar spine pathology. Orthop Nurs 2006;25:415–20 [quiz: 21–2].

38. Carragee EJ, Don AS, Hurwitz EL, et al. 2009 ISSLS Prize Winner: Does discography cause accelerated progression of degeneration changes in the lumbar disc: a ten-year matched cohort study. Spine (Phila Pa 1976) 2009;34:2338–45.

39. Fourney DR, Andersson GB, Arnold PM, et al. Chronic low back pain: a heterogeneous condition with challenges for an evidence-based approach. Spine, in press.

40. Lander ES, Linton LM, Birren B, et al. Initial sequencing and analysis of the human genome. Nature 2001;409:860–921.

41. Frazer KA, Ballinger DG, Cox DR, et al. A second generation human haplotype map of over 3.1 million SNPs. Nature 2007;449:851–61.

42. International HapMap Consortium. The International HapMap Project. Nature 2003;426:789–96.

43. The 1000 Genomes Project Consortium, Durbin RM, Abecasis GR, et al. A map of human genome variation from population-scale sequencing. Nature 2010;467:1061–73.

44. The 1000 Genomes Project Consortium. About the 1000 Genomes Project. 2010. Available at: http://www.1000genomes.org/about. Accessed August 4, 2011.

45. Ragoussis J. Genotyping technologies for genetic research. Annu Rev Genomics Hum Genet 2009;10:117–33.

46. Magi R, Pfeufer A, Nelis M, et al. Evaluating the performance of commercial whole-genome marker sets for capturing common genetic variation. BMC Genomics 2007;8:159.

47. Fakhrai-Rad H, Pourmand N, Ronaghi M. Pyrosequencing: an accurate detection platform for single nucleotide polymorphisms. Hum Mutat 2002;19:479–85.

48. Cardon LR, Bell JI. Association study designs for complex diseases. Nat Rev Genet 2001;2:91–9.

49. Zhang Y, Sun Z, Liu J, et al. Advances in susceptibility genetics of intervertebral degenerative disc disease. Int J Biol Sci 2008;4:283–90.

50. Kalichman L, Hunter DJ. The genetics of intervertebral disc degeneration. Associated genes. Joint Bone Spine 2008;75:388–96.

51. Chan D, Song Y, Sham P, et al. Genetics of disc degeneration. Eur Spine J 2006;15(Suppl 3):S317–25.

52. Ala-Kokko L. Genetic risk factors for lumbar disc disease. Ann Med 2002;34:42–7.

53. Jim JJ, Noponen-Hietala N, Cheung KM, et al. The TRP2 allele of COL9A2 is an age-dependent risk

factor for the development and severity of intervertebral disc degeneration. Spine (Phila Pa 1976) 2005; 30:2735–42.

54. Paassilta P, Lohiniva J, Goring HH, et al. Identification of a novel common genetic risk factor for lumbar disk disease. JAMA 2001;285:1843–9.

55. Annunen S, Paassilta P, Lohiniva J, et al. An allele of COL9A2 associated with intervertebral disc disease. Science 1999;285:409–12.

56. Roughley P, Martens D, Rantakokko J, et al. The involvement of aggrecan polymorphism in degeneration of human intervertebral disc and articular cartilage. Eur Cell Mater 2006;11:1–7 [discussion].

57. Kawaguchi Y, Osada R, Kanamori M, et al. Association between an aggrecan gene polymorphism and lumbar disc degeneration. Spine (Phila Pa 1976) 1999;24:2456–60.

58. Dong DM, Yao M, Liu B, et al. Association between the -1306C/T polymorphism of matrix metalloproteinase-2 gene and lumbar disc disease in Chinese young adults. Eur Spine J 2007;16:1958–61.

59. Takahashi M, Haro H, Wakabayashi Y, et al. The association of degeneration of the intervertebral disc with 5a/6a polymorphism in the promoter of the human matrix metalloproteinase-3 gene. J Bone Joint Surg Br 2001;83:491–5.

60. Goupille P, Jayson MI, Valat JP, et al. Matrix metalloproteinases: the clue to intervertebral disc degeneration? Spine (Phila Pa 1976) 1998;23:1612–26.

61. Le Maitre CL, Freemont AJ, Hoyland JA. The role of interleukin-1 in the pathogenesis of human intervertebral disc degeneration. Arthritis Res Ther 2005;7: R732–45.

62. Solovieva S, Leino-Arjas P, Saarela J, et al. Possible association of interleukin 1 gene locus polymorphisms with low back pain. Pain 2004;109:8–19.

63. Solovieva S, Kouhia S, Leino-Arjas P, et al. Interleukin 1 polymorphisms and intervertebral disc degeneration. Epidemiology 2004;15:626–33.

64. Song YQ, Cheung KM, Ho DW, et al. Association of the asporin D14 allele with lumbar-disc degeneration in Asians. Am J Hum Genet 2008;82:744–7.

65. Torres B, Orozco G, Garcia-Lozano JR, et al. Asporin repeat polymorphism in rheumatoid arthritis. Ann Rheum Dis 2007;66:118–20.

66. Kizawa H, Kou I, Iida A, et al. An aspartic acid repeat polymorphism in asporin inhibits chondrogenesis and increases susceptibility to osteoarthritis. Nat Genet 2005;37:138–44.

67. Ikegawa S, Kawamura S, Takahashi A, et al. Replication of association of the D-repeat polymorphism in asporin with osteoarthritis. Arthritis Res Ther 2006; 8:403 [author reply].

68. Tilkeridis C, Bei T, Garantziotis S, et al. Association of a COL1A1 polymorphism with lumbar disc disease in young military recruits. J Med Genet 2005;42:e44.

69. Kawaguchi Y, Kanamori M, Ishihara H, et al. The association of lumbar disc disease with vitamin-D receptor gene polymorphism. J Bone Joint Surg Am 2002;84: 2022–8.

70. Videman T, Gibbons LE, Battie MC, et al. The relative roles of intragenic polymorphisms of the vitamin D receptor gene in lumbar spine degeneration and bone density. Spine (Phila Pa 1976) 2001;26:E7–12.

71. Videman T, Leppavuori J, Kaprio J, et al. Intragenic polymorphisms of the vitamin D receptor gene associated with intervertebral disc degeneration. Spine (Phila Pa 1976) 1998;23:2477–85.

72. Pluijm SM, van Essen HW, Bravenboer N, et al. Collagen type I alpha1 Sp1 polymorphism, osteoporosis, and intervertebral disc degeneration in older men and women. Ann Rheum Dis 2004;63:71–7.

73. Grant SF, Reid DM, Blake G, et al. Reduced bone density and osteoporosis associated with a polymorphic Sp1 binding site in the collagen type I alpha 1 gene. Nat Genet 1996;14:203–5.

74. Uitterlinden AG, Burger H, Huang Q, et al. Relation of alleles of the collagen type Ialpha1 gene to bone density and the risk of osteoporotic fractures in postmenopausal women. N Engl J Med 1998;338:1016–21.

75. Riggs BL. Vitamin D-receptor genotypes and bone density. N Engl J Med 1997;337:125–6.

76. Morrison NA, Qi JC, Tokita A, et al. Prediction of bone density from vitamin D receptor alleles. Nature 1994;367:284–7.

77. Seki S, Kawaguchi Y, Chiba K, et al. A functional SNP in CILP, encoding cartilage intermediate layer protein, is associated with susceptibility to lumbar disc disease. Nat Genet 2005;37:607–12.

78. Lorenzo P, Bayliss MT, Heinegard D. A novel cartilage protein (CILP) present in the mid-zone of human articular cartilage increases with age. J Biol Chem 1998;273:23463–8.

Biomechanics of Intervertebral Disk Degeneration

Nozomu Inoue, MD, PhD*, Alejandro A. Espinoza Orías, PhD

KEYWORDS

• Biomechanics • Intervertebral disk • Degeneration

The intervertebral disk has a composite structure consisting of a gelatinous proteoglycan-rich nucleus pulposus surrounded by a collagen-rich anulus fibrosus. The proteoglycan in the nucleus pulposus provides high water content within the nucleus pulposus and, in turn, contributes to sustaining large loads applied to the vertebral body. The load is distributed evenly to the anulus fibrosus through hydrostatic pressure. The fiber orientation of the anulus fibrosus is suitable to resist hoop stresses generated by the hydrostatic pressure in healthy conditions (see article by Grunhagen and colleagues elsewhere in this issue).

Degenerative changes in the biomechanical properties can occur in the nucleus pulposus and anulus fibrosus tissues individually. These changes can be shown as changes in material properties of each tissue. Degenerative changes in structural properties may be represented as consequences of these changes in material properties of the substructure of the disk. However, degenerative structural changes in the disk, such as loss of the volume of the nucleus pulposus and fissures in anulus fibrosus, can only be evaluated by analysis of structural parameters. It is important to understand how these changes affect the function of the motion segment and relate to symptoms such as low back pain (LBP) (see article by Karppinen and colleagues elsewhere in this issue).

This article discusses the degenerative changes in the material properties of nucleus pulposus and anulus fibrosus followed by the changes in structural properties of the entire disk, with an emphasis on the degenerative changes in viscoelastic properties of the whole disk. Instability of the motion segment as a consequence of the structural failure associated with the degenerative changes on the disk are also discussed. Instability of the lumbar spine, which has been considered to be one of the significant causes for mechanical LBP, is reviewed.

MATERIAL PROPERTIES OF THE DEGENERATIVE INTERVERTEBRAL DISK COMPONENTS
Nucleus Pulposus

The disk degeneration process affects several of the structures differently, and apparently at different times during its progression. The impaired synthesis of the disk matrix involves all of its components at different time points.[1–4] The process is believed to start in the nucleus pulposus, exhibiting a decrease in its proteoglycan concentration[3,5–9] and gradual change in collagen type that transitions into a more fibrotic tissue.[10] These factors effectively dehydrate the nucleus pulposus down from a peak nucleus water content in the adult disk of approximately 70%–80%.[11] Recently, Murakami and colleagues[12] quantified the difference in water content between old (3 years) and young (6 months) anulus fibrosus and nucleus pulposus tissue of rabbits, showing significant differences among them. In addition, the nucleus

This work was supported by NIH grant P01 AR48152.
Spine Biomechanics Laboratory, Department of Orthopedic Surgery, Rush University Medical Center, 1611 West Harrison Street, Orthopedic Building Suite 201, Chicago, IL 60612, USA
* Corresponding author.
E-mail address: Nozomu_Inoue@rush.edu

Orthop Clin N Am 42 (2011) 487–499
doi:10.1016/j.ocl.2011.07.001

orthopedic.theclinics.com

pulposus glycosaminoglycan (GAG), DNA, aggrecan, and collagen types I and II contents were significantly larger in the younger tissue. Evidence like this shows that the nucleus tissue is the most affected. Its decay constitutes one of the largest enablers of disk degeneration. This transition into a more fibrotic type of tissue produces a stiffer nucleus pulposus and the shock-absorbing properties of the disk are severely limited.

The nucleus pulposus, usually referred to as fluid,[13–17] loses its hydrostatic pressure feature.[1,18–23] A more fibrotic (increased collagen in nucleus pulposus)[10,24] tissue does not behave in the same manner as a fluid/gel nucleus pulposus. The nucleus pulposus tissue undergoes a process of stiffening by means of gradual loss of proteoglycans and change of collagens from type II to type I,[3,24] becoming a more fibrous and solid tissue,[25,26] which was found to amalgamate into one solid phase with the anulus fibrosus in 75% of the cases from the sixth to eighth decade in a cadaveric study by Haefeli and colleagues.[10] The loss of proteoglycans causes the decrease of swelling pressure in the nucleus pulposus,[27] identified as the main load-bearing mechanism in the nondegenerate nucleus pulposus.[28] As a consequence, load mechanics are altered and, for a period during the initial phase of degeneration, the disk is unstable.

Anulus Fibrosus

The mechanical behavior of the anulus fibrosus has been well documented in terms of tensile and compressive tests, but less so in shear. Tensile behavior corresponds with the circumferential direction on the annular wall and was characterized in static and dynamic tests to explain its mechanism to resist hoop stresses produced by the nucleus pulposus hydrostatic pressure.[29] These two loading conditions are commonly accepted to simulate the body weight borne by the spinal column (compression) and the additional stresses seen in outward lateral bending and flexion/extension (tension). The greatest strengths are usually seen when loading the lamellae in the direction of the reinforcing fibers. The arrangement of the elastic fibers plays an important role in the overall mechanical properties of the anulus fibrosus.[30,31] Elastic anisotropy in the anulus[32] is maintained with degeneration, with posterolateral and outer lamellae regions having decreases of about 30% to 50% with advancing degeneration.[33–36]

However, in cases like spondylolisthesis, anterior-posterior shear seems to be the dominant failure mode and this has not been studied, as well as shear within the anulus lamellae in cases of annular failure leading to herniation. In the

degenerate anulus fibrosus, the fiber patterns become disorganized, and the elastic response also varies as a consequence.[37,38] The elastic properties in an intact model are anisotropic and highly nonlinear.[39,40] This nonlinearity, exhibited by a toe region on the stress-strain curves, is common to cartilaginous tissues.[41–46] Moreover, the response of degenerate anulus fibrosus tissue has been shown to be of a twofold increase in the toe region modulus in tensile testing, which was correlated with age, as well as fiber realignment toward the loading direction.[47,48] Dynamic viscoelastic testing has shown that the dynamic modulus of anulus fibrosus increases with degeneration at tensile strains greater than 6%.[49] Earlier quasistatic test results from Acaroglu and colleagues[33,35] described a strong influence of degeneration on elastic properties such as the Poisson ratio, failure stress, and strain energy density of the anulus fibrosus. The work by Guerin and colleagues[47] reports no other significant changes in the elastic properties of the anulus fibrosus tissue.

In addition to elastic anisotropy, permeability also has been shown to vary spatially and is influenced by age, degeneration, and water content in the disk.[50] These values have been incorporated in a finite element model simulation by Natarajan and colleagues,[51] and they showed their effect on disk height and annular failure.

DEGENERATIVE CHANGES IN STRUCTURAL PROPERTIES OF THE MOTION SEGMENT

The function of the motion segment is to provide the spine with axial stability while allowing mobility.[52] The intervertebral disk is responsible for carrying enormous amounts of compressive loading while maintaining flexibility.[53] The load on the disk is mainly compressive, but it is also subjected to other types of loads such as tensile and shear stresses.[26,54] As the compressive load is subjected to the disk, hydrostatic pressure develops within the inner core of gelatinous nucleus pulposus, which pushes outward causing the outer ring of fibrous anulus fibrosus to bulge and experience tensile stress in the fibers.[55] Loads on the lumbar disk (L3/4) of volunteers performing different body postures[19,56,57] as well as disk pressures[58] have been measured in vivo. These studies revealed that the load on the L3/4 level disk in a sitting position and in a standing position with 20° of flexion was 250% of the total body weight, although the portion of the body above the L3/4 level represented only 60%. Such large loads have been validated with mathematical models.[59,60] This finding suggests that the load on the lumbar disk is composed of external and internal inputs.[54] The external load is the weight of the body above the lumbar disk, and the internal load is the muscle force required to stabilize the spine in different postures. Increases in disk pressure should also be expected when a fluid is injected, as Andersson and Schultz[61] showed when they inquired about the effects of injecting saline in a disk, and found varied responses in cases in which the injected fluid was retained, notably the large increases in pressure (up to 83%). In contrast, a decrease in pressure was observed in the degenerated disk.[16]

Several animal models have been established to investigate degenerative changes in structural properties of the lumbar motion segment. A commonly used mechanical damage method to cause disk degeneration is the needle puncture or stab wound. Several researchers have recently arrived at the same conclusions when reporting that the diameter of the wound has to be large enough to create degeneration.[62–64] Korecki and colleagues[65,66] showed that, in an in vitro cyclic testing setting, bovine disks showed immediate and progressive differences in the dynamic modulus and stiffness of the anulus fibrosus tissue after puncture. Aside from the lamellar disturbances, cell viability and matrix remodeling were observed. Another animal model (ovine) of disk degeneration from induced lesions has also shown regeneration in the midwall of the anulus fibrosus.[67] In a different loading condition, a murine tail model has also shown differences in the anulus fibrosus tissue as a consequence of dynamic compression, but did not achieve degenerate disk quality after long cycles of compression.[68] These reports suggest that puncture injuries lead to degenerative remodeling including granulation tissue, which current image-based diagnostics methods might not be able to distinguish.[69]

MacLean and colleagues[70] investigated static viscoelastic behaviors of rat caudal motion segments, vertebrae, and isolated disk explants in different permeability conditions and showed that differences in endplate permeability conditions had a significant effect on the viscoelastic behaviors. Johannessen and colleagues[71] showed a decrease in stress relaxation after 10,000 cycles of compressive loading in adult sheep lumbar motion segments and recovery of the stress relaxation after 18 hours of unloading in phosphate-buffered saline solution, suggesting intervertebral disk fluid transport during loading and unloading.

Boxberger and colleagues[72,73] used a degenerative disk model in rat by injection of chondroitinase-ABC to the disks. In this model, nucleus pulposus degeneration has been successfully induced with GAG loss as a consequence of chondroitinase-ABC injection to the disks, which were tested in a linear viscoelastic tension/compression regime afterward. Results showed that the dynamic stiffness was decreased at low loads. Nucleus pulposus GAG content was shown to be related to the neutral zone properties in the tension-compression cyclic tests. However, the tension and compression extremes of the load displacement curve were not shown to be related. This finding shows that a degenerate nucleus produces hypermobility in addition to low pressures. Such distortion in load sharing leads to the development of hoop stresses in the anulus that resist compressive loads.[72,73]

Kim and colleagues[74–76] used a rabbit degenerative disk model with 18-gauge needle puncture of the disk to investigate changes in dynamic viscoelastic properties of the whole disk associated with the disk degeneration. In this model, the proteoglycan content decreased and collagen content increased 4 weeks after puncture. The dynamic viscoelastic test showed a decrease in elastic and viscous properties in the punctured disk (**Fig. 1**). The correlation study showed that the proteoglycan content positively correlated with the elastic and viscous mechanical properties

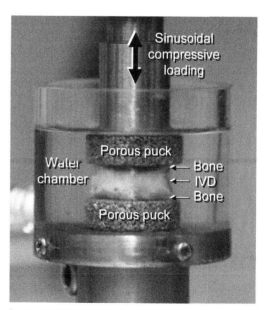

Fig. 1. Experimental test chamber for an unconfined dynamic compression experiment to record viscoelastic properties of a rabbit disk. The bone-disc-bone complex was secured between 2 porous pucks that prevented friction of the endplates with respect to these structures. Disks can be altered chemically to promote and recover from degeneration. Their dynamic viscoelastic properties can be assessed in this way. IVD, intervertebral disk.

and height of the disk; however, there was no correlation with the collagen content. These results suggest that the proteoglycan is a governing factor for viscoelastic properties and structural properties of the disk.

Using the same rabbit degenerative disk model and the dynamic viscoelastic testing method, Miyamoto and colleagues[77] investigated the effects of OP-1 injection in the lumbar disk on the biomechanical and biochemical restoration of the disk. In this study, a significant increase in wet weight and proteoglycan content was observed in both nucleus pulposus and anulus fibrosus tissues of the OP-1-injected disks, compared with the lactose-injected control disks, whereas an increase in collagen content was observed only in the nucleus pulposus. These results suggested that increased proteoglycan content, induced by the injection of OP-1, resulted in tissue hydration in both the nucleus pulposus and anulus fibrosus. The results of the dynamic viscoelastic test showed that the elastic modulus has a significant positive correlation with the proteoglycan content in the nucleus pulposus and the proteoglycan and collagen content in the anulus fibrosus. Similarly, the viscous modulus was shown to have a significant positive correlation with the proteoglycan content in the nucleus pulposus and the proteoglycan and collagen content in the anulus fibrosus.

INSTABILITY OF THE MOTION SEGMENT ASSOCIATED WITH INTERVERTEBRAL DISK DEGENERATION

As disk degeneration progresses, structural failure of the disk is manifested by tears and clefts in the anulus fibrosus. These material disruptions occur in different directions and are the result of a variety of influencing factors, including altered loading of the disk. Potential relationships between osteophytes and peripheral tears were first reported by Schmorl and Junghanns,[78] and also highlighted that, because of the tears, segmental instability would be affected. Farfan[79] and Kirkaldy-Willis[80] concluded that tears were by-products of torsional stresses, implicating them as initiators of the failure of other disk components in the disk degeneration cascade.

Disk fissures have been classified in 3 categories, depending on their morphology and anatomic position in the disk: (1) peripheral tears or rim lesions, parallel to the endplates and exhibiting normal separation of the disk from the subchondral bone of the vertebral body, which, with time, developed (2) circumferential tears that present evidence of delamination as a failure mode; and (3) radial tears that, as the name implies, propagate in a direction perpendicular to an imaginary axis of the disk (if it is considered as a flat cylinder), which usually lead to disk herniations and expulsion of nucleus material. The literature shows few reports that address the crack propagation phenomena involved in disk tears, because it is common to report only the resulting condition (ruptured anulus, herniated disk).[38,81,82] Many of the models consider the anulus as a bulk material but, recently, more advanced models have incorporated annular layers[83] and implemented permeability and porosity,[84–87] as well as the disk's osmoviscoelastic properties.[88,89] The interlamellar structures have been deemed especially sensitive to shear stresses,[25,90,91] and the literature is lacking reports of their allegedly weaker mechanical properties. They are believed to play a predominant role when destructive processes such as delamination occur as part of herniation, as has been attempted in analytical models of the disk,[92] of anulus fibrosus tissue,[93] and of individual lamellae.[94] Schollum and colleagues[67,95] recently analyzed in detail the interface between annular lamellae in an ovine model by subjecting thin slices of immature and mature anulus fibrosus tissue to microtensile tests. Although their studies mostly described the architecture of the interlamellar interface, important differences in the response to tensile forces were shown between young and old tissue, with the older tissue exhibiting a more ordered and uniform lamellar separation than the young tissue; however, the investigators did not report elastic properties.

Fujiwara and colleagues[7,96] studied the effect of disk degeneration graded by magnetic resonance imaging on the segmental motion of the lumbar spine using a total of 106 motion segments obtained from 44 cadaveric lumbar spines taken from 18 women and 25 men with a mean age of 69 years. The investigators found that segmental motion increased with increasing severity of disk degeneration to grade 4, but decreased when the disk degeneration advanced to grade 5. Such segmental motion changes were greater in axial rotation compared with those in lateral bending, flexion, and extension, showing the importance of torsional instability in diagnosing spinal instability. The results of these studies are important for understanding the kinematic property changes in relation to the types or grades of disk degeneration. The results were consistent with the previous reports and the concept of 3 stages of spinal degeneration: dysfunction, instability, and restabilization proposed by Kirkaldy-Willis and Farfan.[97]

INSTABILITY OF THE LUMBAR SPINE ASSOCIATED WITH INTERVERTEBRAL DISK DEGENERATION

Segmental instability of the lumbar spine is frequently considered a cause of LBP, but instability of the spine is poorly defined and understood.[97-105] The basic concept of spinal instability is that excessive motion beyond normal constraints causes either compression or stretching of the neural elements or causes abnormal deformations of ligaments, joint capsules, annular fibers, or endplates, which are known to have a significant number of nociceptors. Even though several studies have indicated that excessive motion on flexion/extension radiographs is associated with LBP or degenerative disk disease,[106,107] other studies cite decreased motion in patients with degenerative changes and such pain.[108,109]

Lumbar segmental instability may be associated with a spectrum of clinical manifestations of degenerative changes in the intervertebral disk.[97,110-114] Intervertebral disk degeneration has been studied using magnetic resonance (MR) imaging, and grades of degeneration have been reported.[111-118] The relationship between the types (or grades) of disk degeneration and kinematic characteristics of the motion segment has been studied using cadaveric spinal motion segments.[96,119-123] Despite some variation in results, likely because different loading conditions and methods of grading degenerative disk changes were used, the overall results of these studies indicate that the biomechanical characteristics of the motion segment can become altered significantly when degenerative changes develop in the intervertebral disk.

In vivo Measurement of Lumbar Segmental Movement

There have been numerous in vivo studies on segmental instability of the lumbar spine in which dynamic flexion/extension radiographs were used.[108,124-133] However, these dynamic radiographic techniques have been found to be inaccurate.[134,135] The errors associated with sagittal plane translational motion measurement reported in the literature range from 1 to 4 mm,[134,136] or 3% to 15% of the vertebral depth.[137-139] Schaffer and colleagues[135] reported high false-positive and false-negative rates (ie, normal translations are categorized outside of the normal range and vice versa) with significant differences between measurement methods despite high reliability across radiographic quality, raters, and measurement. More sophisticated techniques, such as biplanar stereoradiography,[140-145] centrode pattern analysis,[100,137,146-156] and traction-compression radiography,[138,157] have been introduced but have not been widely accepted. More accurate methods involve invasive techniques by inserting metal beads or spinous process wire to determine three-dimension (3-D) motion.[158-160] However, because these methods are invasive, they are not appropriate for routine use in clinical practice or for in vivo human studies. Studies on segmental instability have also been limited by other factors in addition to these problems associated with accurate measurement of segmental motion in vivo. For example, the range of motion measured in most of these studies is affected by the variability in voluntary efforts that the subject applies at the time of examination and can also be limited because of pain.

Other two-dimensional (2-D) imaging methods for measuring axial rotation, as opposed to flexion/extension, have involved MR imaging of subjects in various rotated positions.[161,162] Although these studies were noninvasive and controlled for voluntary motions, they could only determine changes in segmental motion around 1 axis. It has been suggested that coupled motions could play an important role in determining spinal instability. To measure these coupled motions, studies have been conducted to measure 3-D motions in vivo. More invasive techniques involve inserting wires into the spinous process of subjects to determine 3-D motion.[163] Although this method has proved more accurate than radiographs, its invasive nature limits its widespread clinical use. Other studies have used biplanar radiography, in which the radiograms of the spine were taken from 2 directions simultaneously and 3-D motions are calculated by the positions of anatomic landmarks in corresponding images.[142,164-167] There has been some concern about the accuracy in determining anatomic landmarks for biplanar radiography, as well as a lack of equipment for this method in typical clinical settings.

To overcome some of these limitations to 3-D motion measurement, Lim and colleagues[168] developed a 3-D imaging technique using dynamic computed tomography (CT) to determine 6-degree-of-freedom (3 rotations and 3 translations) transformation of individual cadaveric cervical vertebrae during motion by tracking eigenvectors of the individual vertebrae. The investigators showed that accurate measurements (± 1 mm and $\pm 1°$) can be made using CT in vitro. The research group expanded on this technique to measure vertebral segmental movements in human lumbar spines in vivo (**Fig. 2**). Although this method was able to determine the rotations and translations of the lumbar vertebrae during motion in vivo, it was limited in determining

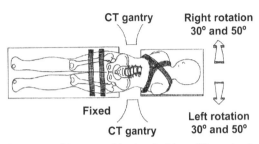

Fig. 2. A subject's positioning inside a CT gantry to study torso rotation. Straps hold subject onto a torso rotation apparatus and CT records evidence of coupled motion during torsion. Segmental movements are level dependent and the pattern of segmental movement is different between healthy subjects and subjects with LBP.

transformation of the sacrum because an entire 3-D CT model of a sacrum is difficult to obtain clinically and the eigenvector analysis using a partial-sacrum 3-D model caused an error of the measurement of the segmental motion at L5 to S1. The same research group developed another method to determine transformation of individual vertebrae including the sacrum during motion using the 3-D CT model and a volume merge method (**Fig. 3**).[169,170] This method can determine the rotations and translations during motion even if the 3-D geometry of the bone is incomplete, as in the case of the sacrum (an assumption of the bone as a rigid body still holds) at each position. Thus, it

is able to determine the transformation of the incomplete sacrum 3-D CT model with an accuracy of less than 0.1 mm in translation and 0.2° in rotation.

Relationship Between Instability and Disk Degeneration

Most patients with segmental instability have disk degeneration, but the relationship between instability and degeneration is not clear. Takeuchi and colleagues[171] presented a study using MR images in which T1 relaxation time was decreased in degenerative disks and the energy dissipated to axial loading was linearly correlated with T1 relaxation time. The investigators attempted to correlate the intrinsic biomechanical properties of the disk with MR imaging findings, but no information could be derived about the segmental motion characteristics from this study. Toyone and colleagues[172] reported that bone marrow adjacent to the disk in patients with symptomatic lumbar segmental instability, defined by flexion more than 5° and dynamic anterior-posterior translation more than 3 mm, had decreased signals on T1-weighted spin-echo MR images or Modic type I changes. Inaccurate flexion/extension radiographs of patients were used in this study by Toyone and colleagues[172] and pathogenesis of the osseous changes with disk degeneration is not known.

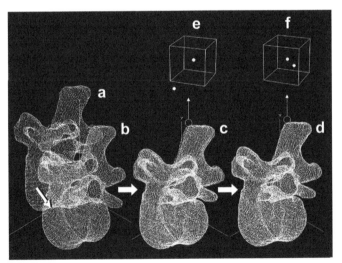

Fig. 3. Description of the volume merge method for analysis of segmental movement. A vertebral body in the neutral position (a) was virtually rotated (b) and translated (c) towards the rotated position. The position was refined with 0.05° and 0.05 mm increments, respectively, until the maximized volume merging was determined (d). A voxel with a dimension of 1.0 × 1.0 × 1.0 mm was created for each point of the stationary target. The number of points of the moving vertebra (*white dots*) that fell within the voxel of the stationary target (*yellow dots*) was determined and the percentage of volume merge was defined: (e) no volume merge, (f) volume merge achieved within the voxel region of interest.

Results of the in vitro studies of segmental motion characteristics and disk degeneration done by Fujiwara and colleagues[96] showed that torsional motion was most significantly affected by the degenerative changes in disk and facet joints. In addition, some investigators advocate the importance of torsional loads and stability on the injuries and degeneration of the motion segments.[173–178] Torsional instability in relation to the degenerative changes in the disk had been investigated in vivo using the aforementioned in vivo 3-D measurement technique.[168] The investigators found that a relationship exists between the severity of intervertebral disk degeneration and increases in the torsional movement in vivo, which was previously shown only in cadaveric studies.[169,170]

SUMMARY

A decrease in proteoglycan content and increased collagen fiber associated with degeneration contribute changes in material properties of nucleus pulposus from a fluid material to a solid material. Changes in material properties of the anulus fibrosus tissue are also affected by water content, which is a direct consequence of proteoglycan content. Degenerative structural changes of the disk are well documented, as are the changes in its viscoelastic properties. Decrease in proteoglycan content in the nucleus pulposus is also considered to be a governing factor affecting the dynamic viscoelastic properties of the disk. The highest correlation between the instability and the severity of the disk degeneration in torsion, among different loading directions, indicates that the fissures in the anulus fibrosus contribute the instability. This result agrees with the concept of degenerative cascade proposed by Kirkaldy-Willis. Increased segmental movement with disk degeneration up to grade 4 has also been measured in vivo. Further investigation is needed to confirm whether LBP is associated with increased segmental motion. To this end, current progress made on image analysis techniques using clinical imaging modalities will be a powerful tool to investigate this challenging problem.

REFERENCES

1. Adams MA, Dolan P, McNally DS. The internal mechanical functioning of intervertebral disks and articular cartilage, and its relevance to matrix biology. Matrix Biol 2009;28:384.
2. Hadjipavlou AG, Tzermiadianos MN, Bogduk N, et al. The pathophysiology of disc degeneration: a critical review. J Bone Joint Surg Br 2008;90:1261.
3. Roughley PJ. Biology of intervertebral disc aging and degeneration: involvement of the extracellular matrix. Spine (Phila Pa 1976) 2004;29:2691.
4. Yoon ST. The potential of gene therapy for the treatment of disc degeneration. Orthop Clin North Am 2004;35:95.
5. Hukins DWL, Meakin JR. Relationship between structure and mechanical function of the tissues of the intervertebral joint. Am Zool 2000;40:42.
6. Antoniou J, Steffen T, Nelson F, et al. The human lumbar intervertebral disc: evidence for changes in the biosynthesis and denaturation of the extracellular matrix with growth, maturation, ageing, and degeneration. J Clin Invest 1996;98:996.
7. Podichetty VK. The aging spine: the role of inflammatory mediators in intervertebral disc degeneration. Cell Mol Biol (Noisy-le-grand) 2007;53:4.
8. Urban JPG, Roberts S, Ralphs J. The nucleus of the intervertebral disc from development to degeneration. Amer Zool 2000;40:53.
9. Coventry MB, Ghormley RK, Kernohan JW. The intervertebral disc: its microscopic anatomy and pathology: part I: anatomy, development, and physiology. J Bone Joint Surg Am 1945;27:105.
10. Haefeli M, Kalberer F, Saegesser D, et al. The course of macroscopic degeneration in the human lumbar intervertebral disc. Spine (Phila Pa 1976) 2006;31:1522.
11. Bibby SR, Jones DA, Lee RB, et al. The pathophysiology of the intervertebral disc. Joint Bone Spine 2001;68:537.
12. Murakami H, Yoon TS, Attallah-Wasif ES, et al. Quantitative differences in intervertebral disc-matrix composition with age-related degeneration. Med Biol Eng Comput 2010;48:469.
13. McNally DS, Adams MA. Internal intervertebral disc mechanics as revealed by stress profilometry. Spine (Phila Pa 1976) 1992;17:66.
14. McNally DS, Adams MA, Goodship AE. Development and validation of a new transducer for intradiscal pressure measurement. J Biomed Eng 1992;14:495.
15. McNally DS, Shackleford IM, Goodship AE, et al. in vivo stress measurement can predict pain on discography. Spine (Phila Pa 1976) 1996;21:2580.
16. Adams MA, McNally DS, Dolan P. 'Stress' distributions inside intervertebral discs. The effects of age and degeneration. J Bone Joint Surg Br 1996;78:965.
17. Iatridis JC, Weidenbaum M, Setton LA, et al. Is the nucleus pulposus a solid or a fluid? Mechanical behaviors of the nucleus pulposus of the human intervertebral disc. Spine (Phila Pa 1976) 1996;21:1174.
18. Nachemson A, Morris J. Lumbar discometry. Lumbar intradiscal pressure measurements in vivo. Lancet 1963;1:1140.

19. Nachemson A, Morris JM. in vivo measurements of intradiscal pressure. Discometry, a method for the determination of pressure in the lower lumbar discs. J Bone Joint Surg Am 1964;46:1077.

20. Nachemson AL. Disc pressure measurements. Spine (Phila Pa 1976) 1981;6:93.

21. Nachemson AL. Intradiscal pressure. J Neurosurg 1995;82:1095.

22. Adams MA, Freeman BJ, Morrison HP, et al. Mechanical initiation of intervertebral disc degeneration. Spine (Phila Pa 1976) 2000;25:1625.

23. McNally DS, Adams MA, Goodship AE. Can intervertebral disc prolapse be predicted by disc mechanics? Spine (Phila Pa 1976) 1993;18:1525.

24. Buckwalter JA. Aging and degeneration of the human intervertebral disc. Spine (Phila Pa 1976) 1995;20:1307.

25. Iatridis JC, Setton LA, Weidenbaum M, et al. Alterations in the mechanical behavior of the human lumbar nucleus pulposus with degeneration and aging. J Orthop Res 1997;15:318.

26. Stokes IA, Iatridis JC. Mechanical conditions that accelerate intervertebral disc degeneration: overload versus immobilization. Spine (Phila Pa 1976) 2004;29:2724.

27. Urban JP, McMullin JF. Swelling pressure of the lumbar intervertebral discs: influence of age, spinal level, composition, and degeneration. Spine (Phila Pa 1976) 1988;13:179.

28. Johannessen W, Elliott DM. Effects of degeneration on the biphasic material properties of human nucleus pulposus in confined compression. Spine (Phila Pa 1976) 2005;30:E724.

29. Nachemson A. Lumbar intradiscal pressure. Experimental studies on post-mortem material. Acta Orthop Scand Suppl 1960;43:1.

30. Smith LJ, Byers S, Costi JJ, et al. Elastic fibers enhance the mechanical integrity of the human lumbar anulus fibrosus in the radial direction. Ann Biomed Eng 2008;36:214.

31. Smith LJ, Fazzalari NL. The elastic fibre network of the human lumbar anulus fibrosus: architecture, mechanical function and potential role in the progression of intervertebral disc degeneration. Eur Spine J 2009;18:439.

32. Skaggs DL, Weidenbaum M, Iatridis JC, et al. Regional variation in tensile properties and biochemical composition of the human lumbar anulus fibrosus. Spine (Phila Pa 1976) 1994;19:1310.

33. Acaroglu ER, Iatridis JC, Setton LA, et al. Degeneration and aging affect the tensile behavior of human lumbar anulus fibrosus. Spine (Phila Pa 1976) 1995;20:2690.

34. Ebara S, Iatridis JC, Setton LA, et al. Tensile properties of nondegenerate human lumbar anulus fibrosus. Spine (Phila Pa 1976) 1996;21:452.

35. Galante JO. Tensile properties of the human lumbar anulus fibrosus. Acta Orthop Scand Suppl 1967;100:1.

36. Wu HC, Yao RF. Mechanical behavior of the human anulus fibrosus. J Biomech 1976;9:1.

37. Schollum ML, Robertson PA, Broom ND. How age influences unravelling morphology of annular lamellae - a study of interfibre cohesivity in the lumbar disc. J Anat 2010;216:310.

38. Schollum ML, Robertson PA, Broom ND. ISSLS prize winner: microstructure and mechanical disruption of the lumbar disc anulus: part I: a microscopic investigation of the translamellar bridging network. Spine (Phila Pa 1976) 2008;33:2702.

39. Guerin HL, Elliott DM. Quantifying the contributions of structure to anulus fibrosus mechanical function using a nonlinear, anisotropic, hyperelastic model. J Orthop Res 2007;25:508.

40. Wagner DR, Lotz JC. Theoretical model and experimental results for the nonlinear elastic behavior of human anulus fibrosus. J Orthop Res 2004;22:901.

41. Wren TA, Carter DR. A microstructural model for the tensile constitutive and failure behavior of soft skeletal connective tissues. J Biomech Eng 1998;120:55.

42. Elliott DM, Narmoneva DA, Setton LA. Direct measurement of the Poisson's ratio of human patella cartilage in tension. J Biomech Eng 2002;124:223.

43. Soltz MA, Ateshian GA. A Conewise Linear Elasticity mixture model for the analysis of tension-compression nonlinearity in articular cartilage. J Biomech Eng 2000;122:576.

44. Woo SL, Simon BR, Kuei SC, et al. Quasi-linear viscoelastic properties of normal articular cartilage. J Biomech Eng 1980;102:85.

45. Li LP, Soulhat J, Buschmann MD, et al. Nonlinear analysis of cartilage in unconfined ramp compression using a fibril reinforced poroelastic model. Clin Biomech (Bristol, Avon) 1999;14:673.

46. Huang CY, Mow VC, Ateshian GA. The role of flow-independent viscoelasticity in the biphasic tensile and compressive responses of articular cartilage. J Biomech Eng 2001;123:410.

47. Guerin HA, Elliott DM. Degeneration affects the fiber reorientation of human anulus fibrosus under tensile load. J Biomech 2006;39:1410.

48. O'Connell GD, Guerin HL, Elliott DM. Theoretical and uniaxial experimental evaluation of human anulus fibrosus degeneration. J Biomech Eng 2009;131:111007.

49. Sen S, Boxberger JI, Schroeder Y, et al. Effect of degeneration on the dynamic viscoelastic properties of human anulus fibrosus in tension. In: Proceedings of the ASME 2008 Summer Bioengineering Conference. Marco Island (FL). New York (NY): American Society of Mechanical Engineers; 2009.

50. Gu WY, Mao XG, Foster RJ, et al. The anisotropic hydraulic permeability of human lumbar anulus

fibrosus. Influence of age, degeneration, direction, and water content. Spine (Phila Pa 1976) 1999;24: 2449.

51. Natarajan RN, Williams JR, Andersson GB. Modeling changes in intervertebral disc mechanics with degeneration. J Bone Joint Surg Am 2006; 88(Suppl 2):36.

52. Adams MA, Dolan P, Hutton WC. The lumbar spine in backward bending. Spine (Phila Pa 1976) 1988; 13:1019.

53. Hirsch C. The reaction of intervertebral discs to compression forces. J Bone Joint Surg Am 1955; 37:1188.

54. White AA, Panjabi M. Clinical biomechanics of the spine. Philadelphia: Lippincott Williams & Wilkins; 1990.

55. Reuber M, Schultz A, Denis F, et al. Bulging of lumbar intervertebral disks. J Biomech Eng 1982; 104:187.

56. Nachemson A. The load on lumbar disks in different positions of the body. Clin Orthop Relat Res 1966;45:107.

57. Nachemson A. Mechanical stresses on lumbar disks. Curr Pract Orthop Surg 1966;3:208.

58. Wilke HJ, Neef P, Caimi M, et al. New in vivo measurements of pressures in the intervertebral disc in daily life. Spine (Phila Pa 1976) 1999; 24:755.

59. Schultz AB, Andersson GB. Analysis of loads on the lumbar spine. Spine (Phila Pa 1976) 1981;6:76.

60. Schultz AB, Andersson GB, Haderspeck K, et al. Analysis and measurement of lumbar trunk loads in tasks involving bends and twists. J Biomech 1982;15:669.

61. Andersson GB, Schultz AB. Effects of fluid injection on mechanical properties of intervertebral discs. J Biomech 1979;12:453.

62. Elliott DM, Yerramalli CS, Beckstein JC, et al. The effect of relative needle diameter in puncture and sham injection animal models of degeneration. Spine (Phila Pa 1976) 2008;33:588.

63. Hsieh AH, Hwang D, Ryan DA, et al. Degenerative anular changes induced by puncture are associated with insufficiency of disc biomechanical function. Spine (Phila Pa 1976) 2009;34:998.

64. Wang JL, Tsai YC, Wang YH. The leakage pathway and effect of needle gauge on degree of disc injury post anular puncture: a comparative study using aged human and adolescent porcine discs. Spine (Phila Pa 1976) 2007;32:1809.

65. Korecki CL, Kuo CK, Tuan RS, et al. Intervertebral disc cell response to dynamic compression is age and frequency dependent. J Orthop Res 2009;27:800.

66. Korecki CL, MacLean JJ, Iatridis JC. Characterization of an in vitro intervertebral disc organ culture system. Eur Spine J 2007;16:1029.

67. Schollum ML, Appleyard RC, Little CB, et al. A detailed microscopic examination of alterations in normal anular structure induced by mechanical destabilization in an ovine model of disc degeneration. Spine (Phila Pa 1976) 2010;35:1965.

68. Wuertz K, Godburn K, MacLean JJ, et al. in vivo remodeling of intervertebral discs in response to short- and long-term dynamic compression. J Orthop Res 2009;27:1235.

69. Korecki CL, Costi JJ, Iatridis JC. Needle puncture injury affects intervertebral disc mechanics and biology in an organ culture model. Spine (Phila Pa 1976) 2008;33:235.

70. MacLean JJ, Roughley PJ, Monsey RD, et al. in vivo intervertebral disc remodeling: kinetics of mRNA expression in response to a single loading event. J Orthop Res 2008;26:579.

71. Johannessen W, Vresilovic EJ, Wright AC, et al. Intervertebral disc mechanics are restored following cyclic loading and unloaded recovery. Ann Biomed Eng 2004;32:70.

72. Boxberger JI, Orlansky AS, Sen S, et al. Reduced nucleus pulposus glycosaminoglycan content alters intervertebral disc dynamic viscoelastic mechanics. J Biomech 2009;42:1941.

73. Boxberger JI, Sen S, Yerramalli CS, et al. Nucleus pulposus glycosaminoglycan content is correlated with axial mechanics in rat lumbar motion segments. J Orthop Res 1906;24:2006.

74. Kim J, An H, Masuda K, et al. Dynamic viscoelastic properties of rabbit lumbar discs. In: Trans Orthop Res Soc; 2005. p. 1280.

75. Kim JG, An HS, Masuda K, et al. Dissimilarity in dynamic viscoelastic properties of lumbar disc levels. New York: The International Society for the Study of the Lumbar Spine; 2005.

76. Kim JG, Miyamoto K, Masuda K, et al. Correlations among biomechanical, biochemical and structural properties of the degenerated intervertebral disc. In 52nd Annual Meeting of the Orthopaedic Research Society. Chicago (IL), March 19–22, 2006. p. 49.

77. Miyamoto K, Masuda K, Kim JG, et al. Intradiscal injections of osteogenic protein-1 restore the viscoelastic properties of degenerated intervertebral discs. Spine J 2006;6:692.

78. Schmorl G, Junghanns H. The human spine in health and disease. New York and London: Grune and Stratton; 1971.

79. Farfan HF. Mechanical disorders of the low back. Philadelphia: Lea & Febiger; 1973.

80. Kirkaldy-Willis WH. The pathology and pathogenesis of low back pain. Managing low back pain. In: Kirkaldy-Willis WH, editor. Managing low back pain. Philadelphia (PA): Churchill Livingstone; 1983. p. 23.

81. Tampier C, Drake JD, Callaghan JP, et al. Progressive disc herniation: an investigation of the

mechanism using radiologic, histochemical, and microscopic dissection techniques on a porcine model. Spine (Phila Pa 1976) 2007;32:2869.

82. Veres SP, Robertson PA, Broom ND. ISSLS prize winner: microstructure and mechanical disruption of the lumbar disc anulus: part II: how the anulus fails under hydrostatic pressure. Spine (Phila Pa 1976) 2008;33:2711.

83. Natarajan RN, Lundberg HJ, Oegema T, et al. A novel multilayered annular model to predict delamination in a lumbar intervertebral disc. In: Proceedings of the ASME 2009 Summer Bioengineering Conference, Resort at Squaw Creek, Lake Tahoe (CA), USA. New York (NY): American Society of Mechanical Engineers; 2010.

84. Fagan AB, Sarvestani G, Moore RJ, et al. Innervation of anulus tears: an experimental animal study. Spine (Phila Pa 1976) 2010;35:1200.

85. Galbusera F, Schmidt H, Neidlinger-Wilke C, et al. The mechanical response of the lumbar spine to different combinations of disc degenerative changes investigated using randomized poroelastic finite element models. Eur Spine J 2011;20(4):563–71.

86. Schmidt H, Shirazi-Adl A, Galbusera F, et al. Response analysis of the lumbar spine during regular daily activities–a finite element analysis. J Biomech 2010;43:1849.

87. Williams JR, Natarajan RN, Andersson GB. Inclusion of regional poroelastic material properties better predicts biomechanical behavior of lumbar discs subjected to dynamic loading. J Biomech 2007;40:1981.

88. Schroeder Y, Elliott DM, Wilson W, et al. Experimental and model determination of human intervertebral disc osmoviscoelasticity. J Orthop Res 2008; 26:1141.

89. Schroeder Y, Huyghe JM, van Donkelaar CC, et al. A biochemical/biophysical 3D FE intervertebral disc model. Biomech Model Mechanobiol 2010;9:641.

90. Costi JJ, Stokes IA, Gardner-Morse M, et al. Direct measurement of intervertebral disc maximum shear strain in six degrees of freedom: motions that place disc tissue at risk of injury. J Biomech 2007;40:2457.

91. Iatridis JC, Mente PL, Stokes IA, et al. Compression-induced changes in intervertebral disc properties in a rat tail model. Spine (Phila Pa 1976) 1999;24:996.

92. Goel VK, Monroe BT, Gilbertson LG, et al. Interlaminar shear stresses and laminae separation in a disc. Finite element analysis of the L3-L4 motion segment subjected to axial compressive loads. Spine (Phila Pa 1976) 1995;20:689.

93. Elliott DM, Setton LA. Anisotropic and inhomogeneous tensile behavior of the human anulus fibrosus: experimental measurement and material model predictions. J Biomech Eng 2001;123:256.

94. Holzapfel GA, Schulze-Bauer CA, Feigl G, et al. Single lamellar mechanics of the human lumbar anulus fibrosus. Biomech Model Mechanobiol 2005;3:125.

95. Schollum ML, Robertson PA, Broom ND. A microstructural investigation of intervertebral disc lamellar connectivity: detailed analysis of the translamellar bridges. J Anat 2009;214:805.

96. Fujiwara A, Lim TH, An HS, et al. The effect of disc degeneration and facet joint osteoarthritis on the segmental flexibility of the lumbar spine. Spine (Phila Pa 1976) 2000;25:3036.

97. Kirkaldy-Willis WH, Farfan HF. Instability of the lumbar spine. Clin Orthop Relat Res 1982;110.

98. Farfan HF, Gracovetsky S. The nature of instability. Spine (Phila Pa 1976) 1984;9:714.

99. Frymoyer JW, Newberg A, Pope MH, et al. Spine radiographs in patients with low-back pain. An epidemiological study in men. J Bone Joint Surg Am 1984;66:1048.

100. Gertzbein SD, Seligman J, Holtby R, et al. Centrode patterns and segmental instability in degenerative disc disease. Spine (Phila Pa 1976) 1985;10:257.

101. Morgan FP, King T. Primary instability of lumbar vertebrae as a common cause of low back pain. J Bone Joint Surg Br 1957;39:6.

102. Nachemson A. Lumbar spine instability. A critical update and symposium summary. Spine (Phila Pa 1976) 1985;10:290.

103. Panjabi M. Low back pain and spinal instability. In: Weinstein J, Gordon SL, editors. Low back pain: a scientific and clinical overview. Rosemont (IL): American Academy of Orthopedic Surgeons; 1996. p. 367.

104. Panjabi MM, Kaigle AM, Pope MH. Degeneration, injury, and spinal instability. In: Wiesel SW, Weinstein JN, Herkowitz H, et al, editors. The lumbar spine. Philadelphia: WB Saunders; 1996. p. 203.

105. Stokes IA, Frymoyer JW. Segmental motion and instability. Spine (Phila Pa 1976) 1987;12:688.

106. Hayes MA, Howard TC, Gruel CR, et al. Roentgenographic evaluation of lumbar spine flexion-extension in asymptomatic individuals. Spine (Phila Pa 1976) 1989;14:327.

107. Knuttson F. The instability associated with disc degeneration in the lumbar spine. Acta Radiol 1944;25:593.

108. Dvorak J, Panjabi MM, Grob D, et al. Clinical validation of functional flexion/extension radiographs of the cervical spine. Spine (Phila Pa 1976) 1993;18:120.

109. Gracovetsky S, Newman N, Pawlowsky M, et al. A database for estimating normal spinal motion derived from noninvasive measurements. Spine (Phila Pa 1976) 1995;20:1036.

110. Boden SD, Davis DO, Dina TS, et al. Abnormal magnetic-resonance scans of the lumbar spine in asymptomatic subjects. A prospective investigation. J Bone Joint Surg Am 1990;72:403.

111. Modic MT, Masaryk TJ, Ross JS, et al. Imaging of degenerative disc disease. Radiology 1988; 168:177.

112. Modic MT, Masaryk TJ, Weinstein MA. Magnetic resonance imaging of the spine. Magn Reson Annu 1986;37.

113. Modic MT, Ross JS. Magnetic resonance imaging in the evaluation of low back pain. Orthop Clin North Am 1991;22:283.

114. Modic MT, Ross JS. Lumbar degenerative disc disease. Radiology 2007;245:43.

115. Modic MT. Advances in spinal imaging. Clin Neurosurg 1992;38:97.

116. Nowicki BH, Haughton VM. Neural foraminal ligaments of the lumbar spine: appearance at CT and MR imaging. Radiology 1992;183:257.

117. Pfirrmann CW, Metzdorf A, Zanetti M, et al. Magnetic resonance classification of lumbar intervertebral disc degeneration. Spine (Phila Pa 1976) 2001;26:1873.

118. Thompson JP, Pearce RH, Schechter MT, et al. Preliminary evaluation of a scheme for grading the gross morphology of the human intervertebral disc. Spine (Phila Pa 1976) 1990;15:411.

119. Haughton VM, Schmidt TA, Keele K, et al. Flexibility of lumbar spinal motion segments correlated to type of tears in the anulus fibrosus. J Neurosurg 2000;92:81.

120. Mimura M, Panjabi MM, Oxland TR, et al. Disc degeneration affects the multidirectional flexibility of the lumbar spine. Spine (Phila Pa 1976) 1994; 19:1371.

121. Nachemson AL, Schultz AB, Berkson MH. Mechanical properties of human lumbar spine motion segments. Influence of age, sex, disc level, and degeneration. Spine (Phila Pa 1976) 1979;4:1.

122. Nowicki BH, Yu S, Reinartz J, et al. Effect of axial loading on neural foramina and nerve roots in the lumbar spine. Radiology 1990;176:433.

123. Schmidt TA, An HS, Lim TH, et al. The stiffness of lumbar spinal motion segments with a high-intensity zone in the anulus fibrosus. Spine (Phila Pa 1976) 1998;23:2167.

124. Boden SD, Wiesel SW. Lumbosacral segmental motion in normal individuals. Have we been measuring instability properly? Spine (Phila Pa 1976) 1990;15:571.

125. Boxall D, Bradford DS, Winter RB, et al. Management of severe spondylolisthesis in children and adolescents. J Bone Joint Surg Am 1979;61:479.

126. Dupuis PR, Yong-Hing K, Cassidy JD, et al. Radiologic diagnosis of degenerative lumbar spinal instability. Spine (Phila Pa 1976) 1985;10:262.

127. Dvorak J, Panjabi MM, Chang DG, et al. Functional radiographic diagnosis of the lumbar spine. Flexion-extension and lateral bending. Spine (Phila Pa 1976) 1991;16:562.

128. Dvorak J, Panjabi MM, Novotny JE, et al. Clinical validation of functional flexion-extension roentgenograms of the lumbar spine. Spine (Phila Pa 1976) 1991;16:943.

129. Lysell E. Motion in the cervical spine. An experimental study on autopsy specimens. Acta Orthop Scand Suppl 1969;123:1–61.

130. Penning L. Normal movements of the cervical spine. AJR Am J Roentgenol 1978;130:317.

131. Posner I, White AA 3rd, Edwards WT, et al. A biomechanical analysis of the clinical stability of the lumbar and lumbosacral spine. Spine (Phila Pa 1976) 1982;7:374.

132. Quinnell RC, Stockdale HR. Flexion and extension radiography of the lumbar spine: a comparison with lumbar discography. Clin Radiol 1983;34:405.

133. Torgerson WR, Dotter WE. Comparative roentgenographic study of the asymptomatic and symptomatic lumbar spine. J Bone Joint Surg Am 1976;58:850.

134. Panjabi M, Chang D, Dvorak J. An analysis of errors in kinematic parameters associated with in vivo functional radiographs. Spine (Phila Pa 1976) 1992;17:200.

135. Shaffer WO, Spratt KF, Weinstein J, et al. 1990 Volvo Award in clinical sciences. The consistency and accuracy of roentgenograms for measuring sagittal translation in the lumbar vertebral motion segment. An experimental model. Spine (Phila Pa 1976) 1990;15:741.

136. Saraste H, Brostrom LA, Aparisi T, et al. Radiographic measurement of the lumbar spine. A clinical and experimental study in man. Spine (Phila Pa 1976) 1985;10:236.

137. Danielson B, Frennered K, Irstam L. Roentgenologic assessment of spondylolisthesis. I. A study of measurement variations. Acta Radiol 1988;29:345.

138. Kalebo P, Kadziolka R, Sward L. Compression traction radiography of lumbar segmental instability. Spine (Phila Pa 1976) 1990;15:351.

139. Wall MS, Oppenheim WL. Measurement error of spondylolisthesis as a function of radiographic beam angle. J Pediatr Orthop 1995;15:193.

140. Bey MJ, Kline SK, Tashman S, et al. Accuracy of biplane x-ray imaging combined with model-based tracking for measuring in-vivo patellofemoral joint motion. J Orthop Surg Res 2008;3:38.

141. Brown RH, Burstein AH, Nash CL, et al. Spinal analysis using a three-dimensional radiographic technique. J Biomech 1976;9:355.

142. Li G, Wuerz TH, DeFrate LE. Feasibility of using orthogonal fluoroscopic images to measure in vivo joint kinematics. J Biomech Eng 2004;126:314.

143. Stokes IA, Wilder DG, Frymoyer JW, et al. 1980 Volvo Award in clinical sciences. Assessment of patients with low-back pain by biplanar radiographic

measurement of intervertebral motion. Spine (Phila Pa 1976) 1981;6:233.

144. Suh CH. The fundamentals of computer aided X-ray analysis of the spine. J Biomech 1974;7:161.

145. Wilder DG, Seligson D, Frymoyer JW, et al. Objective measurement of L4-5 instability. A case report. Spine (Phila Pa 1976) 1980;5:56.

146. Wachowski MM, Mansour M, Lee C, et al. How do spinal segments move? J Biomech 2009;42:2286.

147. Nagerl H, Hawellek T, Lehmann A, et al. Non-linearity of flexion-extension characteristics in spinal segments. Acta Bioeng Biomech 2009;11:3.

148. Rousseau MA, Bradford DS, Hadi TM, et al. The instant axis of rotation influences facet forces at L5/S1 during flexion/extension and lateral bending. Eur Spine J 2006;15:299.

149. Huang RC, Girardi FP, Cammisa FP Jr, et al. The implications of constraint in lumbar total disc replacement. J Spinal Disord Tech 2003;16:412.

150. Resnick DK, Weller SJ, Benzel EC. Biomechanics of the thoracolumbar spine. Neurosurg Clin N Am 1997;8:455.

151. Bogduk N, Amevo B, Pearcy M. A biological basis for instantaneous centres of rotation of the vertebral column. Proc Inst Mech Eng H 1995;209:177.

152. Haher TR, O'Brien M, Felmly WT, et al. Instantaneous axis of rotation as a function of the three columns of the spine. Spine (Phila Pa 1976) 1992;17:S149.

153. Mimura M. Rotational instability of the lumbar spine–a three-dimensional motion study using bi-plane X-ray analysis system. Nippon Seikeigeka Gakkai Zasshi 1990;64:546 [in Japanese].

154. Pearcy MJ, Bogduk N. Instantaneous axes of rotation of the lumbar intervertebral joints. Spine (Phila Pa 1976) 1988;13:1033.

155. Gertzbein SD, Seligman J, Holtby R, et al. Centrode characteristics of the lumbar spine as a function of segmental instability. Clin Orthop Relat Res 1986;208:48–51.

156. Ogston NG, King GJ, Gertzbein SD, et al. Centrode patterns in the lumbar spine. Baseline studies in normal subjects. Spine (Phila Pa 1976) 1986;11:591.

157. Friberg O. Lumbar instability: a dynamic approach by traction-compression radiography. Spine (Phila Pa 1976) 1987;12:119.

158. Panjabi MM, Andersson GB, Jorneus L, et al. in vivo measurements of spinal column vibrations. J Bone Joint Surg Am 1986;68:695.

159. Pope MH, Wilder DG, Jorneus L, et al. The response of the seated human to sinusoidal vibration and impact. J Biomech Eng 1987;109:279.

160. Selvik G. Roentgen stereophotogrammetry. A method for the study of the kinematics of the skeletal system. Acta Orthop Scand Suppl 1989;232:1.

161. Haughton VM, Rogers B, Meyerand ME, et al. Measuring the axial rotation of lumbar vertebrae in vivo with MR imaging. AJNR Am J Neuroradiol 2002;23:1110.

162. Rogers BP, Haughton VM, Arfanakis K, et al. Application of image registration to measurement of intervertebral rotation in the lumbar spine. Magn Reson Med 2002;48:1072.

163. Dickey JP, Pierrynowski MR, Bednar DA, et al. Relationship between pain and vertebral motion in chronic low-back pain subjects. Clin Biomech (Bristol, Avon) 2002;17:345.

164. Anderst W, Donaldson W, Lee J, et al. Fused and adjacent segment motion in the cervical spine 6 months after anterior cervical discectomy and fusion. In 56th Annual Meeting of the Orthopaedic Research Society. New Orleans (LA), March 9–13, 2010. p. 146.

165. Li G, Wang S, Passias P, et al. Segmental in vivo vertebral motion during functional human lumbar spine activities. Eur Spine J 2009;18:1013.

166. Pearcy M, Portek I, Shepherd J. Three-dimensional x-ray analysis of normal movement in the lumbar spine. Spine (Phila Pa 1976) 1984;9:294.

167. Pearcy MJ. Stereo radiography of lumbar spine motion. Acta Orthop Scand Suppl 1985;212:1.

168. Lim TH, Eck JC, An HS, et al. A noninvasive, three-dimensional spinal motion analysis method. Spine (Phila Pa 1976) 1997;22:1996.

169. Ochia RS, Inoue N, Renner SM, et al. Three-dimensional in vivo measurement of lumbar spine segmental motion. Spine (Phila Pa 1976) 2006;31:2073.

170. Ochia RS, Inoue N, Takatori R, et al. in vivo measurements of lumbar segmental motion during axial rotation in asymptomatic and chronic low back pain male subjects. Spine (Phila Pa 1976) 2007;32:1394.

171. Takeuchi T, Shea M, White AA. Correlation of magnetic resonance relaxation times with degeneration and biomechanical properties in human lumbar intervertebral disks. In 38th Annual Meeting of the Orthopaedic Research Society. Washington, DC, February 17–20, 1992. p. 191.

172. Toyone T, Takahashi K, Kitahara H, et al. Vertebral bone-marrow changes in degenerative lumbar disc disease. An MRI study of 74 patients with low back pain. J Bone Joint Surg Br 1994;76:757.

173. Barbir A, Godburn KE, Michalek AJ, et al. Effects of torsion on intervertebral disc gene expression and biomechanics, using a rat tail model. Spine (Phila Pa 1976) 2011;36(8):607–14.

174. Espinoza Orias AA, Malhotra NR. Elliott DM: Rat disc torsional mechanics: effect of lumbar and caudal levels and axial compression load. Spine J 2009;9:204.

175. Veres SP, Robertson PA, Broom ND. The influence of torsion on disc herniation when combined with flexion. Eur Spine J 2010;19:1468.

176. Yang KH, An HS, Ochia RS, et al. in vivo measurement changes in lumbar facet joint width during torsion. In 51st Annual Meeting of the Orthopaedic Research Society. Washington, DC, February 20–23, 2005. p. 690.

177. Adams MA, Hutton WC. The relevance of torsion to the mechanical derangement of the lumbar spine. Spine (Phila Pa 1976) 1981;6:241.

178. Farfan HF, Cossette JW, Robertson GH, et al. The effects of torsion on the lumbar intervertebral joints: the role of torsion in the production of disc degeneration. J Bone Joint Surg Am 1970; 52:468.

Diagnostic Tools and Imaging Methods in Intervertebral Disk Degeneration

Sharmila Majumdar, PhD[a,b,*], Thomas M. Link, MD[a],
Lynne S. Steinbach, MD[a], Serena Hu, MD[b],
John Kurhanewicz, PhD[a]

KEYWORDS

- Spine • Imaging • Disk • Magnetic resonance
- Spectroscopy • T_{1rho} • T_2

The incidence of back pain is ubiquitous in many societies; it has been reported as ranging from 8% to 80%.[1–3] Most people experiencing back pain have self-limited episodes; however, a small proportion of this pain becomes chronic and debilitating (see the article by Karppinen and colleagues elsewhere in this issue for further exploration of this topic). Disorders of the low back have may compromise quality of life and present a tremendous financial impact on society through lost productivity, increased health care, and societal costs.[4,5] In contrast to individuals with spinal degeneration resulting in spinal stenosis and disk herniation, those with disk degeneration have much more variable presentations and responses to treatment. Although aging of individuals inevitably leads to aging and degeneration of the spine, it has been proposed that physiologic degeneration is a different clinical entity from pathologic degeneration, with the implication that chronic back pain is the exception rather than the rule and that those with pathologic degeneration do not have appropriate repair or compensatory mechanisms (see the article by Chan and colleagues elsewhere in this issue for further exploration of this topic).

Intervertebral disks provide stable support to adjacent vertebral bodies and allow movement to the vertebral bodies, thereby affecting spinal flexibility. They absorb and distribute loads during daily activities. Intervertebral disks undergo age-related degeneration, increase in back pain, and stiffness. The connections between pain and disk degeneration are not fully understood (see the articles by Inoue and Espinoza Orias, and Karppinen and colleagues, elsewhere in this issue for further exploration of this topic).

The intervertebral disk is composed of the nucleus pulposus, the annulus fibrosus, and the cartilaginous end-plates (see the article by Grunhagen and colleagues elsewhere in this issue for further exploration of this topic). The nucleus pulposus is a viscous, mucoprotein gel that is approximately centrally located within the disk[6] and is composed of glycosaminoglycans in a loose network of type II collagen. The annulus fibrosus forms the outer boundary of the disk and is made up of type-I collagen fibers arranged in lamellae. The proteoglycans of the nucleus osmotically exert a "swelling pressure" that enables it to support spinal compressive loads. The pressurized nucleus also creates tensile stress within the

[a] Department of Radiology and Biomedical Imaging, University of California San Francisco, Campus Box 2520, QB3 Building, 2nd Floor, Suite 203, 1700 4th Street, San Francisco, CA 94158, USA
[b] Department of Orthopedic Surgery, University of California San Francisco, 1500 Owens Street, San Francisco, CA 94158, USA
* Corresponding author. Department of Radiology and Biomedical Imaging, University of California San Francisco, Campus Box 2520, QB3 Building, 2nd Floor, Suite 203, 1700 4th Street, San Francisco, CA 94158.
E-mail address: Sharmila.Majumdar@ucsf.edu

Orthop Clin N Am 42 (2011) 501–511
doi:10.1016/j.ocl.2011.07.007

collagen fibers of the annulus and ligamentous structures surrounding the nucleus.

Disk degeneration is characterized by a loss of cellularity and degradation of the extracellular matrix resulting in morphologic changes and alterations in biomechanical properties. Changes in proteoglycan content within the nucleus leads to reduced water content, depressurization, and flattening of the disk. Disruption of the collagen network in the annulus ultimately leads to disk rupture and herniation. Disk-height loss also results in narrowing of the vertebral foramen with compression of the nerve roots and may lead to the development of spinal stenosis as well as foraminal narrowing. It has been proposed that biochemical degradation, upregulation of genes associated with collagen matrix degradation, and the cumulative effect of mechanical loading, all stimulate the degenerative disk process and, thus, contribute to functional impairment and pain (see the articles by Chan and colleagues, Kao and colleagues, and Inoue and Espinoza Orias elsewhere in this issue for further exploration of this topic). Thus, biomarkers that may be objectively associated with pain and functional impairment and yet provide noninvasive diagnosis of disk degeneration and its accompanying biochemical and biomechanical changes, are clearly required. It is in this context that MRI and spectroscopy has potential. In the following sections, the authors review the current diagnostic tools and recent developments for assessing disk degeneration.

DIAGNOSTIC IMAGING OF INTERVERTEBRAL DISK

Conventional radiographs have been used to assess degenerative disk disease for many years and are still the first imaging test in patients with suspected disk disease. Radiographic findings, however, provide indirect signs and include disk-space narrowing and reactive end-plate changes with spondylophytes and sclerosis. Associated anterolisthesis and retrolisthesis may also be a sign of degenerative disk disease. Radiographs are limited for assessing early-stage disease and quantifying the amount of disk degeneration. Disk bulges and herniations are not seen on radiographs.

CT scanning was the first line of investigation for suspected lumbar prolapsed intervertebral disk disease in the past, but has been overtaken by MRI. CT scanning exposes the patient to ionizing radiation and does not adequately demonstrate the disk in relation to the surrounding tissues compared with MRI because of inferior soft tissue contrast resolution. Nevertheless, it may be helpful in visualizing posterior osteophytes, which may be important for surgical planning. Although pain provocation using discography or CT discography[7] has been shown to improve the odds of a positive surgical outcome, there a high incidence of false positives has been reported[8,9] and there remains a significant number of severely degenerated disks that have been found to be painless.[10] In part because of the widespread occurrence of abnormal radiographic findings, the use of provocative discography is theorized to determine which disk is the pain generator. Because degenerated disks can develop in-growth of nerve fibers that are sensitive to pain,[11] it is thought that these fibers will be stimulated and irritated by injecting the disk and pressurizing it. Reproduction of the patient's typical pain should signify that the patient's pain is occurring at that disk level. The surgeon may use this test to determine at which levels the patient should have surgery. However, the test is painful, subjective, and can be difficult to interpret, particularly in chronic-pain patients.[12] In addition, although fine needles are used for the injection into the disk (22 g and 25 g), there appears to be a higher incidence in late symptomatic degeneration in normal levels compared with those that were not injected (35% after discography compared with 14% in nondiscogram disks).[13]

It is in this context that nonionizing MRIs, which reflect changes in disk height and morphology, are being used for diagnostic purposes. Using T_1- and T_2-weighted images, structural changes in the disk are visualized, as seen on representative images in **Figs. 1** and **2**. A decrease in T_2-weighted signal intensity with increased lumbar disk degeneration is often seen, as shown in **Fig. 2**. Normal intervertebral disks show a well-defined, oval, high-signal intensity from the nucleus pulposus (see **Fig. 1**) and there is low-signal intensity from the annulus fibrosus, whereas degenerated disks are characterized by a change in the signal from the nucleus pulposus to give an irregular outline and a reduction in signal intensity on longer TE sequences, such as proton density and T_2-weighting (see **Fig. 2**). In advanced cases, there is no clear demarcation between annulus and nucleus.[10] A semiquantitative assessment of morphologic degeneration in intervertebral disk degeneration can be performed using Pfirrmann grading, which is a 5-point scale system and is assessed from T_2-weighted MRIs. **Fig. 3**[14] shows representative disks with the different Pfirrmann grades. MRI is capable of assessing the disk degeneration in terms of signal changes and demonstrates posterior disk bulges, protrusions, extrusions, and

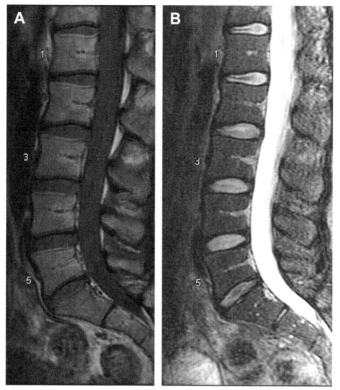

Fig. 1. Sagittal (*A*) T$_1$-weighted and (*B*) fat-saturated T$_2$-weighted fast spin echo sequences of the lumbar spine, showing normal disk spaces with normal disk and adjacent bone marrow signal.

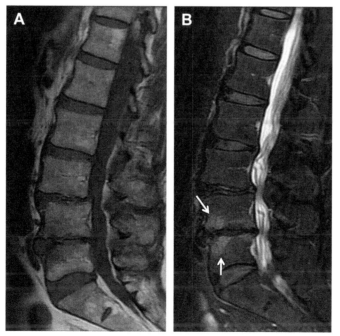

Fig. 2. Sagittal T$_1$-weighted and fat-saturated (*A*) T$_2$-weighted fast spin echo (*B*) sequences of the lumbar spine demonstrate severe degenerative disk disease at L3/4 and L4/5 with disk height loss, disk desiccation, decreased signal, posterior disk bulges, and Modic type 1 reactive end-plate changes at L4/5 (*arrows*). Note substantial spinal canal narrowing from L3-S1.

Grade	Structure	Distinction of Nucleus and Annulus	Signal Intensity	Height of Disc
I	Homogeneous, bright white	Clear	Hyperintense	Normal
II	Inhomogeneous	Clear	Hyperintense	Normal
III	Inhomogeneous, gray	Unclear	Intermediate	Normal to slightly decreased
IV	Inhomogeneous, gray to black	Lost	Intermediate to hypointense	Normal to moderately decreased
V	Inhomogeneous, black	Lost	Hypointense	Collapsed disc space

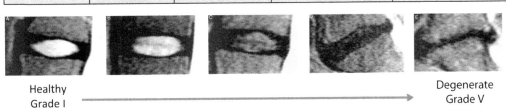

Healthy Grade I → Degenerate Grade V

Fig. 3. Representative images showing disks with varying Pfirrmann grades. (*Courtesy of* Gabby Joseph, Department of Radiology and Biomedical Imaging, UCSF.)

sequestrations, as well as their effect upon the adjacent spinal cord and nerve roots.

Less common findings in MRIs include Modic end-plate changes,[15] which are thought to be a sign of abnormal stresses at the disk and the so-called high intensity zone. This region, usually in the posterior aspect of the disk, with higher signal on T_2 images, may correlate with an annular tear of the disk fibers and the resultant inflammatory response. Studies that have attempted to correlate the presence of these findings[16,17] with positive provocative discography are encouraging but not conclusive.

Investigators have used the uptake of gadolinium triethylene triamine pentaacetic acid enhancement to assess the intervertebral disk. There has been recent interest in the high-signal intensity zone in the posterior annulus seen in T_2-weighted images,[18,19] in which a band-like contrast enhancement of the disk has been correlated with vascularization (often seen as a consequence of annular tears) and which corresponds to pain, even in the absence of stenosis.[20] In follow-up studies, however, these high intensity zones did not correlate with symptoms.[21]

QUANTITATIVE MRI
For Biochemical Assessment

In an effort to improve the capability of MRI techniques to quantitatively assess spinal degeneration (in particular, disk degeneration) surrogate MRI measures of tissue hydration, such as relaxation times (T_1 and T_2) and, more recently, $T_{1\rho}$ are

being studied. In vitro studies have shown that there are highly significant differences between the nucleus and the annulus in both T_1 and T_2 relaxation times. A moderate negative correlation between the reciprocal of T_2 and water content for disk tissue samples suggests that a weakened collagen network could permit a greater degree of swelling (ie, a higher water content in the disk).[22] There are significant differences in T_1 by region, the nucleus having a higher value than the annulus and in the loaded disk versus the unloaded disk. T_2 values also show a significant difference by region. The nucleus is greater than the annulus and T_2 decreases with increasing degeneration.[23] T_1 and water content in the nucleus and annulus are correlated, but the change of relaxation time with water content is significantly higher in the nucleus compared with the annulus.[24] In vivo, the T_1 and T_2 relaxation times and the proton density of the nucleus pulposus was measured in 107 normal and 18 surgically proven degenerate intervertebral disks,[25] showing no age-related dependence of proton density, a marker of hydration, but showing highly significant difference between the T_1 values of normal and degenerate disks. T_2 showed highly significant differences in the younger age groups, but not in older age groups.

Boos and colleagues[26] observed statistically significant ($P = .001$) mean differences between normal (n = 100) and herniated (n = 20) intervertebral disks (difference in T_1 between the groups was 196 millisecond and in T_2 was 15 millisecond). In a subsequent study[27] it was demonstrated that, when matched by age, gender, and occupational risk factors, asymptomatic patients showed a high rate (76%) of disk herniations. This was significantly less than the symptomatic group incidence of 96%. T_1 and T_2[28] in 22 patients with sciatica severe enough to require a discectomy was compared with T_1 and T_2 in asymptomatic volunteers (controls) who were matched according to age, gender, disk level, and the extent of herniation (protrusion or extrusion). The symptomatic subjects exhibited significantly shorter T_1 and T_2 relaxation times than the matched asymptomatic subjects did.

Recent attention has been focused on MRI $T_{1\rho}$ relaxation time measurements that have the potential for assessing changes in the extracellular matrix (ECM), particularly proteoglycan loss in the intervertebral disk. In vivo, using different duration spin-locking pulses, $T_{1\rho}$-weighted images (**Fig. 4**) were obtained. Fitting an exponential to the decay of signal with the time of spin-locking (TSL), a $T_{1\rho}$ map was generated (see **Fig. 4**) and the reproducibility of disk $T_{1\rho}$ was found to be 4.59%.[29] Studies have demonstrated quantitatively that $T_{1\rho}$ correlates with proteoglycan content and water loss in the disk.[30] $T_{1\rho}$ varies between the nucleus and the annulus,[31] with the median $T_{1\rho}$ value for the nucleus being 116.6 ± 21.4 milliseconds and 84.1 ± 11.7 milliseconds for the annulus, and these values between the nucleus and annulus were found to be significantly different ($P<.05$). The correlations between age and $T_{1\rho}$ relaxation time in the nucleus ($r^2 = -0.82$, $P = .0001$) and annulus ($r^2 = -0.37$, $P = .04$) were also significant. $T_{1\rho}$ relaxation times decreased with disk degeneration (**Fig. 5**),[30,31] demonstrating the changes with Pfirrmann grade and T_2 (**Fig. 6**) and showing the correlation to patient-reported physical activity and disability as assessed by clinical questionnaires (short form health survey [SF 36] and Oswestry Disability Index [ODI]).[32]

MRI DIFFUSION MEASUREMENTS

Diffusion of water protons in MRI is modified by the biochemical environment and diffusion-related signal loss signal and has been used to study disk degeneration in vitro. Significant differences are demonstrated in the diffusion coefficient between the nucleus and annulus, the nucleus having a higher value than the annulus. Diffusion decreased with increasing Thompson grade (or increased degeneration), and with loading of the disk.[23] Diffusion in the nucleus decreases with glycosaminoglycan content, water content, and collagen degradation, and shows regional dependence.[33] Diffusion changes in the annulus were not as evident with changes in matrix except in directional diffusion in the anterior annulus. A representative diffusion-weighted image and calculation of the apparent diffusion coefficient is shown in **Fig. 7**.

Kerttula and colleagues[34] showed decreased diffusion in degenerated disks in vivo compared with healthy controls. Kealey and colleagues[35] reported a 9% reduction in the apparent diffusion coefficient in abnormal disks compared with normal disk. The impact of the diurnal loading cycle on the disk diffusion coefficient was investigated[36] and it was found that apparent diffusion coefficient significantly decreased in the annulus (-5.2%) and the intermediate regions (-2.2%) with no significant changes in the nucleus, contrary to the regional changes seen in T_2 values that show changes in the nucleus and annulus. The relationship between diffusion measures and visual degenerative changes in lumbar intervertebral disks as measured by the Pfirrmann grade showed decreases of 4% to 5% in degenerated disks, but there was considerable overlap between normal and degenerated disks.[37]

DIFFUSION OF CONTRAST AGENTS

The diffusion of gadodiamide 24 hours after injection was studied in 150 disks (96 normal and 54 degenerate).[38] The study measured the enhancement percentage, peak enhancement percentage for different regions in the disk, and the time taken to achieve peak enhancement percentage. The

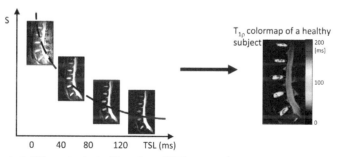

Fig. 4. Images obtained at different spin-locking times (TSL) are used to construct a $T_{1\rho}$ map. (*Courtesy of* Gabby Joseph, Department of Radiology and Biomedical Imaging, UCSF.)

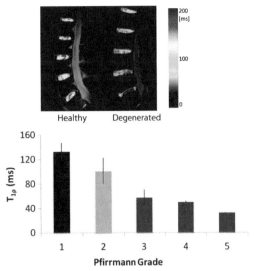

Fig. 5. Representative $T_{1\rho}$ maps in healthy and degenerated disks showing a decrease in $T_{1\rho}$ with degeneration. Bar plot showing the relationship between Pfirrmann grade and $T_{1\rho}$. Groups that are significantly different ($P<.05$) are categorized by different colors. (*Courtesy of* Gabby Joseph, Department of Radiology and Biomedical Imaging, UCSF.)

peak enhancement in the end-plate zone was significantly correlated to the diffusion of contrast agent into the nucleus in the total sample of disks, as well as in degenerated disks. This indicates the possible role of end-plate permeability in disk nutrition.

A recent study[39] investigated the influence of a sustained mechanical load on diffusion of small solutes in and out of the normal disk using serial postcontrast (gadoteridol) enhanced imaging at different time points: precontrast and 1.5, 3, 4.5, 6, and 7.5 hours postcontrast, injection. One month later, the same volunteers were subjected to sustained supine loading for 4.5 hours. MRI scans were performed precontrast (before loading) and postcontrast (after loading) at 1.5, 3, and 4.5 hours. Their spines were then unloaded and recovery scans performed at 6 and 7.5 hours

postcontrast. This study revealed significantly lower signal intensity ratios in the central region of the loaded disk compared with the unloaded disks, This indicates reduction in transport rates for the loaded disks. The behavior of the loaded and unloaded disks were significantly different over the longer time periods, suggesting that sustained supine creep loading (50% of body weight) for 4.5 hours retards transport of small solutes into the center of human disk. Three hours of accelerated diffusion in recovery were required to return to normal.

MRI FOR BIOMECHANICAL ASSESSMENT

Spine kinematics, which has been studied using open-MRI scanners and have revealed relationships between spinal segment motion and facet joint osteoarthritis, will not be reviewed at length in this article. However, in the context of disk degeneration, in a study measuring segmental motion in flexion, extension, and neutral positions, Kong and colleagues[40,41] found that abnormal spinal motion resulted in disk degeneration, in addition to facet joint degeneration, and that increased translational motion of the segments was associated with severe disk degeneration. In the link between the different components and disk degeneration, biomechanical instability clearly is implicated in lower back pain, and warrants thorough investigation (see the article by Inoue and Espinoza Orias elsewhere in this issue for further exploration of this topic).

NUCLEAR MAGNETIC RESONANCE AND MRI SPECTROSCOPY IN INTERVERTEBRAL DISK
High-Resolution Magic-Angle Spinning in Specimens

High-resolution magic angle spinning (HR-MAS) nuclear magnetic resonance (NMR) spectroscopy is a nondestructive technique that has been successfully used to characterize the composition of various intact biologic tissues, such as cartilage (**Fig. 8**).[42] By using high-field strength, one is

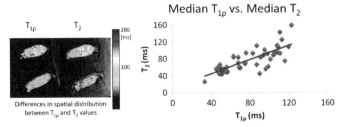

Fig. 6. $T_{1\rho}$ and T_2 maps showing differences in the spatial distribution of $T_{1\rho}$ and T_2. The correlation between $T_{1\rho}$ and T_2 values. (*Courtesy of* Gabby Joseph, Department of Radiology and Biomedical Imaging, UCSF.)

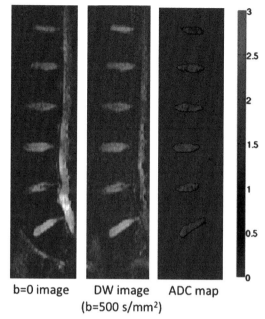

b=0 image   DW image   ADC map
              (b=500 s/mm²)

Fig. 7. Diffusion-weighted images and apparent diffusion coefficient map of intervertebral disks. (*Courtesy of* Dimitrios Karampinos, Department of Radiology and Biomedical Imaging, UCSF.)

able to resolve resonances to a degree that allows identification of chemical markers that may facilitate subtle distinctions between normal and degenerated tissues. HR-MAS spectroscopy has

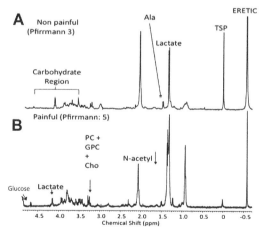

Fig. 8. Representative ^{1}H HR-MAS Carr-Purcell-Meiboom-Gill (CPMG) spectra from the nucleus of (*A*) non-painful (Pfirrmann 3) and (*B*) painful (Pfirrmann 5) degenerative intervertebral disks. Alanine (Ala), the N-acetyl peak (Acetyl) of proteoglycans, phosphocholine (PC), glycerophosphocholine (GPC), choline (Cho), lactate (Lac), and glucose (Glu) could be resolved and quantified in disk spectra. The peak at −0.5 ppm spectra, is the electronic concentration standard (ERETIC).

been applied to intervertebral disks spanning a range of Thompson grades to identify the NMR-observable chemicals and to determine the difference in the ratios of these chemicals between disks at different stages of degeneration.[43] Using data generated from patient tissue samples removed from surgery, it has been demonstrated that MRI spectroscopy at high fields (11) can quantify chemical features specific to painful disks.[44] Specifically, it has been demonstrated that measures of lactate, proteoglycan, choline, and collagen may provide a quantitative discriminator between painful and non-painful disks.

In a repeat study, specimens from 24 patients with discogenic pain, degenerated disk disease, 5 patients with degenerated disk disease but no pain, and 3 deformity patients with scoliosis undergoing anterior and posterior spinal fusion were obtained, and immediately (within minutes of surgery) placed on dry ice and stored at −80°C. In order to classify the tissue, patient sagittal, and axial T_1-weighted and T_2-weighted MRI images were acquired, analyzed, and classified using the Pfirrmann grading scheme.[14] The disk nucleus was pathologically separated from the annulus before the HR-MAS study. HR-MAS data were acquired at 1.0 ± 0.5°C and a 2250 Hz spin rate using a Varian INOVA spectrometer operating at 11.75 T (500 MHz for ^{1}H) and equipped with a 4 mm gHX nanoprobe. A long echo time (echo time = 144 milliseconds) rotor synchronized Carr-Purcell-Meiboom-Gill (CPMG) sequence was used in these studies to filter out short T_2 lipids and accurately quantify lactate doublet at 1.33 ppm from lipids. Unfortunately, as seen in the painful disk spectrum (see **Fig. 8**B), residual lipid often remained, prohibiting the accurate quantification of the lactate doublet in disk samples. However, the lactate quartet was well resolved and of a sufficiently good signal-to-noise ratio to robustly quantify lactate in the CPMG spectra. Also established, is a way to calibrate the spectrum using the Electronic Reference To access In vivo Concentrations (ERETIC) method (see **Fig. 8**).[45] The absolute levels of the individual disk chemicals (chemical peak area to ERETIC peak area) for the nucleus of degenerated painful and non-painful disks are given in **Fig. 9**. The focus was on the HR-MAS spectra of the nucleus because, for in vivo proton spectra of degenerated disks, the selected region of interest is centered on the nucleus.

Visually, both spectra (see **Fig. 6**) demonstrated chemical changes typical of disk degeneration, including an increase in resolution of the resonances in the carbohydrate region of the spectrum, decreased N-acetyl, and increased lactate

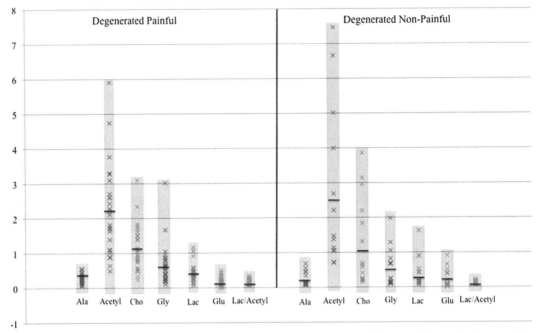

Fig. 9. A plot of the individual (x) and mean (–) disk chemical to ERETIC ratios and lactate to N-acetyl ratio normalized to sample weights from the nucleus of painful (n = 30) and non-painful (n = 16) degenerative intervertebral disks.

peaks.[43,44,46] Quantitatively, there were not any significant differences between individual chemicals from degenerated painful and non-painful disk spectra (see **Fig. 7**). Important to the current study, there was a twofold higher mean lactate in painful versus non-painful disk tissue, but due to the large variability of lactate measurements in the patient cohorts, the difference in lactate levels was not significant (4.14 ± 4.72 vs 2.17 ± 1.11, $P = .19$). Additionally the N-acetyl peak was not different between the painful and non-painful cohorts (23.65 ± 27.05 vs 17.74 ± 8.17, $P = .49$). However, this study confirmed prior published results,[45] demonstrating discrimination between

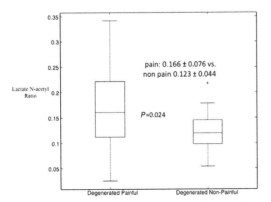

Fig. 10. A box plot of lactate to N-acetyl ratios from the nucleus of painful (n = 30) and non-painful (n = 16) degenerative intervertebral disks.

painful and non-painful disks (**Fig. 10**) using the lactate to N-acetyl ratio. The mean lactate to N-acetyl ratio was significantly different between painful and non-painful degenerated disks (mean = 0.166 ± 0.076 vs 0.123 ± 0.044, $P = .024$); however, there was still overlap of individual ratios.

In Vivo Magnetic Resonance Spectroscopy

Extension of these spectroscopic methods in vivo is limited by the low signal-to-noise ratio, the presence of water in the disk and adjoining tissue, the presence of lipids in adjoining bone marrow, and the broad line widths seen in vivo due to bone susceptibility-induced line broadening. However, at higher field strengths, with spatially selective pulses and improved localized shimming, a recent study using [1]H- magnetic resonance spectroscopy (MRS) in bovine and human cadaver disks reported changes in metabolic concentration with increasing grade of disk degeneration and a relationship between metabolic concentration and proteoglycan content.[47] Representative in vivo spectra in human subjects are shown in **Fig. 11**. For spectroscopy scans, only the N-acetyl resonance (2.04 ppm) that is associated with proteoglycan and the water resonance (4.7 ppm) can be robustly quantified; the other metabolites cannot be accurately quantified because of the limitation of the signal-to-noise ratio in in vivo scans. Furthermore, the lactate peak seen in HR-MAS cannot be separated from lipid or accurately

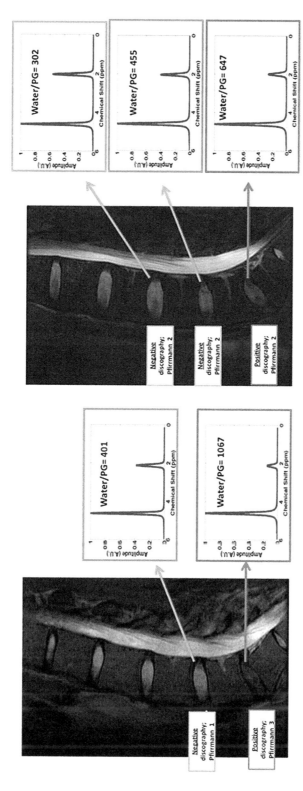

Fig. 11. Water to proteoglycan (PG) peak area ratio is elevated in the disk with positive discography. Although all disks are Pfirrmann grade 2, the disk with positive discography has elevated water to proteoglycan peak area ratio. The amplitude of water was normalized to 1 to illustrate the differences in water to PG peak area ratio between disks. (*Courtesy of Jin Zuo, Department of Radiology and Biomedical Imaging, UCSF.*)

quantified in vivo. Thus, in vivo, the water peak and the N-acetyl peak related to proteoglycans was quantified. It was demonstrated that the water to proteoglycan peak area ratio was significantly elevated in patients (compared with controls) and in disks with positive discography (compared with negative discography). The water to proteoglycan peak area ratio, normalized water, normalized proteoglycans, and Pfirrmann grade were significantly associated with patient self-assessment of disability and physical composite score, although disk height was not. Additional assessments of disk $T_{1\rho}$ demonstrated that there was significant association between $T_{1\rho}$, the water to proteoglycan ratio, and normalized proteoglycan content ($r^2 = 0.61$, $P<.05$), but not between $T_{1\rho}$ and normalized water content ($r^2 = 0.24$, $P>.05$).

SUMMARY

MRI methods provide information pertaining to disk morphology and grading schemes that can be used for clinical assessment of disease status. Biochemical changes are reflected by measures of relaxation times and diffusion, whereas contrast agents may have the potential to be used for the assessment of end-plate permeability. HRMAS techniques provide biochemical signatures relevant to degeneration of the disk and, whereas in-vivo spectroscopy may be a challenge at this point, there is a clear need for investigation and study. In vivo spectroscopic markers that correlate with measures of relaxation times, such as $T_{1\rho}$, may provide a measure of the relative role of proteoglycan and water in disk degeneration. The ability to combine these measures of disk morphology and composition with morphologic measures, including facet joint status, makes MRI a potentially powerful tool for determining the causes of lower back pain, and monitoring disease progression and therapy.

REFERENCES

1. Punnett L, Pruss-Ustin A, Nelson D, et al. Estimating the global burden of low back pain attributable to combined occupational exposures. Am J Ind Med 2005;48(6):59–69.
2. Hagen K, Sveback S, Zwart J. Incidence of musculoskeletal complaints in a large adult Norwegian county population: the HUNT study. Spine (Phila Pa 1976) 2006;31(18):2146–50.
3. Liao Z, Pan Y, Huang J, et al. An epidemiological survey of low back pain and axial spondyloarthritis in a Chinese Han population. Scand J Rheumatol 2009;38(6):455–9. [Epub ahead of print].
4. Frymoyer JW, Cats-Baril WL. An overview of the incidences and costs of low back pain. Orthop Clin North Am 1991;22(2):263–71.
5. Vanharanta H, Sachs BL, Spivey M, et al. A comparison of CT/discography, pain response and radiographic disc height. Spine 1988;13(3):321–4.
6. Inoue H. Three-dimensional architecture of lumbar intervertebral discs. Spine 1981;6(2):139–46.
7. Patrick BS. Lumbar discography: a five year study. Surg Neurol 1973;1(5):267–73.
8. Walsh TR, Weinstein JN, Spratt KF, et al. Lumbar discography in normal subjects. A controlled, prospective study. J Bone Joint Surg Am 1990;72(7):1081–8.
9. Wiesel SW, Tsourmas N, Feffer HL, et al. A study of computer-assisted tomography. I. The incidence of positive CAT scans in an asymptomatic group of patients. Spine 1984;9(6):549–51.
10. Modic MT, Pavlicek W, Weinstein MA, et al. Magnetic resonance imaging of intervertebral disc disease: clinical and pulse sequence considerations. Radiology 1984;152:103–11.
11. Coppes M, Marani E, Thomeer R, et al. Innervation of "painful" lumbar discs. Spine (Phila Pa 1976) 1997;22(20):2342–9.
12. Carragee EJ, Lincoln T, Parmar VS, et al. A gold standard evaluation of the "discogenic pain" diagnosis as determined by provocative discography. Spine 2006;31(18):2115–23.
13. Carragee EJ, Don AS, Hurwitz EL, et al. 2009 ISSLS Prize Winner: Does discography cause accelerated progression of degeneration changes in the lumbar disc: a ten-year matched cohort study. Spine (Phila Pa 1976) 2009;34:2338–45.
14. Pfirrmann CW, Metzdorf A, Zanetti M, et al. Magnetic resonance classification of lumbar intervertebral disc degeneration. Spine 2001;26(17):1873–8.
15. Modic MT, Masaryk TJ, Ross JS, et al. Imaging of degenerative disc disease. Radiology 1988;168:177–86.
16. O'Neill C, Kurgansky M, Kaiser J, et al. Accuracy of MRI for diagnosis of discogenic pain. Pain Physician 2008;11:311–26.
17. Kang C, Kim Y, Lee S, et al. Can magnetic resonance imaging accurately predict concordant pain provocation during provocative disc injection? Skeletal Radiol 2009;38(9):877–85.
18. Peng B, Hou S, Wu W, et al. The pathogenesis and clinical significance of a high-intensity zone (HIZ) of lumbar intervertebral disc on MR imaging in the patient with discogenic low back pain. Eur Spine J 2005;15(5):583–7.
19. Peng B, Wu W, Hou S, et al. The pathogenesis of discogenic low back pain. J Bone Joint Surg Br 2005; 87(1):62–7.
20. Stabler A, Weiss M, Scheidler J, et al. Degenerative disk vascularization on MRI: correlation with clinical and histopathologic findings. Skeletal Radiol 1996; 25(2):119–26.

21. Mitra D, Cassar-Pullicino VN, McCall IW. Longitudinal study of high intensity zones on MR of lumbar intervertebral discs. Clin Radiol 2004;59(11):1002–8.

22. Weidenbaum M, Foster RJ, Best BA, et al. Correlating magnetic resonance imaging with the biochemical content of the normal human intervertebral disc. J Orthop Res 1992;10:552–61.

23. Chiu EJ, Newitt DC, Segal MR, et al. Magnetic resonance imaging measurement of relaxation and water diffusion in the human lumbar intervertebral disc under compression in vitro. Spine 2001;26(19):E437–44.

24. Chatani K, Kusaka Y, Mifune T, et al. Topographic differences of 1H-NMR relaxation times (T1, T2) in the normal intervertebral disc and its relationship to water content. Spine 1993;18(15):2271–5.

25. Jenkins JPR, Hickey DS, Zhu XP, et al. Imaging of the intervertebral disc: a quantitative study. Br J Radiol 1985;58:705–9.

26. Boos N, Wallin A, Schmucker T, et al. Quantitative MR imaging of lumbar intervertebral discs and vertebral bodies: Methodology, reproducibility, and preliminary results. Magn Reson Imaging 1994;12(4):577–87.

27. Boos N, Rieder R, Schade V, et al. 1995 Volvo Award in clinical sciences. The diagnostic accuracy of magnetic resonance imaging, work perception, and psychosocial factors in identifying symptomatic disc herniations. Spine 1995;20(24):2613–25.

28. Boos N, Dreier D, Hilfiker E, et al. Tissue characterization of symptomatic and asymptomatic disc herniations by quantitative magnetic resonance imaging. J Orthop Res 1997;15(1):141–9.

29. Blumenkrantz G, Li X, Han ET, et al. A feasibility study of in vivo T1rho imaging of the intervertebral disk. Magn Reson Imaging 2006;24(8):1001–7.

30. Johannessen W, Auerbach JD, Wheaton AJ, et al. Assessment of human disc degeneration and proteoglycan content using T1rho-weighted magnetic resonance imaging. Spine 2006;31(11):1253–7.

31. Auerbach JD, Johannessen W, Borthakur A, et al. In vivo quantification of human lumbar disc degeneration using T(1rho)-weighted magnetic resonance imaging. Eur Spine J 2006;15(Suppl 3):S338–44.

32. Blumenkrantz G, Zuo J, Li X, et al. In vivo 3.0-tesla magnetic resonance T1rho and T2 relaxation mapping in subjects with intervertebral disc degeneration and clinical symptoms. Magn Reson Med 2010;63(5):1193–2000.

33. Antoniou J, Demers CN, Beaudoin G, et al. Apparent diffusion coefficient of intervertebral discs related to matrix composition and integrity. Magn Reson Imaging 2004;22(7):963–72.

34. Kerttula L, Kurunlahti M, Jauhiainen J, et al. Apparent diffusion coefficients and T2 relaxation time measurements to evaluate disc degeneration. A quantitative MR study of young patients with previous vertebral fracture. Acta Radiol 2001;42(6):585–91.

35. Kealey SM, Aho T, Delong D, et al. Assessment of apparent diffusion coefficient in normal and degenerated intervertebral lumbar discs: initial experience. Radiology 2005;235(2):569–74.

36. Ludescher B, Effelsberg J, Martirosian P, et al. T2- and diffusion-maps reveal diurnal changes of intervertebral disc composition: an in vivo MRI study at 1.5 Tesla. J Magn Reson Imaging 2008;28(1):252–7.

37. Niinimaki J, Korkiakoski A, Ojala O, et al. Association between visual degeneration of intervertebral discs and the apparent diffusion coefficient. Magn Reson Imaging 2009;27(5):641–7.

38. Rajasekaran S, Babu JN, Arun R, et al. ISSLS prize winner: a study of diffusion in human lumbar discs: a serial magnetic resonance imaging study documenting the influence of the endplate on diffusion in normal and degenerate discs. Spine 2004;29(23):2654–67.

39. Arun R, Freeman BJ, Scammell BE, et al. 2009 ISSLS Prize Winner: What influence does sustained mechanical load have on diffusion in the human intervertebral disc? an in vivo study using serial postcontrast magnetic resonance imaging. Spine (Phila Pa 1976) 2009;34(21):2324–37.

40. Kong MH, Hymanson HJ, Song KY, et al. Kinetic magnetic resonance imaging analysis of abnormal segmental motion of the functional spine unit. J Neurosurg Spine 2009;10(4):357–65.

41. Kong MH, Morishita Y, He W, et al. Lumbar segmental mobility according to the grade of the disc, the facet joint, the muscle, and the ligament pathology by using kinetic magnetic resonance imaging. Spine (Phila Pa 1976) 2009;34(23):2537–44.

42. Schiller J, Naji L, Huster D, et al. 1H and 13C HR-MAS NMR investigations on native and enzymatically digested bovine nasal cartilage. MAGMA 2001;13:19–27.

43. Keshari KR, Zektzer AS, Swanson MG, et al. Characterization of intervertebral disc degeneration by high-resolution magic angle spinning (HR MAS) spectroscopy. Magn Reson Med 2005;53(3):519–27.

44. Keshari KR, Lotz JC, Link TM, et al. Lactic acid and proteoglycans as metabolic markers for discogenic back pain. Spine 2008;33(3):312–7.

45. Albers MJ, Butler TN, Rahwa I, et al. Evaluation of the ERETIC method as an improved quantitative reference for (1)H HR-MAS spectroscopy of prostate tissue. Magn Reson Med 2009;61(3):525–32.

46. Keshari KR, Lotz JC, Kurhanewicz J, et al. Correlation of HR-MAS spectroscopy derived metabolite concentrations with collagen and proteoglycan levels and Thompson grade in the degenerative disc. Spine (Phila Pa 1976) 2005;30(23):2683–8.

47. Zuo J, Saadat E, Romero A, et al. Assessment of intervertebral disc degeneration with magnetic resonance single-voxel spectroscopy. Magn Reson Med 2009;62(5):1140–6.

Management of Degenerative Disk Disease and Chronic Low Back Pain

Jaro Karppinen, MD, PhD[a],*, Francis H. Shen, MD[b],
Keith D.K. Luk, MCh(Orth), FRCSE, FRCSG, FRACS, FHKAM(Orth)[c],
Gunnar B.J. Andersson, MD, PhD[d],
Kenneth M.C. Cheung, MBBS(UK), MD (HK), FRCS,
FHKCOS, FHKAM(Orth)[c], Dino Samartzis, DSc[c],*

KEYWORDS

- Disk • Degeneration • Chronic • Low back • Pain
- Conservative • Surgery • Genetic

Low back pain (LBP) affects every population and is one of the world's foremost debilitating conditions.[1] Such pain may lead to diminished function and quality of life, psychological distress, and loss of wages.[2] LBP is one of the most common conditions motivating individuals to seek medical care and often results in prolonged therapeutic interventions.[2,3] Therefore, LBP is a global burden associated with severe socioeconomic and health care consequences.[4–6]

LBP can be divided into several groups based on cause: 80% to 90% mechanical (eg, degenerative disk or joint disease, vertebral fracture, deformity); 5% to 15% neurogenic (eg, herniated disk, spinal stenosis), 1% to 2% nonmechanical conditions (eg, neoplastic disease, infection, inflammatory), 1% to 2% referred visceral pain (eg, gastrointestinal disease, renal disease, abdominal aortic aneurysm), and 2% to 4% other (eg, fibromyalgia, somatoform disorder, malingering).[7] Typically, patients with LBP complain of local pain aggravated by mechanical loading, usually at worst when being upright, and they have no or minimal symptoms at rest. It is generally agreed that intervertebral disks are a major tissue source in chronic LBP.[8,9] Typically, chronic LBP has been defined as pain occurring for 3 months or more, frequently recurring, or lasting beyond the normal healing period for a low back injury.[10,11] If, in case of prolonged LBP, magnetic resonance imaging (MRI) is obtained and a common finding is disk degeneration at the 2 or 3 lowest lumbar levels (**Figs. 1–3**).[12,13]

This work was supported by an Area of Excellence grant from the University Grants Committee of Hong Kong (AoE/M-04/04).

Disclosure: The investigators have no financial or competing interests in relation to this work.

[a] Institute of Clinical Sciences, Department of Physical and Rehabilitation Medicine, University of Oulu, Box 5000, Oulu 90014, Finland

[b] Department of Orthopaedic Surgery, University of Virginia, 400 Ray C. Hunt Drive, Suite 330, Charlottesville, VA 22908, USA

[c] Department of Orthopaedics and Traumatology, Division of Spine Surgery, Li Ka Shing Faculty of Medicine, The University of Hong Kong, Professorial Block, 5th Floor, 102 Pokfulam Road, Pokfulam, Hong Kong SAR, China

[d] Department of Orthopaedic Surgery, Rush University Medical Center, 1611 West Harrison Street, Chicago, IL 60612, USA

* Corresponding authors.

E-mail addresses: Jaro.Karppinen@ttl.fi; dsamartzis@msn.com

Orthop Clin N Am 42 (2011) 513–528
doi:10.1016/j.ocl.2011.07.009
0030-5898/11/$ – see front matter © 2011 Elsevier Inc. All rights reserved.

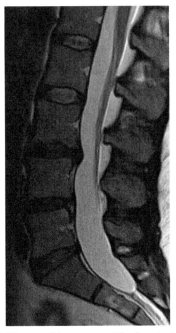

Fig. 1. A 33-year-old woman with chronic LBP for 1 year and left-sided sciatica for 4 months. T2-weighted sagittal MRI images showed disk degeneration from L3 to S1. An L4/5 discectomy was performed, and on last follow-up the patient was asymptomatic.

According to international clinical guidelines, treatment of acute LBP (ie, <3 months) is straightforward in the absence of red flags (**Table 1**) or sciatica symptoms. Often, pain medication is provided and the patient is advised to stay active.[14] However, in the context of chronic LBP, there are several treatment options, but no clear answer exists as to how the physician should plan the treatment process. This article reviews treatment options for the management of chronic LBP and assesses the evidence on their effectiveness, with particular emphasis on degenerative disk disease.

THE ROLE OF DISK DEGENERATION IN CHRONIC LBP

MRI is not recommended early in the disease course unless red flags or signs of nerve root entrapment are present. The reason is that MRI in acute LBP increases medical costs without giving additional information influencing clinical decision making.[15–17] Furthermore, MRI in the current form is not useful in diagnosing discogenic pain when compared with discography.[9] However, discography per se has been found to enhance progression of disk degeneration,[18] and therefore recently published guidelines were not in favor for discography.[19] According to Ohtori and colleagues,[20] injection of a small amount of

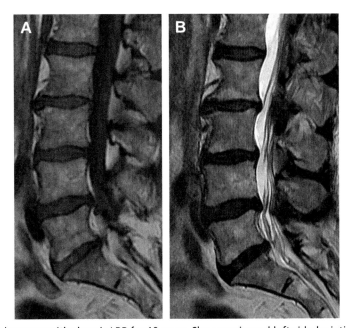

Fig. 2. A 52-year-old woman with chronic LBP for 10 years. She experienced left-sided sciatica for 1 year with no relief with conservative treatment, including physiotherapy and nerve root blockade. (A) T1- and (B) T2-weighted MRI sagittal images showed disk degeneration from L1 to S1 with mixed type I/II Modic lesion at L5/S1. She eventually underwent an L4/5 discectomy and decompression.

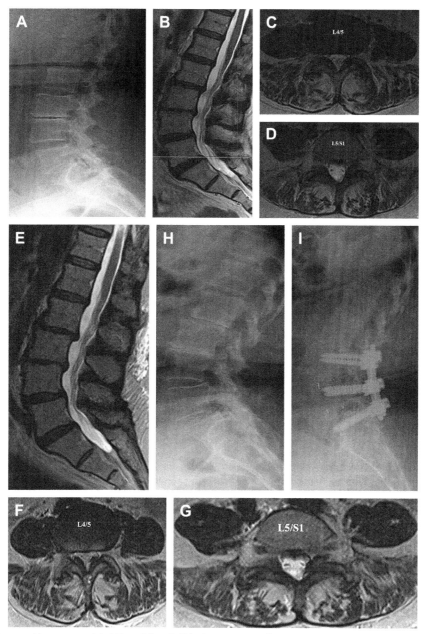

Fig. 3. A 71-year-old woman with (*A*) multilevel disk degeneration from L2 to S1 and a (*B*) grade 1 degenerative spondylolisthesis at L4/5 and L5/S1 (standing radiograph), resulting in (*C, D*) both central and neuroforaminal stenosis. Conservative measures were instituted with good initial results. However, 3.5 years later she presented with recurrent leg, greater than back, symptoms. A second round of conservative treatment yielded only temporary relief. Updated imaging revealed progression of the (*E–G*) degeneration changes at all levels, particularly at L3/4 with (*H*) progression of the degenerative slip (standing radiograph). Surgical intervention was performed for decompression, realignment, and stabilization. Because her main complaint was leg pain, only the stenotic levels from L4 to S1 were addressed. (*I*) A transforaminal lumbar interbody fusion with instrumentation from L4 to S1 was performed with interbody cages and local autograft to restore neuroforaminal height and alignment.

bupivacaine into the painful disk may be a better test for discogenic LBP than discography.[20] However, this procedure is also invasive and may accelerate disk degeneration. Therefore, in most cases of chronic LBP the true tissue origin has remained unknown. In most randomized trials focused on patients with chronic LBP, the tissue source of pain has not been speculated.

Table 1
LBP red flags that contraindicate nonsurgical treatment

Condition	History	Physical Examination
Fracture	Major trauma Minor trauma (older patient)	Kyphosis
Tumor	Age <15 or >50 y Known cancer Unexplained weight loss Night pain	—
Infection	Recent fever or chills Recent bacterial infection (urinary tract infection) Intravenous drug use Immune suppression Unrelenting pain	Fever
Cauda equina syndrome	Saddle numbness Urinary retention, incontinence Severe (progressive) lower extremity neurologic deficit	Weak anal sphincter Perianal sensory loss Flaccid motor weakness Hyporeflexia

Data from Shen FH, Samartzis D, Andersson GB. Nonsurgical management of acute and chronic low back pain. J Am Acad Orthop Surg 2006;14:478.

According to a systematic review by Hancock and colleagues,[21] MRI findings, such as endplate changes and presence of disk degeneration, were found to increase the likelihood of the discogenic origin from discography. Several recent studies support the concept that disk degeneration is associated with low back symptoms.[22–26] All these studies indicate that a higher degree of lumbar disk degeneration is related to a higher likelihood of symptoms, and moreover the presence of moderate disk degeneration or degenerative changes at multiple levels increases the likelihood of pain.[23,26] According to Samartzis and colleagues,[24] the global severity of disk degeneration increases the likelihood of LBP, with a potential dose-response exposure of degenerative changes implicated in the association.

The role of disk degeneration in the development of chronic LBP has received considerable attention; nonetheless, few large-scale studies have addressed the relationship. According to studies by Kjaer and colleagues,[13] Visuri and colleagues,[27] and Paajanen and colleagues,[28,29] disk degeneration on MRI is significantly associated with chronic LBP, whereas Savage and colleagues[30] contend otherwise. More recently, a systematic review by Chou and colleagues[31] assessing degenerative spine findings on MRI in relation to chronic LBP, noted a significant association between the presence of disk degeneration and back pain. However, because of clinical heterogeneity between studies, the investigators hesitated in making any robust conclusions of a direct association or causal

pathway between disk changes and LBP. Nonetheless, a recent study by DePalma and colleagues[32] using numerous diagnostic injections concluded that intervertebral disk degeneration is the most common tissue source of chronic LBP. The likelihood of the intervertebral disk implicated in chronic LBP was highest in young and middle-aged individuals, whereas the probability of pain related to facet or sacroiliac joints was highest in older individuals. In addition, new imaging modalities, such as T1-ρ, T2-relaxation mapping, and chemical exchange saturation transfer, are being developed that are more sensitive to disk changes and could further elaborate more quantitatively on the disk degeneration phenotype as well as possess the potential to image pain (see article by Majumdar and colleagues elsewhere in this issue).[33–38]

In this article, presumed discogenic origin of chronic LBP is referred to as degenerative disk disease. The pathophysiologic mechanism leading to the development of pain in the disk is described elsewhere in this focus issue (see articles by Chan and colleagues, Grunhagen and colleagues, Inoue and Espinoza Orias, and Bae and Masuda). In general, mechanical and chemical mediators brought on by the degenerative process irritate sensory nerve endings (nociceptive fibers) located in the annulus fibrosus, which contribute to pain (**Fig. 4**). As the degenerative process progresses, this situation may further affect the kinematics and load transmission throughout the motion segment, thereby stimulating nociceptive fibers in the facet joints as well.

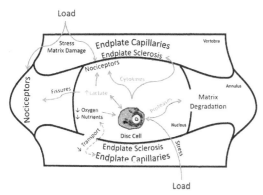

Fig. 4. Numerous risk factors, such as age, abnormal physical loading, and genetics, may lead to the development of intervertebral disk degeneration. Disk cells are adversely influenced by mechanical load (pressure), hypoxia, and nutrient/metabolite deprivation (*red*). In response, they can secrete lactate, cytokines, and proteases (*green*). The damaged matrix may cause endplate sclerosis, sensitize nociceptors, and exacerbate the adverse effects of load and diminished nutrient/metabolite transport (*blue*). Sensitized nociceptors can, in turn, be stimulated by tissue stress and mediators to cause pain. (*Modified from* Masuda K, Lotz JC. New challenges for intervertebral disk treatment using regenerative medicine. Tissue Eng Part B Rev 2010;16:148; with permission.)

THE ROLE OF CENTRAL SENSITIZATION IN CHRONIC LBP

Nociceptive stimuli from peripheral tissue, such as in the intervertebral disk, are transmitted mainly via the spinothalamic tract to the cerebral cortex. In case of persistent injury, C fibers fire repetitively to the dorsal horn, which may lead to central sensitization.[39] Central sensitization is characterized by altered pain sensibility both peripherally and centrally.[40] Even although intervertebral disks are the original pain generators in degenerative disk disease, central sensitization may obscure a peripheral nociceptive tissue source in chronic LBP. The central areas activated by pain include almost constantly secondary somatosensory cortex, insular regions and anterior cingulate cortex, and with slightly less consistency contralateral thalamus and primary somatosensory cortex.[41] There is reasonable evidence that chronic LBP is associated with abnormal brain anatomy and function, especially in the dorsolateral prefrontal cortex, thalamus, brainstem, primary somatosensory cortex, and posterior parietal cortex.[42,43] According to a study by Ruscheweyh and colleagues[44] that assessed structural MRI of the brain and pain status in 205 German subjects, regional brain matter reduction (mainly in cingulate, prefrontal, and motor/premotor regions) was present in chronic LBP sufferers with

symptoms greater than 12 months. However, a recent Canadian study by Seminowicz and colleagues[45] indicated that brain abnormalities in chronic pain may be reversible.[45] These investigators reported that successful treatment of patients with chronic LBP either with spine surgery (n = 8) or with a facet joint injection (n = 6) resulted in restoration of both structure and function of the left dorsolateral prefrontal cortex, which correlated with reduction of both pain and disability.

TREATMENT OF CHRONIC LBP

Existing clinical guidelines list several treatment options for chronic LBP, which include pain medication, exercises, behavioral therapy, multidisciplinary rehabilitation, and surgery (**Box 1**).[14,46]

Box 1
Factors associated with the development and persistence of LBP

Previous episode of back pain[a,c]

Poor job satisfaction or low pay[a,c]

Inadequate coping skills[c]

Fear-avoidance behavior[a,c,d]

Manual labor or physically stressful job[a,c]

Obesity[a,c]

Somatization[a,c]

Smoking[a,c]

Low baseline activity levels[a,c]

Ongoing litigation[c]

Older age[a,c]

Low educational level[c]

Higher pain intensity or disability[c]

Neurologic symptoms[c]

Anxiety[a,c]

Depressed mood[c]

Emotional distress[a,c]

Pain genes[b]

Association does not imply causality. Evidence is mixed for some factors, including smoking, obesity, and low educational level.

[a] Associated with development of LBP in some studies.
[b] Associated with pain severity after surgery. Limited studies exist.
[c] Associated with persistence of LBP in some studies.
[d] The avoidance of physical activities that stems from patients' fears that their pain will worsen.
Modified from Cohen SP, Argoff CE, Carragee EJ. Management of low back pain. BMJ 2008;337:103; with permission.

Patient information is not reviewed in detail here. Yet, patient advice is an integral part of care at all stages. Such advice should preferably be given early in the disease course, because 2.5-hour sessions of individual oral education were found to be more effective than no intervention in return to work in subacute LBP, whereas in chronic LBP education was less effective on back-related function than more intensive interventions.[47] Advice includes information on the benign nature of nonspecific LBP and encourages the patient to be physically active and continue with normal activities as possible.[46]

Some new promising biologic treatment alternatives have been introduced recently. They include stem cell regeneration, gene therapy, tissue engineering, and molecular therapy. All these treatments are reviewed elsewhere in this issue (see articles by Sakai, Woods and colleagues, Leung and colleagues, and Bae and Masuda). This article pays special attention to the following treatment domains: pain medication, exercise therapy, behavioral therapy, multidisciplinary rehabilitation, injection therapy, and surgery.

Initial Clinical Assessment

In the initial assessment, primary health care services, which include occupational health care in those countries where it is available, are of importance. A thorough clinical examination is paramount because it serves both the needs of diagnostics, and is also a part of evidence-based pain treatment.[48] It is generally recommended that every patient with LBP should be examined carefully, with follow-up visits in case of prolonged or recurrent pain (**Table 2**).[49] Degree of baseline disability (rather than pain intensity) is an important prognostic factor for recovery of LBP.[50] Functional impairment can be best evaluated with thorough clinical examination. In addition, patient-reported disability indices, such as the Oswestry Disability Index[51] and the Roland-Morris Questionnaire,[52] are helpful and widely used in the clinical assessment. A further tool in the initial assessment of patients with LBP is pain drawing, which is a simple and inexpensive diagnostic measure to characterize an abnormal psychological profile.[53]

Pain Medication

The clinical guidelines recommend paracetamol as the first medication choice and nonsteroidal antiinflammatory drugs (NSAIDs) or weak opioids, or both, if paracetamol alone does not provide sufficient pain relief.[14,46] NSAIDs are effective for short-term symptom relief in patients with chronic LBP without sciatica, but the effect sizes are small

Table 2
Nonsurgical treatment alternatives for LBP

Nonsurgical Treatment Alternatives

Treatment	Subclassification
Education	–
Medication	Analgesics Nonnarcotic Narcotic Topical NSAIDs Muscle relaxants Corticosteroids Antidepressants
Cognitive behavioral therapy	Operant Cognitive Respondent
Multidisciplinary rehabilitation	–
Immobilization and supports	–
Exercise therapy	–
Massage therapy/physical therapy	–
Acupuncture/dry needling	–
Manipulation	–
Traction	–
Injections	Epidural Facet Trigger point Sacroiliac Intradiscal Prolotherapy
Orthoses	Braces Corsets Unloading corset
Transcutaneous electrical nerve stimulation	–
Acupuncture	–

Data from Shen FH, Samartzis D, Andersson GB. Nonsurgical management of acute and chronic low back pain. J Am Acad Orthop Surg 2006;14:480.

and the various types of NSAID are equally effective.[54,55] In addition, the clinician should evaluate the risk of side-effects in each individual case and take into account the patient's preference as well. In case of persistent pain, strong opioids can be used for short-term management. Overall, the benefits of opioids for long-term management of chronic LBP remain questionable.[56] In addition, early use of opioids for LBP patients increases risk of work disability and leads to overall poor outcomes.[57,58] Tricyclic antidepressants may be offered if other drugs are insufficient in pain relief[46]; however, there is no evidence on their efficacy in chronic LBP.[54,59]

Exercise Therapy

Exercise therapy is the key element in the treatment of chronic LBP. Exercise therapy is effective at decreasing pain and improving function.[60] However, exercise therapy was noted to have only a modest effect size[61] and most statistically significant trial results on the efficacy of exercise in chronic LBP were not of clinical importance.[62,63]

Selecting the type of exercise therapy for optimum effectiveness for chronic LBP is of importance. According to a meta-regression analysis by Hayden and colleagues,[64] exercise therapy should consist of individually designed programs, include stretching or strengthening, and should be delivered with supervision. In addition, high-dose exercise programs fared better than low-dose exercise programs. In general, no specific exercise type was superior to other types.[60] However, patient populations in the trials have been heterogeneous, whereas treatment interventions based on validated classification systems may result in larger effect sizes for the given treatments.[65] Moreover, exercise therapy may not be tolerated by all patients with degenerative disk disease (at least at advanced degenerative disease). Patients with type I and mixed types I/II Modic changes do not respond well to exercise therapy.[66,67]

The role of exercise therapy is supported by a review on the effectiveness of exercises for prevention of recurrences of LBP.[68] The review found moderate-quality evidence that posttreatment exercise programs can prevent recurrences of LBP. Additional exercise programs after formal treatment of LBP has been completed are beneficial. However, evidence on treatment interventions, defined as treatment of a current episode of LBP with the aim to prevent new episodes of pain, was conflicting.[68]

Behavioral Therapy

The main behavioral treatment approaches in chronic LBP are operant, cognitive, or respondent therapies (see **Table 3**).[69–71] There is moderate evidence that operant therapy is more effective than waiting list, and that behavioral therapy in general is more effective than usual care in short-term pain relief in chronic LBP.[72] The strength of evidence on the efficacy of behavioral therapy was found to be mostly of low quality.[63,72]

Two high-quality trials, published after the systematic reviews, suggest that cognitive therapy is an essential part in the treatment of chronic LBP.

Table 3	
Various behavioral approaches for the treatment of LBP	
Behavioral Treatment Approaches	
Type	**Definition**
Operant	Removes positive reinforcement of pain behaviors and promotes healthy behaviors
Cognitive	Identifies and modifies harmful cognitions, such as maladaptive thoughts, feelings, and beliefs about LBP, using cognitive restructuring techniques (eg, imagery and attention diversion)
Respondent	Modifies the physiologic responses to pain through reduction of muscular tension using different relaxation techniques

In a Danish pragmatic trial,[73] a cognitive, educational intervention for chronic LBP resulted in at least as good outcomes as exercise therapy despite fewer treatment sessions. Moreover, they used a classification system in which the delivery of specific exercise therapy was based on assessment findings. According to a British multicenter study by Lamb and colleagues,[74] cognitive behavioral therapy was found to significantly improve back-specific function compared with the usual care in subacute or chronic LBP. Furthermore, the effect was sustained over the 1-year follow-up period. In the intervention group, participants attended a program that targeted behaviors and beliefs about physical activity and avoidance of activity and consisted of individual assessment (up to 1.5 hours in duration) and 6 sessions of group therapy (1.5 hours per session).

Multidisciplinary Rehabilitation

Multidisciplinary rehabilitation has been defined to include multidisciplinary biopsychosocial rehabilitation coupled with a minimum of 1 physical dimension (ie, psychological or social or occupational).[75] There is strong evidence that intensive multidisciplinary biopsychosocial rehabilitation with functional restoration improves function, and there is moderate evidence that multidisciplinary rehabilitation with functional restoration reduces LBP when compared with less intensive treatments.[75] More recently, moderate evidence of multidisciplinary rehabilitation compared with other kinds of active treatment on pain intensity in the short-term was found[63]; however, no effect on pain intensity in the long-term was observed.[63]

The optimal content of multidisciplinary rehabilitation remains to be defined. Behavioral therapy is widely considered to be an essential part of multidisciplinary rehabilitation, but the addition of behavioral therapy to inpatient rehabilitation did not seem to increase the effect of inpatient rehabilitation alone.[72] Similarly, the addition of cognitive behavioral therapy did not increase the efficacy of physical conditioning.[76] Multidisciplinary rehabilitation can be performed as outpatient rehabilitation as well. Based on a study by Lambeek and colleagues[77] addressing a Dutch population, multidisciplinary outpatient work-related intervention was effective in return to work.

Based on systematic reviews by Guzman and colleagues[75] and Ravenek and colleagues,[78] there is contradictory evidence regarding vocational outcomes after multidisciplinary rehabilitation. In addition to multidisciplinary rehabilitation, physical conditioning programs, sometimes referred to as work conditioning, work hardening, or functional restoration/exercise programs, have a small effect on sickness absence at long-term follow-up in workers with chronic LBP.[76] Return to work should be a feasible and realistic outcome of multidisciplinary rehabilitation according to Buijs and colleagues,[79] who used a multidisciplinary outpatient care program, including workplace intervention and graded activity aiming at function restoration (instead of pain elimination) and return to work. Their program was well accepted by patients. Patient expectations were low at the start but the program was successful in changing patients' goal setting from pain-oriented toward function restoration and return to work. In support of the positive effect of multidisciplinary rehabilitation on vocational outcomes, a high-quality Dutch trial by Lambeek and colleagues[77] addressing patients who were on sick leave because of chronic LBP reported significantly less median duration of days until sustainable return to work in the so-called integrated care group (88 days) compared with to the usual care group (208 days). The integrated care intervention included a workplace intervention based on participatory ergonomics and a graded activity program based on cognitive behavioral principles, whereas the multidisciplinary team consisted only of a clinical occupational physician, a medical specialist, an occupational therapist, and a physiotherapist.

Injection Therapy

There is insufficient evidence to support epidural and facet joint injections, or local trigger point injections, in subacute and chronic LBP.[80] A recent practice guideline by Chou and colleagues[81] recommended against facet joint steroid injections, prolotherapy, and intradiscal steroid injections in nonradicular LBP, and strongly recommends against provocative discography. Epidural or transforaminal steroid injection is recommended in patients with persistent radiculopathy caused by a herniated lumbar disk because there is evidence for moderate short-term benefits. Furthermore, the benefits of botulinum and epidural steroid injection, intradiscal electrothermal therapy, therapeutic medial branch block, radiofrequency denervation, intrathecal therapy with opioids or other medications, and sacroiliac joint steroid injection are questionable in nonradicular LBP.[81]

It could be argued that intradiscal injections with other more potent antiinflammatory drugs than steroids could be beneficial in nonradicular LBP. Tumor necrosis factor α (TNF-α) antagonists are eagerly evaluated in the treatment of sciatica.[82] However, the current evidence does not support their use in degenerative disk disease.[83] Fibrin injection in the experimentally damaged disks resulted in reduced TNF-α synthesis.[84] No in vivo human studies have been performed. In addition, various growth factors and stem cell therapies that entail direct injection into the disk for repair/regeneration have been studied, largely in animal models and in disks with mild to moderate degeneration (see articles elsewhere in this issue by Sakai, Woods and colleagues, Leung and colleagues, and Bae and Masuda).[85–93] Although their effectiveness for pain management in symptomatic degenerated disks has not been fully addressed, such disk therapies could serve as a viable option in the future and warrant further investigation.

Peng and colleagues[94] reported their findings based on their randomized controlled trial (RCT) assessing the efficacy of methylene blue intradiscal injection (n = 36) compared with a placebo group (n = 36) in 72 patients with chronic discogenic LBP lasting longer than 6 months. These investigators noted at 24-month postinjection follow-up that intradiscal injection of methylene blue significantly reduced mean pain and Oswestry Disability Index scores by 41 and 35, respectively, among patients with chronic discogenic pain compared with 1% and 2%, respectively, in the placebo group. The investigators concluded that methylene blue acts to denervate the nociceptive fibers found in annular fissures. However, the study has not been replicated. Thus, the benefit of methylene blue injection remains speculative. Alternatively, although Peng and colleagues[94] reported their procedure to be safe, an animal study performed by O'Neill and colleagues[95] noted that methylene blue if leaked out of the disk and into the epidural space may prove extremely neurotoxic, resulting in paralysis in their animal models. O'Neill and colleagues[95] have advocated that until the exact mechanism of toxicity and dose response of the relation are determined, the use of methylene blue to address symptomatic degenerative disk disease should be avoided or at least used in the setting of an intact annulus fibrosus that may diminish the risk of leakage of the injected agent.

Surgery

Surgery is an option for patients with degenerative disk disease nonresponsive to conservative treatment (see **Figs. 1–3**). Although controversial, in the carefully selected patient, lumbar spinal fusion may be regarded as the gold standard of surgical treatment of degenerative disk disease. Spinal fusions are a relatively common spine procedure that continues to grow in popularity. According to Rajaee and colleagues,[96] the rate of spinal fusion has increased 2.4-fold from 1998 to 2008 in the United States.

Because pain relief has been achieved in other arthritic joints of the body through the elimination of painful motion, it has been assumed that analogous relief can be achieved through a successful spinal fusion. In a multicenter randomized trial, Fritzell and colleagues[97] compared 3 common surgical techniques (posterior only, anterior only, and combined anterior posterior approaches) used to achieve a lumbar fusion. In this study, all fusion techniques were found to reduce pain and improve function, but there was no difference among the techniques used to achieve fusion. The investigators concluded that immobilization of the motion segment appeared to be the important component, whereas the surgical technique used appeared to be less important.[97] Similarly, the use of instrumentation also remains unclear. Meta-analysis[98] and randomized, prospective studies[99] have suggested that although fusion rates are increased with pedicle screw fixation, an improvement in clinical outcomes may not be noted. Conversely, several have advocated that specific appropriateness criteria may improve surgical outcomes in patients with LBP.[100] Nonetheless, according to a systematic review by Chou and colleagues,[101] fusion is no more effective than intensive conservative rehabilitation for degenerative disk disease. Furthermore, fusion was associated with small to moderate benefits compared with standard (nonintensive) conservative therapy. Moreover, based on the Medical

Research Council Spine Stabilization RCT assessing patients with chronic LBP at a minimum of 1-year duration who were randomized to undergo lumbar fusion or an intensive rehabilitation program based on cognitive behavioral principles, no difference in disability and functional outcome was noted in both treatment groups.[102]

The efficacy of total disk replacement (TDR) has been scrutinized throughout the years (see article by Mayer and Siepe elsewhere in this issue). Based on a systematic review by van den Eerenbeemt and colleagues,[103] it was concluded that studies assessing the efficacy of TDR lacked proper control groups and were generally of low quality. The results indicate that TDR is at best only of similar efficacy to lumbar fusion. In clinical practice, TDR is used mostly for single-level disk disease and not for multilevel disease. Nevertheless, the investigators concluded that the existing evidence, specifically regarding long-term effectiveness or safety, is considered insufficient to justify the widespread use of TDR for single-level degenerative disease. Furthermore, the correlation between radiographic evidence of motion preservation and clinical improvement in pain intensity has not been completely supported.[104] In a recent prospective study addressing TDR by Blondel and colleagues,[105] superior clinical outcomes based on Oswestry Disability Index and pain scales were observed in individuals with Modic type I endplate changes on MRI compared with Modic type II or no Modic changes. The findings from this study have stressed the importance of proper patient selection in individuals undergoing TDR to maximize surgical outcomes.

In general, rehabilitation is needed after disk surgery. Exercise programs starting 4 to 6 weeks after surgery seem to lead to a faster decrease in pain and disability than no treatment. Moreover, high-intensity exercise programs seem to lead to a faster decrease in pain and disability than low-intensity programs.[106] No systematic reviews are available to assess the efficacy of rehabilitation regime after lumbar fusion surgery, but 1 recent RCT by Abbott and colleagues[107] found a beneficial effect for rehabilitation after lumbar fusion surgery. However, the investigators concluded that in addition to neuromuscular exercises, rehabilitation should also address maladaptive pain coping.

Newer surgical techniques focusing on the use of dynamic stabilization have been described for the management of degenerative disk disease. Several systems currently exist and can be subdivided into 4 groups: (1) dynamic interspinous spacers, (2) static interspinous spacers, (3) pedicle screw/rod-based posterior dynamic stabilizing system, and (4) total facet replacement systems. Theoretically, they all attempt to address the degenerative segment through either direct distraction forces to unload the disk, or to shield the disk and facet joints from motion, or reduce facet contact and pressure. High-quality RCTs and systematic reviews on the role and outcomes of these systems on the management of degenerative disk disease are absent.

PROGNOSTIC FACTORS

According to a systematic review, maladaptive pain coping behavior, in addition to baseline disability, is an important prognostic factor for poor recovery of LBP.[50] Throughout the past decade, genetic analysis has been used to screen and identify risk factors for various spine-related conditions (eg, disk degeneration),[108–112] and to prognosticate the development of disease progression (eg, scoliosis).[113–115]

Maladaptive Pain Coping

Recent studies uniformly suggest that abnormal fear-avoidance behavior predicts prolonged LBP.[50,116,117] Similarly, low expectations on return to work and abnormal fear-avoidance behavior predicted slow recovery after disk surgery.[118] A nonorganic pain drawing is defined as one with poorly defined pain patterns, pain with expansion to other parts of the body, and pain with a bizarre or nonanatomic appearance. In a recent study by Andersen and colleagues,[119] a nonorganic pain drawing was a significant risk factor for inferior outcome after spinal fusion surgery.

Genetic Factors

Strong evidence, primarily based on twin studies, has suggested that LBP may have a genetic predisposition.[120–123] Some investigators, such as Karppinen and colleagues,[124] have noted that prognostic genotypes (eg, interleukin 6 haplotype

Table 4
Pain genes

Gene	Protein	Mutation	Phenotype	Reference
ABCB1	ATP-binding cassette, B1	SNP	Altered morphine sensitivity	Campa et al[129]
COMT[a]	Catechol-O-methyltransferase	Multiple SNPs	Increased/decreased pain sensitivity	Dai et al[125]; Diatchenko et al[130]
CYP2D6	Cytochrome P450 2D6	Multiple SNPs	Altered analgesic efficacy	Stamer and Stuber[131]
FAAH	Fatty acid amide hydrolase	Multiple SNPs	Increased pain sensitivity	Kim et al[132]
GCH1[a]	GTP cyclohydrolase	Multiple SNPs	Partial analgesia	Kim et al[126]; Tegeder et al[133]
IL-6[a]	Interleukin 6 GGGA haplotype	SNP	Increased pain sensitivity	Karppinen et al[124]
MC1R	Melanocortin 1 receptor	SNP	Partial analgesia, increased analgesic responsiveness	Mogil et al[134]
OPRM1	Opioid receptor μ1	Multiple SNPs	Decreased pain sensitivity, decreased opioid analgesia	Fillingim et al[135]
OPRD1	Opioid receptor δ1	Multiple SNPs	Increased/decreased pain sensitivity	Kim et al[136]
SCN9A[a]	α-subunit, voltage-gated $Na_v1.7$	Multiple SNPs	Increased/decreased pain sensitivity	Reimann et al[127]; Yang et al[137]
TRPA1	Transient receptor potential A1	Multiple SNPs	Increased pain sensitivity	Kim et al[132]
TRPV1	Transient receptor potential V1	SNP	Decreased pain sensitivity	Kim et al[132]

Abbreviation: SNP, single nucleotide polymorphism.
 [a] Reported investigation in spine patients.
Modified from Foulkes T, Wood JN. Pain genes. PLoS Genet 2008;4:e1000086; with permission.

GGGA) may predict the duration of pain and may have an interaction effect with certain modifiable risk factors of pain in adults (eg, physical work load). In the setting of spine surgery outcomes, the implications of pain genes, and their role in sensitivity and processing of pain, may predict surgical outcomes in patients undergoing spine fusion for degenerative disk disease. According to Dai and colleagues,[125] who prospectively assessed 69 patients undergoing instrumented spine fusion for chronic discogenic LBP and their 1-year postoperative clinical outcomes, polymorphisms in the catechol-O-methyltransferase (COMT) gene were found to improve postoperative 1-year Oswestry Disability Index and pain scores. Based on the same group of patients, Kim and colleagues[126] also showed that polymorphic variations of the guanosine triphosphate cyclohydrolase 1 (GCH1) gene, specifically the T allele at rs998259 of GCH1, was found to improve postoperative clinical outcomes. Another interesting pain gene is SCN9A, which encodes the α-subunit of the voltage-gated sodium channel $Na_v1.7$. A common polymorphism in the gene was associated with increased likelihood of pain among patients and lowered pain threshold among healthy females.[127] Additional known pain genes are noted in **Table 4**. Others have contended that the presence of chronic LBP may act to potentiate genetic susceptibility to the pain experience through epigenetic modification.[128]

Although additional, larger studies are warranted to assess the detailed role and mechanism of pain genes in individuals suffering from degenerative disk disease and chronic LBP in addition to the need to replicate previous findings in different populations, this field of pain genetics provides a new direction in understanding the pain experience and perception and may be useful for identifying individuals susceptible to LBP or who would benefit most from spine surgery. Furthermore, identification of pain genes may lead to gene therapy to treat LBP conditions. Although promising, the role of pain genes in such settings needs to account for the complex biopsychosocial factors, pain history, and gender differences that may also play a role in the patient's pain profile and that may dictate management and prognostic outcomes.

SUMMARY

Conservative decisions in the treatment of degenerative disk disease are based on interventions made for patients with chronic LBP. There is convincing evidence that patient education, exercise therapy, and cognitive behavioral therapy are the cornerstones for the treatment of chronic LBP. However, the effect sizes of these treatments are modest. Furthermore, these therapies work best in a multidisciplinary rehabilitation context. Pain medication is needed for most patients with degenerative disk disease, and surgery may be needed for a minority only.

In the future, more research should focus on strategies of early recognition and treatment of high-risk patients. These high-risk patients should perhaps be offered treatment(s) based on their clinical profile (ie, current and past symptoms and clinical finding) or genetic predisposition to pain. For example, a patient with an abnormal psychosocial profile may benefit most from cognitive therapy, whereas exercise therapy may be of lesser importance. Similarly, an individual susceptible to pain sensitivity because of genetic factors may not benefit from surgical intervention and alternative means should be pursued. For those with problems in workability more intensive multidisciplinary outpatient approaches may be needed. Recent evidence suggests that these interventions should include workplace intervention in combination with progressive exercise therapy based on cognitive principles. In addition, biologic therapies for disk repair and regeneration may show promise for the treatment of discogenic LBP.

REFERENCES

1. Andersson GB. Epidemiological features of chronic low-back pain. Lancet 1999;354:581–5.
2. Deyo RA, Tsui-Wu YJ. Descriptive epidemiology of low-back pain and its related medical care in the United States. Spine 1987;12:264–8.
3. Hart LG, Deyo RA, Cherkin DC. Physician office visits for low back pain. Frequency, clinical evaluation, and treatment patterns from a U.S. national survey. Spine 1995;20:11–9.
4. Dagenais S, Caro J, Haldeman S. A systematic review of low back pain cost of illness studies in the United States and internationally. Spine J 2008;8:8–20.
5. Ekman M, Jonhagen S, Hunsche E, et al. Burden of illness of chronic low back pain in Sweden: a cross-sectional, retrospective study in primary care setting. Spine 2005;30:1777–85.
6. Wenig CM, Schmidt CO, Kohlmann T, et al. Costs of back pain in Germany. Eur J Pain 2008;13(3):280–6.
7. Deyo RA, Weinstein JN. Low back pain. N Engl J Med 2001;344:363–70.
8. Hurri H, Karppinen J. Discogenic pain. Pain 2004; 112:225–8.
9. Manchikanti L, Glaser SE, Wolfer L, et al. Systematic review of lumbar discography as a diagnostic test for chronic low back pain. Pain Physician 2009;12:541–59.

10. Jayson MI. Why does acute back pain become chronic? BMJ 1997;314:1639–40.

11. Shen FH, Samartzis D, Andersson GB. Nonsurgical management of acute and chronic low back pain. J Am Acad Orthop Surg 2006;14:477–87.

12. Bendix T, Kjaer P, Korsholm L. Burned-out discs stop hurting: fact or fiction? Spine (Phila Pa 1976) 2008;33:E962–7.

13. Kjaer P, Leboeuf-Yde C, Korsholm L, et al. Magnetic resonance imaging and low back pain in adults: a diagnostic imaging study of 40-year-old men and women. Spine (Phila Pa 1976) 2005;30:1173–80.

14. Koes BW, van Tulder M, Lin CW, et al. An updated overview of clinical guidelines for the management of non-specific low back pain in primary care. Eur Spine J 2010;19:2075–94.

15. Gilbert FJ, Grant AM, Gillan MG. Does early imaging influence management and improve outcome in patients with low back pain? A pragmatic randomised controlled trial. Health Technol Assess 2004;8:1–131.

16. Jarvik JG, Hollingworth W, Martin B, et al. Rapid magnetic resonance imaging vs radiographs for patients with low back pain: a randomized controlled trial. JAMA 2003;289:2810–8.

17. Modic MT, Obuchowski NA, Ross JS, et al. Acute low back pain and radiculopathy: MR imaging findings and their prognostic role and effect on outcome. Radiology 2005;237:597–604.

18. Carragee EJ, Don AS, Hurwitz EL, et al. 2009 ISSLS Prize Winner: Does discography cause accelerated progression of degeneration changes in the lumbar disc: a ten-year matched cohort study. Spine (Phila Pa 1976) 2009;34:2338–45.

19. Chou R, Loeser JD, Owens DK, et al. Interventional therapies, surgery, and interdisciplinary rehabilitation for low back pain: an evidence-based clinical practice guideline from the American Pain Society. Spine (Phila Pa 1976) 2009;34:1066–77.

20. Ohtori S, Kinoshita T, Yamashita M, et al. Results of surgery for discogenic low back pain: a randomized study using discography versus discoblock for diagnosis. Spine (Phila Pa 1976) 2009;34:1345–8.

21. Hancock MJ, Maher CG, Latimer J, et al. Systematic review of tests to identify the disc, SIJ or facet joint as the source of low back pain. Eur Spine J 2007;16:1539–50.

22. Cheung KM, Karppinen J, Chan D, et al. Prevalence and pattern of lumbar magnetic resonance imaging changes in a population study of one thousand forty-three individuals. Spine (Phila Pa 1976) 2009;34:934–40.

23. de Schepper EI, Damen J, van Meurs JB, et al. The association between lumbar disc degeneration and low back pain: the influence of age, gender, and individual radiographic features. Spine (Phila Pa 1976) 2010;35:531–6.

24. Samartzis D, Karppinen J, Chan D, et al. The association of disc degeneration based on magnetic resonance imaging and the presence of low back pain. Presented at: World Forum for Spine Research: Intervertebral Disc. Montreal, Canada, July 5–8, 2010.

25. Samartzis D, Karppinen J, Mok F, et al. A population-based study of juvenile disc degeneration and its association with overweight and obesity, low back pain, and diminished functional status. J Bone Joint Surg Am 2011;93:662–70.

26. Takatalo J, Karppinen J, Niinimäki J, et al. Does lumbar disc degeneration on MRI associate with low back symptom severity in young Finnish adults? Spine (Phila Pa 1976) 2011. [Epub ahead of print].

27. Visuri T, Ulaska J, Eskelin M, et al. Narrowing of lumbar spinal canal predicts chronic low back pain more accurately than intervertebral disc degeneration: a magnetic resonance imaging study in young Finnish male conscripts. Mil Med 2005;170:926–30.

28. Paajanen H, Erkintalo M, Kuusela T, et al. Magnetic resonance study of disc degeneration in young low-back pain patients. Spine (Phila Pa 1976) 1989;14:982–5.

29. Paajanen H, Erkintalo M, Parkkola R, et al. Age-dependent correlation of low-back pain and lumbar disc regeneration. Arch Orthop Trauma Surg 1997;116:106–7.

30. Savage RA, Whitehouse GH, Roberts N. The relationship between the magnetic resonance imaging appearance of the lumbar spine and low back pain, age and occupation in males. Eur Spine J 1997;6:106–14.

31. Chou D, Samartzis D, Bellabarba C, et al. Degenerative MRI changes in patients with chronic low back pain: a systematic review. Spine 2011. [Epub ahead of print].

32. DePalma MJ, Ketchum JM, Saullo T. What is the source of chronic low back pain and does age play a role? Pain Med 2011;12:224–33.

33. Blumenkrantz G, Zuo J, Li X, et al. In vivo 3.0-tesla magnetic resonance T1rho and T2 relaxation mapping in subjects with intervertebral disc degeneration and clinical symptoms. Magn Reson Med 2010;63:1193–200.

34. Borthakur A, Maurer PM, Fenty M, et al. T1rho MRI and discography pressure as novel biomarkers for disc degeneration and low back pain. Spine (Phila Pa 1976) 2011. [Epub ahead of print].

35. Kim M, Chan Q, Anthony MP, et al. Assessment of glycosaminoglycan distribution in human lumbar intervertebral discs using chemical exchange saturation transfer at 3 T: feasibility and initial experience. NMR Biomed 2011. [Epub ahead of print].

36. Mellon EA, Beesam RS, Kasam M, et al. Single shot T1rho magnetic resonance imaging of

metabolically generated water in vivo. Adv Exp Med Biol 2009;645:279–86.

37. Witschey WR 2nd, Borthakur A, Elliott MA, et al. Artifacts in T1 rho-weighted imaging: compensation for B(1) and B(0) field imperfections. J Magn Reson 2007;186:75–85.

38. Zuo J, Joseph GB, Li X, et al. In-vivo intervertebral disc characterization using magnetic resonance spectroscopy and T1rho imaging: association with discography and Oswestry Disability Index and SF-36. Spine (Phila Pa 1976) 2011. [Epub ahead of print].

39. DeLeo JA. Basic science of pain. J Bone Joint Surg Am 2006;88(Suppl 2):58–62.

40. Latremoliere A, Woolf CJ. Central sensitization: a generator of pain hypersensitivity by central neural plasticity. J Pain 2009;10:895–926.

41. Peyron R, Laurent B, Garcia-Larrea L. Functional imaging of brain responses to pain. A review and meta-analysis (2000). Neurophysiol Clin 2000;30: 263–88.

42. Apkarian AV, Sosa Y, Sonty S, et al. Chronic back pain is associated with decreased prefrontal and thalamic gray matter density. J Neurosci 2004;24: 10410–5.

43. Schmidt-Wilcke T, Leinisch E, Ganssbauer S, et al. Affective components and intensity of pain correlate with structural differences in gray matter in chronic back pain patients. Pain 2006;125:89–97.

44. Ruscheweyh R, Deppe M, Lohmann H, et al. Pain is associated with regional grey matter reduction in the general population. Pain 2011;152:904–11.

45. Seminowicz DA, Wideman TH, Naso L, et al. Effective treatment of chronic low back pain in humans reverses abnormal brain anatomy and function. J Neurosci 2011;31:7540–50.

46. Savigny P, Watson P, Underwood M. Early management of persistent non-specific low back pain: summary of NICE guidance. BMJ 2009;338:b1805.

47. Engers A, Jellema P, Wensing M, et al. Individual patient education for low back pain. Cochrane Database Syst Rev 2008;1:CD004057.

48. Chou R, Qaseem A, Snow V, et al. Diagnosis and treatment of low back pain: a joint clinical practice guideline from the American College of Physicians and the American Pain Society. Ann Intern Med 2007;147:478–91.

49. Pohjolainen T, Karppinen J, Kumpulainen T, et al. Low back and neck disorders. In: Facultas, evaluation of functional ability. Helsinki (Finland): Suomalainen Lääkäriseura Duodecim ja Työeläkevakuuttajat TELA; 2008 [in Finnish].

50. Chou R, Shekelle P. Will this patient develop persistent disabling low back pain? JAMA 2010;303: 1295–302.

51. Fairbank JC, Couper J, Davies JB, et al. The Oswestry low back pain disability questionnaire. Physiotherapy 1980;66:271–3.

52. Stratford PW, Binkley JM. Measurement properties of the RM-18. A modified version of the Roland-Morris Disability Scale. Spine (Phila Pa 1976) 1997;22:2416–21.

53. Ransford AO, Cairns D, Mooney V. The pain drawing as an aid to the psychologic evaluation of patients with low-back pain. Spine (Phila Pa 1976) 1976;1: 127–34.

54. Kuijpers T, van Middelkoop M, Rubinstein SM, et al. A systematic review on the effectiveness of pharmacological interventions for chronic non-specific low-back pain. Eur Spine J 2011;20:40–50.

55. Roelofs PD, Deyo RA, Koes BW, et al. Non-steroidal anti-inflammatory drugs for low back pain. Cochrane Database Syst Rev 2008;1:CD000396.

56. Deshpande A, Furlan A, Mailis-Gagnon A, et al. Opioids for chronic low-back pain. Cochrane Database Syst Rev 2007;3:CD004959.

57. Franklin GM, Stover BD, Turner JA, et al. Early opioid prescription and subsequent disability among workers with back injuries: the Disability Risk Identification Study Cohort. Spine (Phila Pa 1976) 2008;33:199–204.

58. Webster BS, Verma SK, Gatchel RJ. Relationship between early opioid prescribing for acute occupational low back pain and disability duration, medical costs, subsequent surgery and late opioid use. Scand J Work Environ Health 2007;32: 2127–32.

59. Urquhart DM, Hoving JL, Assendelft WW, et al. Antidepressants for non-specific low back pain. Cochrane Database Syst Rev 2008;1:CD001703.

60. Hayden JA, van Tulder MW, Malmivaara A, et al. Exercise therapy for treatment of non-specific low back pain. Cochrane Database Syst Rev 2005;3:CD000335.

61. Keller A, Hayden J, Bombardier C, et al. Effect sizes of non-surgical treatments of non-specific low-back pain. Eur Spine J 2007;16:1776–88.

62. van Tulder M, Malmivaara A, Hayden J, et al. Statistical significance versus clinical importance: trials on exercise therapy for chronic low back pain as example. Spine (Phila Pa 1976) 2007;32:1785–90.

63. van Middelkoop M, Rubinstein SM, Kuijpers T, et al. A systematic review on the effectiveness of physical and rehabilitation interventions for chronic non-specific low back pain. Eur Spine J 2011;20:19–39.

64. Hayden JA, van Tulder MW, Tomlinson G. Systematic review: strategies for using exercise therapy to improve outcomes in chronic low back pain. Ann Intern Med 2005;142:776–85.

65. Fersum KV, Dankaerts W, O'Sullivan PB, et al. Integration of subclassification strategies in randomised controlled clinical trials evaluating manual therapy treatment and exercise therapy for non-specific chronic low back pain: a systematic review. Br J Sports Med 2010;44:1054–62.

66. Jensen TS, Karppinen J, Sorensen JS, et al. Vertebral endplate signal changes (Modic change): a systematic literature review of prevalence and association with non-specific low back pain. Eur Spine J 2008;17:1407–22.

67. Modic MT, Steinberg PM, Ross JS, et al. Degenerative disk disease: assessment of changes in vertebral body marrow with MR imaging. Radiology 1988;166:193–9.

68. Choi BK, Verbeek JH, Tam WW, et al. Exercises for prevention of recurrences of low-back pain. Cochrane Database Syst Rev 2010;1:CD006555.

69. Fordyce WE. Behavioral methods for chronic pain and illness. St Louis (MO): Mosby; 1976.

70. Pincus T, Vogel S, Burton AK, et al. Fear avoidance and prognosis in back pain: a systematic review and synthesis of current evidence. Arthritis Rheum 2006;54:3999–4010.

71. Turk DC, Flor H. Etiological theories and treatments for chronic back pain. II. Psychological models and interventions. Pain 1984;19:209–33.

72. Henschke N, Ostelo RW, van Tulder MW, et al. Behavioural treatment for chronic low-back pain. Cochrane Database Syst Rev 2010;7:CD002014.

73. Sorensen PH, Bendix T, Manniche C, et al. An educational approach based on a non-injury model compared with individual symptom-based physical training in chronic LBP. A pragmatic, randomised trial with a one-year follow-up. BMC Musculoskelet Disord 2010;11:212.

74. Lamb SE, Hansen Z, Lall R, et al. Group cognitive behavioural treatment for low-back pain in primary care: a randomised controlled trial and cost-effectiveness analysis. Lancet 2010;375: 916–23.

75. Guzman J, Esmail R, Karjalainen K, et al. Multidisciplinary rehabilitation for chronic low back pain: systematic review. BMJ 2001;322:1511–6.

76. Schaafsma F, Schonstein E, Whelan KM, et al. Physical conditioning programs for improving work outcomes in workers with back pain. Cochrane Database Syst Rev 2010;1:CD001822.

77. Lambeek LC, van Mechelen W, Knol DL, et al. Randomised controlled trial of integrated care to reduce disability from chronic low back pain in working and private life. BMJ 2010;340: c1035.

78. Ravenek MJ, Hughes ID, Ivanovich N, et al. A systematic review of multidisciplinary outcomes in the management of chronic low back pain. Work 2010;35:349–67.

79. Buijs PC, Lambeek LC, Koppenrade V, et al. Can workers with chronic back pain shift from pain elimination to function restore at work? Qualitative evaluation of an innovative work related multidisciplinary programme. J Back Musculoskeletal Rehabil 2009; 22:65–73.

80. Staal JB, de Bie R, de Vet HC, et al. Injection therapy for subacute and chronic low-back pain. Cochrane Database Syst Rev 2008;3:CD001824.

81. Chou R, Atlas SJ, Stanos SP, et al. Nonsurgical interventional therapies for low back pain: a review of the evidence for an American Pain Society clinical practice guideline. Spine (Phila Pa 1976) 2009;34: 1078–93.

82. Karppinen J. New perspectives on sciatica. In: DeLeo JA, Sorkin LS, Watkins LR, editors. Immune and glial regulation of pain. Seattle (WA): IASP Press; 2007. p. 385–406.

83. Cohen SP, Wenzell D, Hurley RW, et al. A double-blind, placebo-controlled, dose-response pilot study evaluating intradiscal etanercept in patients with chronic discogenic low back pain or lumbosacral radiculopathy. Anesthesiology 2007;107:99–105.

84. Buser Z, Kuelling F, Liu J, et al. Biological and biomechanical effects of fibrin injection into porcine intervertebral discs. Spine (Phila Pa 1976) 2011;36: E1201–9.

85. Serigano K, Sakai D, Hiyama A, et al. Effect of cell number on mesenchymal stem cell transplantation in a canine disc degeneration model. J Orthop Res 2010;28:1267–75.

86. Sakai D, Mochida J, Iwashina T, et al. Differentiation of mesenchymal stem cells transplanted to a rabbit degenerative disc model: potential and limitations for stem cell therapy in disc regeneration. Spine (Phila Pa 1976) 2005;30:2379–87.

87. Sakai D, Mochida J, Iwashina T, et al. Regenerative effects of transplanting mesenchymal stem cells embedded in atelocollagen to the degenerated intervertebral disc. Biomaterials 2006;27: 335–45.

88. Sakai D, Mochida J, Yamamoto Y, et al. Transplantation of mesenchymal stem cells embedded in Atelocollagen gel to the intervertebral disc: a potential therapeutic model for disc degeneration. Biomaterials 2003;24:3531–41.

89. An HS, Masuda K. Relevance of in vitro and in vivo models for intervertebral disc degeneration. J Bone Joint Surg Am 2006;88(Suppl 2):88–94.

90. An HS, Takegami K, Kamada H, et al. Intradiscal administration of osteogenic protein-1 increases intervertebral disc height and proteoglycan content in the nucleus pulposus in normal adolescent rabbits. Spine (Phila Pa 1976) 2005;30:25–31 [discussion: 2].

91. Zhang Y, An HS, Song S, et al. Growth factor osteogenic protein-1: differing effects on cells from three distinct zones in the bovine intervertebral disc. Am J Phys Med Rehabil 2004;83:515–21.

92. Takegami K, Thonar EJ, An HS, et al. Osteogenic protein-1 enhances matrix replenishment by intervertebral disc cells previously exposed to interleukin-1. Spine (Phila Pa 1976) 2002;27:1318–25.

93. Yang F, Leung VY, Luk KD, et al. Mesenchymal stem cells arrest intervertebral disc degeneration through chondrocytic differentiation and stimulation of endogenous cells. Mol Ther 2009;17:1959–66.

94. Peng B, Pang X, Wu Y, et al. A randomized placebo-controlled trial of intradiscal methylene blue injection for the treatment of chronic discogenic low back pain. Pain 2010;149:124–9.

95. O'Neill C, Thullier D, Buser Z, et al. Toxicity of methylene blue in the epidural space. Presented at: International Society for the Study of the Lumbar Spine. Gothenburg, Sweden, June 14–18, 2011.

96. Rajaee SS, Bae HW, Kanim LE, et al. Spinal fusion in the United States: analysis of trends from 1998 to 2008. Spine (Phila Pa 1976) 2011. [Epub ahead of print].

97. Fritzell P, Hagg O, Wessberg P, et al. Chronic low back pain and fusion: a comparison of three surgical techniques: a prospective multicenter randomized study from the Swedish lumbar spine study group. Spine (Phila Pa 1976) 2002;27:1131–41.

98. Mardjetko SM, Connolly PJ, Shott S. Degenerative lumbar spondylolisthesis. A meta-analysis of literature 1970-1993. Spine (Phila Pa 1976) 1994;19: 2256S–65S.

99. France JC, Yaszemski MJ, Lauerman WC, et al. A randomized prospective study of posterolateral lumbar fusion. Outcomes with and without pedicle screw instrumentation. Spine (Phila Pa 1976) 1999;24:553–60.

100. Danon-Hersch N, Samartzis D, Wietlisbach V, et al. Appropriateness criteria for surgery improve clinical outcomes in patients with low back pain and/or sciatica. Spine (Phila Pa 1976) 2010. [Epub ahead of print].

101. Chou R, Baisden J, Carragee EJ, et al. Surgery for low back pain: a review of the evidence for an American Pain Society Clinical Practice Guideline. Spine (Phila Pa 1976) 2009;34:1094–109.

102. Fairbank J, Frost H, Wilson-MacDonald J, et al. Randomised controlled trial to compare surgical stabilisation of the lumbar spine with an intensive rehabilitation programme for patients with chronic low back pain: the MRC spine stabilisation trial. BMJ 2005;330:1233.

103. van den Eerenbeemt KD, Ostelo RW, van Royen BJ, et al. Total disc replacement surgery for symptomatic degenerative lumbar disc disease: a systematic review of the literature. Eur Spine J 2010;19:1262–80.

104. Putzier M, Funk JF, Schneider SV, et al. Charité total disc replacement–clinical and radiographical results after an average follow-up of 17 years. Eur Spine J 2006;15:183–95.

105. Blondel B, Tropiano P, Gaudart J, et al. Clinical results of lumbar total disc arthroplasty in accordance with Modic signs, with a 2 year minimum follow-up. Spine (Phila Pa 1976) 2011. [Epub ahead of print].

106. Ostelo RW, Costa LO, Maher CG, et al. Rehabilitation after lumbar disc surgery: an update Cochrane review. Spine (Phila Pa 1976) 2009;34:1839–48.

107. Abbott AD, Tyni-Lenne R, Hedlund R. Early rehabilitation targeting cognition, behavior, and motor function after lumbar fusion: a randomized controlled trial. Spine (Phila Pa 1976) 2010;35:848–57.

108. Karppinen J, Daavittila I, Solovieva S, et al. Genetic factors are associated with Modic changes in endplates of lumbar vertebral bodies. Spine (Phila Pa 1976) 2008;33:1236–41.

109. Sambrook PN, MacGregor AJ, Spector TD. Genetic influences on cervical and lumbar disc degeneration: a magnetic resonance imaging study in twins. Arthritis Rheum 1999;42:366–72.

110. Song YQ, Cheung KM, Ho DW, et al. Association of the asporin D14 allele with lumbar-disc degeneration in Asians. Am J Hum Genet 2008;82:744–7.

111. Videman T, Saarela J, Kaprio J, et al. Associations of 25 structural, degradative, and inflammatory candidate genes with lumbar disc desiccation, bulging, and height narrowing. Arthritis Rheum 2009;60:470–81.

112. Videman T, Battie MC, Ripatti S, et al. Determinants of the progression in lumbar degeneration: a 5-year follow-up study of adult male monozygotic twins. Spine (Phila Pa 1976) 2006;31:671–8.

113. Ogilvie JW. Update on prognostic genetic testing in adolescent idiopathic scoliosis (AIS). J Pediatr Orthop 2011;31:S46–8.

114. Ward K, Ogilvie JW, Singleton MV, et al. Validation of DNA-based prognostic testing to predict spinal curve progression in adolescent idiopathic scoliosis. Spine (Phila Pa 1976) 2010;35:E1455–64.

115. Wang S, Qiu Y, Ma Z, et al. Expression of Runx2 and type X collagen in vertebral growth plate of patients with adolescent idiopathic scoliosis. Connect Tissue Res 2010;51:188–96.

116. Helmhout PH, Staal JB, Heymans MW, et al. Prognostic factors for perceived recovery or functional improvement in non-specific low back pain: secondary analyses of three randomized clinical trials. Eur Spine J 2010;19:650–9.

117. Jensen JN, Albertsen K, Borg V, et al. The predictive effect of fear-avoidance beliefs on low back pain among newly qualified health care workers with and without previous low back pain: a prospective cohort study. BMC Musculoskelet Disord 2009; 10:117.

118. Johansson AC, Linton SJ, Rosenblad A, et al. A prospective study of cognitive behavioural factors as predictors of pain, disability and quality of life one year after lumbar disc surgery. Disabil Rehabil 2010;32:521–9.

119. Andersen T, Christensen FB, Hoy KW, et al. The predictive value of pain drawings in lumbar spinal fusion surgery. Spine J 2010;10:372–9.

120. Livshits G, Popham M, Malkin I, et al. Lumbar disc degeneration and genetic factors are the main risk factors for low back pain in women: the UK Twin Spine Study. Ann Rheum Dis 2011. [Epub ahead of print].

121. Williams FM, Spector TD, MacGregor AJ. Pain reporting at different body sites is explained by a single underlying genetic factor. Rheumatology (Oxford) 2010;49:1753–5.

122. El-Metwally A, Mikkelsson M, Stahl M, et al. Genetic and environmental influences on non-specific low back pain in children: a twin study. Eur Spine J 2008;17:502–8.

123. Battie MC, Videman T, Levalahti E, et al. Heritability of low back pain and the role of disc degeneration. Pain 2007;131:272–80.

124. Karppinen J, Daavittila I, Noponen N, et al. Is the interleukin-6 haplotype a prognostic factor for sciatica? Eur J Pain 2008;12:1018–25.

125. Dai F, Belfer I, Schwartz CE, et al. Association of catechol-O-methyltransferase genetic variants with outcome in patients undergoing surgical treatment for lumbar degenerative disc disease. Spine J 2010;10:949–57.

126. Kim DH, Dai F, Belfer I, et al. Polymorphic variation of the guanosine triphosphate cyclohydrolase 1 gene predicts outcome in patients undergoing surgical treatment for lumbar degenerative disc disease. Spine (Phila Pa 1976) 2010;35:1909–14.

127. Reimann F, Cox JJ, Belfer I, et al. Pain perception is altered by a nucleotide polymorphism in SCN9A. Proc Natl Acad Sci U S A 2010;107:5148–53.

128. Vossen H, Kenis G, Rutten B, et al. The genetic influence on the cortical processing of experimental pain and the moderating effect of pain status. PLoS One 2010;5:e13641.

129. Campa D, Gioia A, Tomei A, et al. Association of ABCB1/MDR1 and OPRM1 gene polymorphisms with morphine pain relief. Clin Pharmacol Ther 2008;83:559–66.

130. Diatchenko L, Nackley AG, Slade GD, et al. Catechol-O-methyltransferase gene polymorphisms are associated with multiple pain-evoking stimuli. Pain 2006;125:216–24.

131. Stamer UM, Stuber F. Codeine and tramadol analgesic efficacy and respiratory effects are influenced by CYP2D6 genotype. Anaesthesia 2007; 62:1294–5 [author reply: 5–6].

132. Kim H, Mittal DP, Iadarola MJ, et al. Genetic predictors for acute experimental cold and heat pain sensitivity in humans. J Med Genet 2006;43:e40.

133. Tegeder I, Costigan M, Griffin RS, et al. GTP cyclohydrolase and tetrahydrobiopterin regulate pain sensitivity and persistence. Nat Med 2006;12:1269–77.

134. Mogil JS, Ritchie J, Smith SB, et al. Melanocortin-1 receptor gene variants affect pain and mu-opioid analgesia in mice and humans. J Med Genet 2005;42:583–7.

135. Fillingim RB, Kaplan L, Staud R, et al. The A118G single nucleotide polymorphism of the mu-opioid receptor gene (OPRM1) is associated with pressure pain sensitivity in humans. J Pain 2005;6:159–67.

136. Kim H, Neubert JK, San Miguel A, et al. Genetic influence on variability in human acute experimental pain sensitivity associated with gender, ethnicity and psychological temperament. Pain 2004;109:488–96.

137. Yang Y, Wang Y, Li S, et al. Mutations in SCN9A, encoding a sodium channel alpha subunit, in patients with primary erythermalgia. J Med Genet 2004;41: 171–4.

Adjacent Level Disk Disease—Is it Really a Fusion Disease?

Teija Lund, MD, PhD[a],*, Thomas R. Oxland, PhD[b,c]

KEYWORDS

- Spine • Fusion • Motion-preserving • Adjacent segment
- Biomechanics

A century ago, Albee[1] and Hibbs[2] independently described spinal fusion to treat Pott's disease and spinal deformity. Anecdotal case reports on adjacent segment degeneration (ASD) as an uncommon complication of lumbosacral fusion started to emerge a few decades later.[3,4] Since the time of Albee and Hibbs, indications for spinal fusion have expanded considerably and, especially in the last 20 years, we have witnessed an increasing number of spine fusions performed for degenerative conditions of the lumbosacral spine. Operative treatment of these inherently benign conditions has evoked discussions about the long-term sequelae of spinal fusions. The fate of the adjacent segment after rigid fusion of the lumbosacral spine has been increasingly studied and reported.

Although the predisposing factors for developing adjacent segment problems after spinal fusion are largely unknown, altered biomechanics of the adjacent segments has been emphasized. Biomechanical studies have shown that spinal fusion increases intervertebral motion, intradiscal pressure, and facet joint stresses of the adjacent levels. The rationale behind the more recent motion-preserving technologies is to protect the adjacent levels from these adverse consequences, thus preventing the development of ASD by preserving motion of the operated levels. However, some recent biomechanical and clinical studies have suggested that the biomechanics of the adjacent segments after a fusion procedure may not be altered as much as previously thought and that, instead, ASD is a sign of continued progression of the degenerative process.

This article summarizes the existing literature on the ASD, both biomechanical and clinical, to provide the reader with our current understanding of the pathogenesis of and the possible risk factors for this increasingly common clinical problem. Moreover, the clinical impact of ASD is discussed. Finally, the question whether the current literature supports the theoretical rationale behind motion-preserving technologies that also aim to protect the adjacent segments will be addressed.

INCIDENCE

The rate of radiologically verified ASD after lumbar and lumbosacral fusions reported in the literature since late 1980s (**Table 1**) has varied from 11% to 100%.[5–29] The true rate of ASD is difficult to define because of the retrospective nature of most of the studies and variable follow-up times. Moreover, the incidence of ASD varies according to the definition applied.[12] Most clinical evidence suggests that the level cranial to the previous fusion is more susceptible to subsequent degeneration compared with levels below the fusion.[5,6,11,15,19,22,27,29–31] This clinical observation

The authors have nothing to disclose.
[a] ORTON Orthopaedic Hospital, Tenholantie 10, PL 29, 00280 Helsinki, Finland
[b] Department of Orthopaedics, University of British Columbia, 566-828 West 10th Avenue, Vancouver, BC V5Z 1L8, Canada
[c] Department of Mechanical Engineering, University of British Columbia, 566-828 West 10th Avenue, Vancouver, BC V5Z 1L8, Canada
* Corresponding author.
E-mail address: teija.lund@orton.fi

Orthop Clin N Am 42 (2011) 529–541
doi:10.1016/j.ocl.2011.07.006

Table 1
Clinical studies on ASD after a lumbosacral fusion

Author	Study Design	Number of Potential Patients	Number of Included Patients	Diagnosis	Type of Surgery	Age at Time of Surgery	Length of FU	Incidence of ASD	Incidence of Reoperations During FU	Significant Risk Factors
Lehmann et al,[5] 1987	Retrospective	94	33	Mixed	Noninstrumented posterior fusion	NA	33 y	Stenosis 42% Instability 45%	15%	—
Kumar et al,[6] 2001	Retrospective	54	28	DDD	Posterior fusion	NA	>30 y	Loss of disk height 36% Instability 14%	NA	—
Hambly et al,[7] 1998	Retrospective	148	42	Mixed	Noninstrumented posterolateral fusion	NA	22.6 y	Disk space ossification 62% Facet joint arthrosis 52%	—	—
Remes et al,[8] 2005	Retrospective	129	102	Isthmic spondylolisthesis	Noninstrumented posterior or posterolateral fusion	15.9 y	21.0 y	DDD 54% Loss of disk height 21% Facet joint degeneration 79%	—	—
Wai et al,[9] 2006	Retrospective	64	39	Discogenic LBP	Noninstrumented ALIF	NA	20.5 y	74 % (advanced in 31%)	6%	—
Seitsalo et al,[10] 1997	Retrospective	175	145	Isthmic spondylolisthesis	Posterior or posterolateral noninstrumented fusion	14.3 y	15.4 y	Loss of disk height 17–32 %	—	—
Disch et al,[11] 2008	Retrospective	102	102	Isthmic spondylolisthesis, DDD	ALIF with or without posterior fusion	54 y	13.8 y	26%	12%	Floating L4/L5 fusion
Ekman et al,[12] 2009	RCT	111	80	Isthmic spondylolisthesis	Posterolateral fusion with or without instrumentation	39 y	12.6 y	Disk height loss (UCLA grading scale) 38%	—	Concomitant laminectomy (UCLA criteria) Instrumentation NS

Study	Type			Indication	Procedure	Age	Follow-up	ASD		Risk factors
Schulte et al,[13] 2007	NA	65	40	DDD, Isthmic spondylolisthesis	360° fusion	32.6 y (Isthmic) 45.1 y (DDD)	114 mo	Disk height reduction 11%–12% (Isthmic) 23%–25% (DDD)	—	Older age; Multilevel fusion
Videbaek et al,[14] 2010	RCT	148	95	DDD, Isthmic spondylolisthesis	ALIF + instrumented posterolatera fusion vs instrumented posterolateral fusion	45 y	8–13 y	89% with MRI evidence of ASD	9%	Older age
Cheh et al,[15] 2007	Retrospective	188	188	Degenerative	Circumferential or posterior instrumented fusion	55 y	7.8 y	43% (56% symptomatic)	—	Age >50 y; Multilevel fusion; Level of proximal instrumented vertebra
Gillet,[16] 2003	Retrospective	149	106	Degenerative	Instrumented posterolateral fusion	55 y	2–15 y	41%	20%	—
Ghiselli et al,[34] 2003	Retrospective	NA	32	75% degenerative spondylolisthesis	Posterolateral fusion with or without instrumentation	56 y	7.3 y	NA	3%	
Ahn et al,[17] 2010	Retrospective	NA	3188	Mixed	45% PLIF 55% other	57 y	NA	80% (in the proximal segments)	3.5 %	Age >61 y; Degenerative disease; Multilevel fusion; Male gender
Ghiselli et al,[18] 2004	Retrospective	NA	215	Mixed	Posterolateral fusion with or without instrumentation	50 y	6.7 y	NA	28%	Single-level fusion; Fusion level
Lai et al,[19] 2004	Retrospective	107	101	Spondylolisthesis	Instrumented posterolateral fusion	61 y	6–7 y	23%	—	Decompression technique
Miyakoshi et al,[20] 2000	Retrospective	74	45	Spondylolisthesis	PLIF + posterior fixation	58 y	6 y	100%	—	—

(continued on next page)

Table 1
(continued)

Author	Study Design	Number of Potential Patients	Number of Included Patients	Diagnosis	Type of Surgery	Age at Time of Surgery	Length of FU	Incidence of ASD	Incidence of Reoperations During FU	Significant Risk Factors
Kumar et al,[21] 2001	Retrospective	NA	83	Degenerative disease	Mixed	51.6 y	5 y	36% above the fusion	17%	Abnormal sacral inclination
Chou et al,[22] 2002	Retrospective	44	32	Degenerative	Decompression and posterolateral instrumented fusion	70.5 y	56 mo	Instability 19%	—	—
Min et al,[23] 2008	Retrospective	NA	48	Mixed	Interbody fusion	51.6 y – 56.2 y	45 mo	63%	7%	Loss of preoperative lumbar lordosis Younger age
Etebar and Cahill[24] 1999	Retrospective	125	125	Degenerative	Posterolateral instrumented fusion	NA	44.8 mo	Symptomatic ASD 14%	—	Multilevel fusion
Throckmorton et al,[25] 2003	Retrospective	148	25	Degenerative	Posterior fusion	56	>2 y	Disk degeneration 80%	—	—
Okuda et al,[26] 2004	Retrospective	NA	87	Degenerative spondylolisthesis	PLIF	64 y	43 mo	29%	4%	—
Aota et al,[27] 1995	NA	72	65	Mixed	Mixed	55.8 y	39 mo	Instability 25%	—	Age >55 y
Kaito et al,[28] 2010	Retrospective	97	85	Spondylolisthesis	PLIF + posterior fixation	64.1 y	38.8 mo	28%	13%	Distraction of the disk space
Park et al,[29] 2007	Retrospective	132	34	Isthmic spondylolisthesis	PLIF + posterior fixation	48.9 y	24.7 mo	21%	0%	—

Abbreviations: ALIF, anterior lumbar interbody fusion; DDD, degenerative disk disease; FU, follow-up; LBP, low back pain; NA, not announced; NS, non-significant; PLIF, posterior lumbar interbody fusion; RCT, randomized controlled trial; UCLA, University of California, Los Angeles.

has further been corroborated by in vitro biomechanical studies.[32,33] Degenerative changes do not appear to be limited to the first adjacent cranial segment but have also been observed at multiple levels above a previous fusion.[18,22,31]

Symptomatic ASD (ie, adjacent segment disease) is relatively rare compared with radiologically verified degenerative changes of the adjacent levels after a lumbosacral fusion, with reported incidence between 0% and 28%.[5,9,11,14–18,21,23,24,26,28,29,34] Ghiselli and colleagues[18] performed a retrospective analysis of 215 fusion patients at an average 6.7 years after a posterior lumbar fusion with or without instrumentation. In their series, new symptoms related to ASD, severe enough to warrant reoperation, developed at a fairly constant rate of 3.9% per year starting from the first postoperative year. Disease-free survival (ie, no reoperation for ASD) was 83.5% and 63.9% at 5 and 10 years after the index surgery, respectively. Another analysis of 3,188 thoracolumbar fusion patients showed an annual decrease of 0.6% in the survival rate when reoperation was defined as the end point.[17] Most clinical data suggest that functional outcomes after lumbar fusion surgery seem to be unaffected by radiographic, asymptomatic ASD,[5,6,8,10,12,13,20,26] although some studies have reported less favorable outcomes in patients with ASD.[15,19] A long-term follow-up of two randomized surgical groups correlated adjacent segment disk degeneration, foraminal compromise, and spinal stenosis to a worse clinical outcome.[14]

CAUSES

To date, most investigators have emphasized the role of biomechanical alterations induced by lumbosacral fusion, namely increased intervertebral motion, intradiscal pressure, and facet joint loads at the adjacent segments, in the pathogenesis of ASD. The literature, however, provides controversial and conflicting evidence. The following will outline the present knowledge on the biomechanical behavior of the adjacent segments and correlate it to clinical data where available and applicable.

Adjacent Segment Intervertebral Motion

Changes induced by rigid fixation and simulated one-level to three-level fusion have been examined extensively using in vitro human cadaveric and animal models, as well as validated finite element models (FEM). Several of these studies have demonstrated significant changes in the intersegmental rotation of the first cranial segment above a simulated fusion, most notably in flexion-extension motion.[35–44] Specifically, the percent increases of the motions of the first adjacent segment after a simulated fusion have ranged from 17% to 103% for flexion, from 17% to 67% for extension, from 6% to 94% for lateral bending, and from 6% to 20% for axial rotation.[36,37,42–44] Some studies have shown that extending the length of the fixation leads to more distinct increases in the intervertebral motions.[39,42,43] On the other hand, several studies have demonstrated only minor changes in the intervertebral rotations of the adjacent segment after a simulated fusion.[45–50] With a specific hybrid testing protocol introduced by Panjabi,[51] significant increases have been demonstrated, not only at the immediate adjacent level to a simulated fusion, but spread across multiple cranial levels.[42]

The large variation observed in the intervertebral rotation of the adjacent segment is at least partly explained by different biomechanical testing modes. One mode is based on the assumption that, postoperatively, the fused patients will try to move their spines to the same extent as preoperatively. By definition, this would demand higher loads, which would then cause the remaining mobile segments to compensate for the lost motion of the fused segment by demonstrating increased range of motion. In biomechanics, this assumption would require displacement-controlled testing protocols and, specifically, a hybrid set-up for identification of adjacent segment changes.[51] Another possibility is that, after a fusion procedure, the patient settles with the restricted lumbar motion, thus applying the same load to the unfused segments as before the operation. Biomechanically, this hypothesis could be tested by load-controlled protocols. In the first scenario, adjacent segment alterations after a fusion can be expected but, in the second one, they should be practically nonexistent.

From a biomechanical perspective, the best way to test for adjacent segment changes has not been worked out. The hybrid protocol[51] is probably the best technique, but it has not been used extensively to date. Furthermore, it is of concern that some load-controlled experiments have observed significant displacement changes at adjacent levels, against the theoretical basis of this testing protocol (see previous discussion). Thus, proper interpretation of the results of biomechanical research calls for careful consideration of the methods used.

in vitro laboratory results are difficult to corroborate in in vivo conditions. In one such study on adult canines, Dekutoski and colleagues[37] found increased motion at the adjacent segment to a spinal fusion with physiologic loading and

concluded that the animals attempted to reproduce the preoperative range of lumbar motion.
The results of this study would support the hypothesis that the adjacent levels after a spinal fusion
are subjected to increased loads with physiologic
loading conditions.

Lumbar spine in vivo kinematics in patients after
spinal fusion operations have been examined
using functional flexion-extension radiography,
videofluoroscopy, and radiostereometry. Luk and
colleagues[52] compared the lumbar spine range
of motion between clinically asymptomatic and
completely pain-free patients with an anterior
one-level or two-level fusion and asymptomatic
volunteers using standardized flexion-extension
radiographs. According to their results, the lumbar
spine of the fusion patients was significantly less
mobile than in the control subjects, which would
suggest that the adjacent segments do not
compensate for the lost motion at the fused
segments. However, the percent contribution of
the unfused segments to the total lumbar motion
was increased because the total lumbar range of
motion decreased proportionally more than that
of the individual levels. Similar results regarding
reduced total lumbar range of motion and no
compensatory increase in the motion of the levels
adjacent to a fusion have been reported by
other investigators using flexion-extension radiography.[7,22,53] Functional radiography on patients
from the US Food and Drug Administration Investigational Device Exemption randomized controlled trials (RCTs) comparing fusion and disk
arthroplasty show that fusion patients have slightly
reduced total lumbar motion postoperatively with
a significant increase in the segmental contribution
of the first cranial adjacent level to the total range
of motion.[54,55] Axelsson and colleagues[56,57] used
the radiostereometry method to study the lumbar
kinematics of fusion patients. Their results showed
that, although hypermobility of the adjacent
segment was seen in individual patients after
a spinal fusion, it was relatively infrequent. At
five-years after lumbar fusion, no significant differences between the preoperative and postoperative motions were detected in the nine fusion
patients included in the study.[55] Interindividual
differences were significant, with the adjacent
segments showing either unchanged, increased
or decreased motion compared with the preoperative situation.[56] Auerbach and colleagues[58] used
videofluoroscopy in five patients after circumferential lumbar fusion and noticed that the angular
motion of the proximal adjacent segment was
significantly more than in asymptomatic controls.
However, because they did not have information
on the preoperative range of motion of their fusion

patients, the results of this small group of patients
might reflect the interindividual variability shown
by Axelsson and colleagues.[56,57] In conclusion,
whether fusion patients will try to maintain their
preoperative lumbar range of motion postoperatively or are content with a restricted mobility is still
a matter of debate.

Alterations in the lumbar muscle function probably play a significant role in the in vivo kinematics
and kinetics of the spine after a fusion procedure.
Damage to these muscles undoubtedly happens
but, to date, this has been an understudied effect.

Adjacent Segment Intradiscal Pressure

Most in vitro biomechanical studies have demonstrated significant changes in the intradiscal
pressure (IDP) of the adjacent disks after simulated fusion suggesting altered anterior column
stresses.[38,45,47,49,59,60] The superior adjacent
segment IDP increased with flexion loading, and
increased and decreased IDP has been noted
with extension loading.[38,45,47,59,60] With flexion
loading, increases in IDP seem more marked after
longer fusions.[38,59] Specifically, an in vitro study
on human cadaveric spines found the IDP to be
increased by 30% after one-level fusion, and by
82% after two-level fusion.[59] Again, changes in
IDP have been shown in all unfused levels.[38]
Contrary to the previous studies, a validated
FEM detected only slight changes in the IDP by
rigid fixation.[49] in vivo IDPs after lumbar fusion
are difficult to measure and remain unknown.

These results must be interpreted with caution in
light of the previous discussion on biomechanical
testing methods used in the assessment of
adjacent segment changes. If a load-controlled
strategy is used there will not be substantial pressure changes in the adjacent segment intervertebral disks. However, if a displacement-controlled
strategy is adopted, then the loading across the
adjacent segment will increase and this will result
in increased intradiscal pressures. As outlined
previously, it is not known which protocol is more
germane to the clinical scenario.

Adjacent Segment Facet Joint Loads

Increased facet joint forces at the level above
a fusion, suggesting increased posterior column
stresses, have been demonstrated by Lee and
Langrana[35] using human cadaveric specimens
and by Rohlmann and colleagues[49] in a validated
FEM, especially with flexion loading. Corrobo-
rating these data with physiologic in vivo loading
is difficult. The previous discussion regarding the
link between the biomechanical methodology
used and the observed load changes at the

adjacent segment applies here for the facet joint contact forces.

RISK FACTORS FOR ASD
Individual Patient Characteristics

The age of the patient at the time of surgery seems to play a role in the development of ASD. Some clinical studies have shown that older patients have a significantly higher risk of developing ASD after a lumbar fusion.[17,27] In a systematic review on ASD and adjacent segment disease after lumbar fusion and disk arthroplasty, Harrop and colleagues[61] identified older age as a risk factor for radiographic ASD changes but, for the development of symptomatic adjacent segment problems, age was no longer a significant factor. However, several retrospective series have not been able to identify age as a significant risk factor for the development of ASD.[16,18,26,30] Clinical experience suggests that ASD would be more common in postmenopausal osteoporotic female patients. The literature has not been able to define gender as a significant risk factor for ASD changes,[18,27,61] although male gender seems to increase the risk of symptomatic ASD and reoperation.[17,61] Of patient-specific anatomic features, lamina inclination of the vertebra above and tropism of the adjacent facet joints have gained most attention. Facet tropism does not seem to be an independent risk factor for ASD[26,28]; however, significantly more asymmetry of the adjacent facet joints has been shown in those patients with earlier reoperations after the index surgery.[62] The role of the lamina inclination angle of the superior adjacent vertebra is controversial with some studies suggesting it is a possible risk factor for ASD[62] and others finding it nonsignificant.[28]

General Surgery-Related Risk Factors

Length of follow-up seems to be a significant risk factor for identifying adjacent level changes; the longer the follow-up the higher the incidence of ASD.[16,28] Interestingly, a recent systematic review identified a shorter follow-up as a risk factor for symptomatic ASD,[61] suggesting that those adjacent segment changes developing relatively soon after the index surgery have a higher risk of being symptomatic.

Whether the end vertebra of a fusion should be selected, such that the first adjacent segment is not degenerated, or whether the fusion can be ended below a degenerated, but presumably asymptomatic segment, remains a clinical problem. In retrospective clinical studies, preexisting disk degeneration of the first unfused segment has not been a significant risk factor for the development of symptomatic ASD.[25,26] It has been suggested that dynamic fixation of radiologically degenerated segments adjacent to rigid fusion might be beneficial for the long-term survival of that segment. However, no significant biomechanical[50] or clinical[63] benefit of this approach has been shown.

Multilevel fusions have been reported to present with a higher risk of ASD compared with one-level fusions,[13–17,27] although the length of the fusion has not unequivocally predicted the emergence of ASD.[31] Moreover, in a survival analysis of 215 fusion patients with 6.7-year follow-up, patients with single-level fusion had a three times higher reoperation risk for ASD than those with a multilevel fusion.[18] In another survival analysis of 3,188 fusion patients, male patients over 61 years-old operated on for degenerative conditions with a multilevel fusion had a 6.6 times higher risk of reoperation compared with those patients who did not have these four risk factors (gender, age, diagnosis, and extent of fusion). They had only a 61% survival rate at 10 years compared with the 94% of the whole patient group.[17] Biomechanical studies give some support to the premise that multilevel fusions increase the risk of ASD; with longer fixations and simulated fusions, the adjacent level changes have been more pronounced.[39,43]

Role of Fusion Technique

In a mathematical analysis on the effects of different fusion types on the adjacent segment, Lee and Langrana[35] showed that, although all types of fusion increased the adjacent segment stresses, the effect of the posterior fusion was significantly greater than that of either an anterior or intertransverse posterolateral fusion. The latter induced the least amount of adversary effects to the adjacent segment. Construct stiffness seems to be an important factor in the development of ASD. An in vitro biomechanical study on human cadaveric spines suggested that an anterior or circumferential fusion might pose the adjacent segment to a greater risk of degenerative changes compared with a posterolateral fusion.[64] Moreover, Sudo and colleagues[60] showed in an in vitro study on bovine spines that an additional posterior interbody fusion may lead to higher adjacent segment stresses than a posterolateral fusion alone owing to significantly increased stiffness of the fusion construct.

It is claimed that instrumented posterior fusions increase the risk of ASD compared with noninstrumented fusions, partly because of the immediate rigidity and increased stiffness of the fusion construct, and partly due to the risk of violating the integrity of the adjacent facet joints of the upper-most instrumented vertebra. Postoperative CT scans have shown the superior segment facet joint violation to occur in 15% to 25% of the screws, and in 24% to 35% of the patients.[65–67] With the Roy-Camille technique of pedicle screw inser-tion,[68] the facet joint violation happens inevitably as part of the technique.[67] Whether the facet joint violation contributes to the origin of ASD remains unknown. In in vitro conditions, superior segment unilateral facet joint violation did not affect the adjacent level range of motion and, after bilateral facet joint violation, only axial rotation increased significantly.[43]

Clinical evidence on the role of the fusion tech-nique in ASD is scarce because, to date, most of the relevant data are based on retrospective patient series. Two RCTs have compared the rate of ASD after lumbar fusions using different techniques. Ekman and colleagues[12] published a follow-up of an RCT comparing conservative and surgical treatment of low-grade isthmic spon-dylolisthesis. Their surgical patients were further randomized into either a noninstrumented or in-strumented posterolateral fusion. At a 12.6-year follow-up, no significant difference in the preva-lence of ASD was seen between these two surgical groups. Another RCT comparing posterolateral in-strumented fusion with a circumferential fusion in the surgical treatment of isthmic spondylolisthesis and degenerative disk disease could not show any significant difference in the ASD between the surgical groups at 8-year to 13-year follow-ups.[14] Thus, such recent clinical data seem to be in conflict with the earlier biomechanical studies.

Role of Laminectomy

In a significant number of surgical procedures for degenerative conditions, a concomitant decom-pression is performed with the fusion. The decom-pression technique may significantly affect the later occurrence of ASD. Chen and colleagues[69] compared three different decompression techni-ques in an in vitro biomechanical study on porcine lumbar spines. They performed the decompres-sion by either preserving the cranial part of the spinous process of the uppermost level or by total laminectomy. With flexion-extension loading, the intervertebral motion of the superior adjacent segment after complete laminectomy was signifi-cantly larger than in the specimens where the posterior tension band (ie, the spinous process, supraspinous and interspinous ligaments) of the adjacent segment was preserved. The motion pattern of the partial laminectomy specimens

was identical to that of those specimens where the integrity of the posterior structures was fully preserved. In another biomechanical study on human cadaveric spines, superior segment disruption of the posterior tension band by lami-nectomy significantly increased the adjacent seg-ment flexion-extension motion.[43] Some clinical evidence further suggests an important role for the decompressive technique in the prevention of ASD. In a retrospective review of 101 spondylolis-thesis patients, Lai and colleagues[19] found a signif-icant difference in the incidence of ASD whether the attachment of the supraspinous ligament of the first superior adjacent segment was preserved (integrity) or not (nonintegrity). Specifically, the incidence of ASD was 6.5% in the integrity group and 24.3% in the nonintegrity group after a mini-mum 6-year follow-up. In a 12.6-year follow-up of 80 patients randomized to either conservative or surgical treatment (posterolateral fusion with or without laminectomy) of low-grade isthmic spon-dylolisthesis, accelerated ASD was noticed in fusion patients, especially when fusion was combined with laminectomy.[12] When laminectomy was performed at the time of fusion, the preva-lence of ASD at 12.6 years postoperatively was 47%. In patients with only a fusion, the prevalence of ASD was 12.5%. In conclusion, sacrificing the posterior tension band complex of the first adja-cent segment may lead to acceleration of ASD.

Role of Sagittal Balance

Unfavorable postoperative sagittal balance has been advocated as a risk factor for accelerated ASD. In an in vitro study on human cadaveric spines, Akamaru and colleagues[32] showed that a simulated hypolordotic fusion resulted in signifi-cant percentage increase of the flexion-extension motion of the superior adjacent segment. The percentage increase of the superior adjacent segment flexion-extension motion compared with the intact segment was −15% for the hyperlordotic fixation, +100% for the in situ fixation, and +225% for the hypolordotic fixation. However, the biome-chanical testing methodology used was load-controlled and, by definition, should not have caused alterations in the biomechanical perfor-mance of the adjacent segments. Hence, these results need to be interpreted with caution. Never-theless, their findings have been corroborated by others.[33,60,70] However, in one in vitro study, the configuration of the immobilized segment had minimal effect on the biomechanical behavior of the adjacent segment.[36] In an in vivo study with skeletally mature sheep, fusion of the index level in kyphosis induced compensatory hyperlordosis, especially at the upper adjacent level, as well as significant degenerative changes of the superior facet joints and lordotic contracture of the posterior ligaments.[71] A compensatory hyperlordosis in the superior mobile levels adjacent to a hypolordotic instrumented segment has also been verified clinically.[70]

Several clinical studies have shown increased incidence of postoperative sagittal balance problems in patients with ASD, specifically loss of preoperative standing lumbar lordosis and a lower postoperative sacral inclination angle (ie, so-called vertical sacrum).[11,23,72] The vertical sacrum seems to be an especially important factor because it has significantly increased the incidence of ASD, even in the presence of normal C7 plumb line.[21] Again, controversy exists because some clinical studies have found the sagittal balance parameters to be of minimal significance in the development of ASD.[26,31]

DOES NONFUSION TECHNOLOGY PROTECT THE ADJACENT SEGMENT?

Proponents of nonfusion technology hypothesize that, by preserving the motion of the index level, the adjacent segments will be protected from subsequent degenerative changes. A recent systematic review reported significantly higher incidence of radiographic and symptomatic ASD after fusion compared with disk arthroplasty.[61] Specifically, fusion patients were 4.7-times more likely to develop radiographic ASD, and 13.9-times more likely to represent with symptomatic ASD than disk arthroplasty patients. However, the meta-analysis is based on grade III and IV data only, so the results have to be interpreted with caution. Furthermore, clinical studies have not demonstrated any significant benefit of different dynamic fixation devices compared with fusion procedures.[53,73,74] However, in one study, symptomatic ASD developed significantly later with dynamic fixation compared with fusion.[73] This minor clinical benefit is reflected in the biomechanical studies, which have shown no difference in the adjacent segment behavior after either a dynamic or a rigid fixation.[46,49,75] In the recent literature on disk arthroplasty, incidences of ASD have varied between 4.3% and 29% with follow-ups ranging from 32 months to 8.7 years.[76–79] The protective effect of index level motion would be reinforced by a connection between the motion of the total disk replacement and the radiographic incidence of ASD. In one clinical series, no patients with more than 5° of motion at the disk arthroplasty level developed ASD during the 8.7-year follow-up, whereas the incidence of ASD was 34% in

those patients with less than 5° of segmental motion at the arthroplasty level.[76] However, Siepe and colleagues[79] did not notice any significant correlation between the mean postoperative index level mobility and the development of ASD at 53 months after disk arthroplasty. In conclusion, the current evidence is not sufficient to confirm the protective effect of the motion-preserving technology to the adjacent segment compared with fusion surgery.

IS ASD A FUSION DISEASE?

An in vivo animal study has demonstrated degenerative changes on MRI at the adjacent levels 12 months after a posterolateral lumbar fusion.[80] However, with a shorter 6-month follow-up no degenerative changes in adjacent disks were seen.[81]

Several clinical case series with long-term follow-up up to 33 years have compared the incidence of ASD after a lumbar fusion to the incidence of degenerative changes in the asymptomatic population. Higher frequency of both disk and facet joint degeneration has been demonstrated after fusion surgery.[5,6,8] Specifically, a 12.6-year follow-up of two cohorts of an RCT, one randomized to conservative treatment for low-grade isthmic spondylolisthesis and the other to posterolateral fusion, reported accelerated ASD in the fusion group.[12] However, none of the studies found any relationship between radiographic ASD and clinical outcome. In similar long-term follow-ups, Seitsalo and colleagues[10] reporting on patients with surgical treatment for isthmic spondylolisthesis, and Wai and colleagues[9] reporting 20.5 years after anterior interbody fusion, noted no significant difference in the rate of degenerative changes in the surgical patients compared with findings in an asymptomatic population. Indeed, MRI studies on asymptomatic populations have shown progression of disk degeneration in up to 46% of the subjects in 5-year follow-up.[82,83] Also, a 16-year follow-up of a low back pain population showed significant progression of disk degeneration on MRI, such that 60% of the lumbar disks of the on an average 37-year old subjects were degenerated.[84]

Finally, if the muscles are damaged because of the surgery, which we know that they are, then the spine will not be functioning in the same way postoperatively as compared with the preoperative clinical situation. The loading on the disk may be increased—for reasons other than those addressed in the previously discussed in vitro studies—not because of the rigidity of the fused segments alone but because of a more comprehensive alteration in the kinematics and kinetics of the lumbar spine.

SUMMARY

Radiographic ASD is a common finding after a lumbar spine fusion. Literature suggests that most patients with ASD remain asymptomatic and a surgical intervention is indicated in relatively few patients. The true incidence of ASD and its clinical impact, however, are difficult to define because most of our knowledge is based on retrospective clinical series with different methodologies and definitions of ASD, heterogeneous patient populations, and variable lengths of follow-up.

In vitro and in vivo studies on the effects of spinal fusion on the adjacent segment behavior have reported controversial results. The challenges the lumbar spine confronts after a fusion procedure remain largely unknown. If the patient attempts to reproduce the same amount of lumbar motion after fusion surgery as before, the adjacent segments might be subjected to increased demands and, therefore, be more susceptible to accelerated degeneration. On the other hand, if the patient is content with less lumbar motion, which presumably loads the adjacent segments to a level comparable to that of the preoperative situation, no significant changes in the adjacent segment stresses should be expected. This raises the question of whether activity restrictions after lumbar fusion would be beneficial in protecting the adjacent segments from subsequent degeneration.

Based on the current evidence, the causes of ASD remain unknown. Proponents of a mechanical explanation to ASD, as well as those who see it as a natural progression of an underlying degenerative disease, will find support for their view in the literature. Probably, the most plausible explanation for the origin of degenerative changes at the adjacent segments is multifactorial, consisting of both mechanical and functional consequences of the fusion procedure itself, and of the individual characteristics of the patient. While waiting for the ultimate answer, the spine surgeon should take into consideration several aspects to minimize the risk of subsequent ASD in an individual patient; namely, meticulous preservation of the superior facet joints in case of instrumented posterior fusion, careful consideration of the decompression technique, and maintenance of the patient's individual sagittal alignment.

REFERENCES

1. Albee FH. Transplantation of a portion of the tibia into the spine for Pott's disease. JAMA 1911;57:885.

2. Hibbs RA. An operation for progressive spinal deformities. NY Med J 1911;93:1013.

3. Anderson CE. Spondyloschisis following spine fusion. J Bone Joint Surg Am 1956;38:1142–6.

4. Unander-Scharin L. A case of spondylolisthesis lumbalis aquisita. Acta Orthop Scand 1950;19:536–44.

5. Lehmann TR, Spratt KF, Tozzi JE, et al. Long-term follow-up of lower lumbar fusion patients. Spine 1987;12:97–104.

6. Kumar MN, Jacquot F, Hall H. Long-term follow-up of functional outcomes and radiographic changes at adjacent levels following lumbar spine fusion for degenerative disc disease. Eur Spine J 2001;10: 309–13.

7. Hambly MF, Wiltse LL, Raghavan N, et al. The transition zone above a lumbosacral fusion. Spine 1998;23:1785–92.

8. Remes VM, Lamberg TS, Tervahartiala PO, et al. No correlation between patient outcome and abnormal lumbar MRI findings 21 years after posterior or posterolateral fusion for isthmic spondylolisthesis in children and adolescents. Eur Spine J 2005;14:833–42.

9. Wai EK, Santos ER, Morcom R, et al. Magnetic resonance imaging 20 years after anterior lumbar interbody fusion. Spine 2006;31:1952–6.

10. Seitsalo S, Schlenzka D, Poussa M, et al. Disc degeneration in young patients with isthmic spondylolisthesis treated operatively or conservatively: a long-term follow-up. Eur Spine J 1997;6:393–7.

11. Disch AC, Schmoelz W, Matziolis G, et al. Higher risk of adjacent segment degeneration after floating fusions: long-term outcome after low lumbar spine fusions. J Spinal Disord Tech 2008;21:79–85.

12. Ekman P, Möller H, Shalabi A, et al. A prospective randomized study on the long-term effect of lumbar fusion on adjacent disc degeneration. Eur Spine J 2009;18:1175–86.

13. Schulte TL, Leistra F, Bullmann V, et al. Disc height reduction in adjacent segments and clinical outcome 10 years after lumbar 360° fusion. Eur Spine J 2007;16:2152–8.

14. Videbaek T, Egund N, Christensen FB, et al. Adjacent segment degeneration after lumbar spinal fusion: the impact of anterior column support. A randomized clinical trial with an eight- to thirteen-year magnetic resonance imaging follow-up. Spine 2010;35:1955–64.

15. Cheh G, Bridwell KH, Lenke LG, et al. Adjacent segment disease following lumbar/thoracolumbar fusion with pedicle screw instrumentation. A minimum 5-year follow-up. Spine 2007;32:2253–7.

16. Gillet P. The fate of the adjacent motion segments after lumbar fusion. J Spinal Disord Tech 2003;16: 338–45.

17. Ahn DK, Park HS, Choi DJ, et al. Survival and prognostic analysis of adjacent segments after spinal fusion. Clin Orthop Surg 2010;2:140–7.

18. Ghiselli G, Wang JC, Bhatia NN, et al. Adjacent segment degeneration in the lumbar spine. J Bone Joint Surg Am 2004;86:1497–503.
19. Lai PL, Chen LH, Niu CC, et al. Relation between laminectomy and development of adjacent segment instability after lumbar fusion with pedicle fixation. Spine 2004;29:2527–32.
20. Miyakoshi N, Abe E, Shimada Y, et al. Outcome of one-level posterior lumbar interbody fusion for spondylolisthesis and postoperative intervertebral disc degeneration adjacent to the fusion. Spine 2000; 25:1837–42.
21. Kumar MN, Baklanov A, Chopin D. Correlation between sagittal plane changes and adjacent segment degeneration following lumbar spine fusion. Eur Spine J 2001;10:314–9.
22. Chou WY, Hsu CJ, Chang WN, et al. Adjacent segment degeneration after lumbar spinal posterolateral fusion with instrumentation in elderly patients. Arch Orthop Trauma Surg 2002;122:39–43.
23. Min JH, Jang JS, Jung BJ, et al. The clinical characteristics and risk factors for the adjacent segment degeneration in instrumented lumbar fusion. J Spinal Disord Tech 2008;21:305–9.
24. Etebar S, Cahill DW. Risk factors for adjacent-segment failure following lumbar fixation with rigid instrumentation for degenerative instability. J Neurosurg 1999;90:163–9.
25. Throckmorton TW, Hilibrand AS, Mencio GA, et al. The impact of adjacent level disc degeneration on health status outcomes following lumbar fusion. Spine 2003;28:2546–50.
26. Okuda S, Iwasaki M, Miyauchi A, et al. Risk factors for adjacent segment degeneration after PLIF. Spine 2004;29:1535–40.
27. Aota Y, Kumano K, Hirabayashi S. Postfusion instability at the adjacent segments after rigid pedicle screw fixation for degenerative lumbar spinal disorders. J Spinal Disord 1995;8:464–73.
28. Kaito T, Hosono N, Mukai Y, et al. Induction of early degeneration of the adjacent segment after posterior lumbar interbody fusion by excessive distraction of lumbar disc space. J Neurosurg Spine 2010;12: 671–9.
29. Park JY, Cho YE, Kuh SU, et al. New prognostic factors for adjacent segment degeneration after one-stage 360° fixation for spondylolytic spondylolisthesis: special reference to the usefulness of pelvic incidence angle. J Neurosurg Spine 2007;7: 139–44.
30. Lee CH, Hwang CJ, Lee SW, et al. Risk factors for adjacent segment disease after lumbar fusion. Eur Spine J 2009;18:1637–43.
31. Pellisé F, Hernández A, Vidal X, et al. Radiologic assessment of all unfused lumbar segments 7.5 years after instrumented posterior spinal fusion. Spine 2007;32:574–9.
32. Akamaru T, Kawahara N, Yoon ST, et al. Adjacent segment motion after a simulated lumbar fusion in different sagittal alignments. A biomechanical analysis. Spine 2003;28:1560–6.
33. Chen WJ, Lai PL, Tai CL, et al. The effect of sagittal alignment on adjacent joint mobility after lumbar instrumentation—a biomechanical study of lumbar vertebrae in a porcine model. Clin Biomech 2004; 19:763–8.
34. Ghiselli G, Wang JC, Hsu WK, et al. L5-S1 segment survivorship and clinical outcome analysis after L4-L5 isolated fusion. Spine 2003;28:1275–80.
35. Lee CK, Langrana NA. Lumbosacral spinal fusion. A biomechanical study. Spine 1984;9:574–81.
36. Ha KY, Schendel MJ, Lewis JL, et al. Effect of immobilization and configuration on lumbar adjacent-segment biomechanics. J Spinal Disord 1993;6: 99–105.
37. Dekutoski MB, Schendel MJ, Ogilvie JW, et al. Comparison of in vivo and in vitro adjacent segment motion after lumbar fusion. Spine 1994;19:1745–51.
38. Chow DH, Luk KD, Evans JH, et al. Effects of short anterior lumbar interbody fusion on biomechanics of neighboring unfused segments. Spine 1996;21: 549–55.
39. Shono Y, Kaneda K, Abumi K, et al. Stability of posterior spinal instrumentation and its effects on adjacent motion segments in the lumbosacral spine. Spine 1998;23:1550–8.
40. Bastian L, Lange U, Knop C, et al. Evaluation of the mobility of adjacent segments after posterior thoracolumbar fixation: a biomechanical study. Eur Spine J 2001;10:295–300.
41. Nohara H, Kanaya F. Biomechanical study of adjacent intervertebral motion after lumbar spinal fusion and flexible stabilization using polyethylene-terephthalate bands. J Spinal Disord Tech 2004;17: 215–9.
42. Panjabi M, Malcolmson G, Teng F, et al. Hybrid testing of lumbar CHARITÉ Discs versus fusions. Spine 2007;32:959–66.
43. Cardoso MJ, Dmitriev AE, Helgeson M, et al. Does superior-segment facet violation or laminectomy destabilize the adjacent level in lumbar transpedicular fixation? An in vitro human cadaveric assessment. Spine 2008;33:2868–73.
44. Ingalhalikar AV, Reddy CG, Lim TH, et al. Effect of lumbar total disc arthroplasty on the segmental motion and intradiscal pressure at the adjacent level: an in vitro biomechanical study. J Neurosurg Spine 2009;11:715–23.
45. Rohlmann A, Neller S, Bergmann G, et al. Effect of an internal fixator and a bone graft on intersegmental spinal motion and intradiscal pressure in the adjacent regions. Eur Spine J 2001;10:301–8.
46. Schmoelz W, Huber JF, Nydegger T, et al. Dynamic stabilization of the lumbar spine and its effects on

adjacent segments. An in vitro experiment. J Spinal Disord Tech 2003;16:418–23.

47. Rao RD, David KS, Wang M. Biomechanical changes at adjacent segments following anterior lumbar interbody fusion using tapered cages. Spine 2005;30:2772–6.

48. Denozière G, Ku DN. Biomechanical comparison between fusion of two vertebrae and implantation of an artificial intervertebral disc. J Biomech 2006; 39:766–75.

49. Rohlmann A, Burra NK, Zander T, et al. Comparison of the effects of bilateral posterior dynamic and rigid fixation devices on the loads in the lumbar spine: a finite element analysis. Eur Spine J 2007;16: 1223–31.

50. Strube P, Tohtz S, Hoff E, et al. Dynamic stabilization adjacent to single-level fusion: part I. Biomechanical effects on lumbar spinal motion. Eur Spine J 2010; 19(12):2171–80.

51. Panjabi MM. Hybrid multidirectional test method to evaluate spinal adjacent-level effects. Clin Biomech 2007;22:257–65.

52. Luk KD, Chow DH, Evans JH, et al. Lumbar spinal mobility after short anterior interbody fusion. Spine 1995;20(7):813–8.

53. Cakir B, Carazzo C, Schmidt R, et al. Adjacent segment mobility after rigid and semirigid instrumentation of the lumbar spine. Spine 2009;34: 1287–91.

54. Cunningham BW, McAfee PC, Geisler FH, et al. Distribution of in vivo and in vitro range of motion following 1-level arthroplasty with the CHARITÉ artificial disc compared with fusion. J Neurosurg Spine 2008;8:7–12.

55. Auerbach JD, Jones KJ, Milby AH, et al. Segmental contribution toward total lumbar range of motion in disc replacement and fusions. A comparison of operative and adjacent levels. Spine 2009;34:2510–7.

56. Axelsson P, Johnsson R, Strömqvist B. The spondylolytic vertebra and its adjacent segment: mobility measured before and after posterolateral fusion. Spine 1997;22:414–7.

57. Axelsson P, Johnsson R, Strömqvist B. Adjacent segment hypermobility after lumbar spine fusion. No association with progressive degeneration of the segment 5 years after surgery. Acta Orthop 2007;78:834–9.

58. Auerbach JD, Wills BP, McIntosh TC, et al. Evaluation of spinal kinematics following lumbar total disc replacement and circumferential fusion using in vivo fluoroscopy. Spine 2007;32:527–36.

59. Weinhoffer SL, Guyer RD, Herbert M, et al. Intradiscal pressure measurements above an instrumented fusion. A cadaveric study. Spine 1995;20:526–31.

60. Sudo H, Oda I, Abumi K, et al. in vitro biomechanical effects of reconstruction on adjacent motion segment: comparison of aligned/kyphotic posterolateral fusion with aligned posterior lumbar interbody fusion/posterolateral fusion. J Neurosurg Spine 2003;99:221–8.

61. Harrop JS, Youssef JA, Maltenfort M, et al. Lumbar adjacent segment degeneration and disease after arthrodesis and total disc arthroplasty. Spine 2008; 33:1701–7.

62. Okuda S, Oda T, Miyauchi A, et al. Lamina horizontalization and facet tropism as the risk factors for adjacent segment degeneration after PLIF. Spine 2008;33:2754–8.

63. Putzier M, Hoff E, Tohtz S, et al. Dynamic stabilization adjacent to single-level fusion: part II. No clinical benefit for asymptomatic, initially degenerated adjacent segments after 6 years follow-up. Eur Spine J 2010;19(12):2181–9.

64. Esses SI, Doherty BJ, Crawford MJ, et al. Kinematic evaluation of lumbar fusion techniques. Spine 1996; 21:676–84.

65. Shah RR, Mohammed S, Saifuddin A, et al. Radiologic evaluation of adjacent superior segment facet joint violation following transpedicular instrumentation of the lumbar spine. Spine 2003;28:272–5.

66. Moshirfar A, Jenis LG, Spector LR, et al. Computed tomography evaluation of superior-segment facet-joint violation after pedicle instrumentation of the lumbar spine with a midline surgical approach. Spine 2006;31:2624–9.

67. Chen Z, Zhao J, Xu H, et al. Technical factors related to the incidence of adjacent superior segment facet joint violation after transpedicular instrumentation in the lumbar spine. Eur Spine J 2008;17:1476–80.

68. Roy-Camille R, Roy-Camille M, Demeulenaere C. Osteosynthesis of dorsal, lumbar, and lumbosacral spine with metallic plates screwed into vertebral pedicles and articular apophyses. Presse Med 1970;78:1447–8 [in French].

69. Chen LH, Lai PL, Tai CL, et al. The effect of interspinous ligament integrity on adjacent segment instability after lumbar instrumentation and laminectomy—an experimental study in porcine model. Biomed Mater Eng 2006;16:261–7.

70. Umehara S, Zindrick MR, Patwardhan AG, et al. The biomechanical effect of postoperative hypolordosis in instrumented lumbar fusion on instrumented and adjacent spinal segments. Spine 2000;25:1617–24.

71. Oda I, Cunningham BW, Buckley RA, et al. Does spinal kyphotic deformity influence the biomechanical characteristics of the adjacent motion segments? An in vivo animal model. Spine 1999;24: 2139–46.

72. Djurasovic M, Carreon LY, Glassman SD, et al. Sagittal alignment as a risk factor for adjacent level degeneration: a case-control study. Orthopedics 2008;31:546.

73. Kanayama M, Togawa D, Hashimoto T, et al. Motion-preserving surgery can prevent early breakdown of

adjacent segments. Comparison of posterior dynamic stabilization with spinal fusion. J Spinal Disord Tech 2009;22:463–7.

74. Kumar A, Beastall J, Hughes J, et al. Disc changes in the bridged and adjacent segments after Dynesys dynamic stabilization system after two years. Spine 2008;33:2909–14.

75. Schmoelz W, Huber JF, Nydegger T, et al. Influence of a dynamic stabilisation system on load bearing of a bridged disc: an in vitro study of intradiscal pressure. Eur Spine J 2006;15:1276–85.

76. Huang RC, Tropiano P, Marnay T, et al. Range of motion and adjacent level degeneration after lumbar total disc replacement. Spine J 2006;6:242–7.

77. Shim CS, Lee SH, Shin HD, et al. CHARITÉ versus ProDisc: a comparative study of a minimum 3-year follow-up. Spine 2007;32:1012–8.

78. Park CK, Ryu KS, Jee WH. Degenerative changes of disks and facet joints in lumbar total disc replacement using ProDisc II: minimum two-year follow-up. Spine 2008;33:1755–61.

79. Siepe CJ, Zelenkov P, Sauri-Barraza JC, et al. The fate of facet joint and adjacent level disc degeneration following total lumbar disc replacement. A prospective clinical, x-ray, and magnetic resonance imaging investigation. Spine 2010;35:1991–2003.

80. Higashino K, Hamasaki T, Kim JH, et al. Do the adjacent level intervertebral discs degenerate after a lumbar spinal fusion? An experimental study using a rabbit model. Spine 2010;35:E1144–52.

81. Hoogendoorn RJ, Helder MN, Wuisman PI, et al. Adjacent segment degeneration. Observations in a goat spinal fusion study. Spine 2008;33(12): 1337–43.

82. Elfering A, Semmer N, Birkhofer D, et al. Risk factors for lumbar disc degeneration: a 5-year prospective MRI study in asymptomatic individuals. Spine 2002;27:125–34.

83. Videman T, Battié MC, Ripatti S, et al. Determinants of the progression in lumbar degeneration: a 5-year follow-up study of adult male monozygotic twins. Spine 2006;31:671–8.

84. Waris E, Eskelin M, Hermunen H, et al. Disc degeneration in low back pain. A 17-year follow-up study using magnetic resonance imaging. Spine 2007; 32:681–4.

Prosthetic Total Disk Replacement—Can We Learn from Total Hip Replacement?

H. Michael Mayer, MD, PhD[a,b,*],
Christoph J. Siepe, MD, PhD[a,b]

KEYWORDS

- Total disk replacement • Spine arthroplasty • Clinical
- Outcomes • Prospective

Surgical fusion of lumbar motion segments has been widely accepted as a treatment option for degenerative low back pain in patients who fail to respond to conservative therapy (see the article by Fritzell and colleagues for further exploration of this topic).[1] Various fusion methods have resulted in acceptable clinical outcomes for a variety of degenerative pathologies.[2–11] Improvements in implant technologies (eg, pedicle screws, cages), access techniques (eg, open, mini-open, percutaneous, navigation), as well as the use of osteoconductive (eg, bone substitutes) and/or osteoinductive (eg, bone morphogenetic proteins [BMP]) have facilitated recent advancements in lumbar fusion technology. However, the influence on the expected improvement in surgical outcome remains unclear.

Although it took more than 90 years from the first written report on instrumented spinal fusion to the first randomized controlled study,[1,12] spinal fusion has always been accepted as a surgical "gold standard." In 2006, Weinstein and colleagues[13] reported more than 200,000 lumbar fusion procedures were performed annually in the United States between 1992 and 2003. Reoperation rates following lumbar fusion reach 11.9% to 27.4% in follow-up periods between 3 to 15 years.

Complication rates up to 70% have been reported, as well as adjacent segment alterations in 31% to 66% of cases.[14–23] These significant disadvantages, however, have not led to a significant reconsideration of fusion procedures because, for many years, it was the only option surgeons had for the treatment of degenerative low back pain. The worldwide introduction of lumbar total disk replacement (TDR) since the end of the 1990s has produced paradoxic, controversial, and occasionally irrational reactions among surgeons, regulatory institutions, health care insurance companies, and health care providers.

In most European countries, lumbar TDR has become a well established and well accepted therapeutic option (which has not led to an increase in total lumbar surgical procedures) with good-to-excellent midterm results.[24–31] Several studies have proven the usefulness of this procedure, its noninferiority or superiority to lumbar fusion in selected patients, and its safety when it comes to reoperations or complications.[32–36] Other studies have shown the cost-effectiveness compared with fusion.[37–40] The fact that this scientific data are not accepted by health care administrations and insurance companies in some health care systems around the world suggests that these

Disclosure: There was no financial support for this article. HMM and CJS are consultants to Synthes Inc, Oberdorf, Switzerland.

[a] Paracelsus Medical School, Srrubergasse 21, A- 5020, Salzburg, Austria
[b] Spine Center, Schön Klinik Muenchen-Harlaching, Harlachinger Street 51, D-81547 Munich, Germany
* Corresponding author. Spine Center, Schön Klinik München Harlaching, Harlachinger Street 51, D-81547 Munich, Germany.
E-mail address: MMayer@schoen-kliniken.de

orthopedic.theclinics.com

processes are not driven by the needs of the patient. Assuming that it is neither a lack of knowledge nor a lack of common sense, nor ignorance of sound scientific work, the reasons for this are obviously political and economic.

To give an update of prosthetic lumbar disk replacement at the beginning of the second decade of this century, it is helpful to have a look into the past and learn from similar developments. In 2009, there were two anniversaries: (1) 50 years since the first implantation of a prosthetic total hip by Sir John Charnley (**Fig. 1**) and (2) 25 years since the first implantation of an artificial disk by Buettner and Schellnack (**Fig. 2**).[41,42] William H. Harris published an article in 2009 in which he reviewed the first 50 years of total hip replacement (THR).[41] Over the years, five observations were made ("skunk works," Pasteur's motto, totally unexpected, research solutions, and the role of alternatives), which more or less characterize the process that THR underwent from the very early attempts and failures to become one of the most successful procedures in orthopedic surgery. In fact, these observations have become a paradigm for what we have experienced in the 25 years since the introduction of lumbar TDR.

SKUNK WORKS

The "very non-traditional effort, which is offline, off-budget, remarkably innovative, driven by creative zealots, uninhibited by failure, and relentless." This is how Harris[41] characterized "skunk work" in the

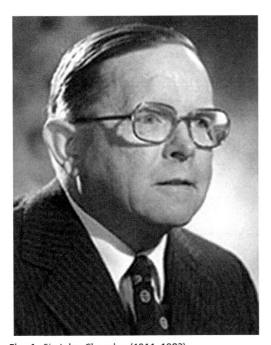

Fig. 1. Sir John Charnley (1911–1982).

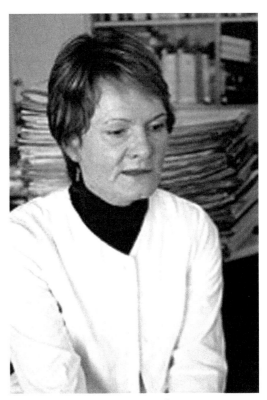

Fig. 2. Karin Büttner-Janz, MD, PhD, 1952.

early days of THR. It was the early failure of Teflon-on-Teflon interfaces, problems with indications, and surgical technique. Looking at some examples of early lumbar disk replacements, we can observe similar "skunk works" such as wrong indications, subsiding of the implant, or spontaneous fusion after disk replacement (**Fig. 3**A, B). Once a technique works, the risk of over-use increases, especially if the indications are not yet standardized or proven. Some typical examples of so-called off-label use of TDR are shown in **Fig. 3**C, D. Interestingly, and sometimes fortunately, these applications did not always lead to an unsatisfactory clinical outcome. In summary, there is an analogy between what happened in the early years of THR and TDR. It reflects the surgeons' attempts to push a technology to its limits.

PASTEUR'S MOTTO

"Chance favors the prepared mind" was one of Louis Pasteur's favorite mottos. It was by chance that Sir John Charnley met Dennis Smith, Chemist at Turner Dental Hospital in Manchester. Smith suggested the use methylmethacrylate for the fixation of hip implants and triggered the development of cemented hip arthroplasty. The history of prosthetic disk replacement is coupled to a historical

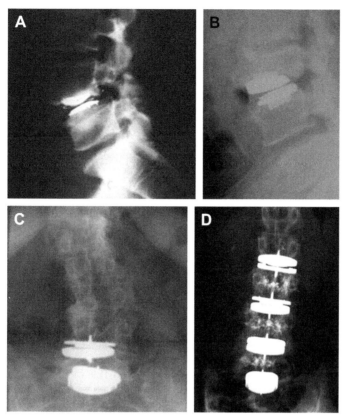

Fig. 3. "Skunk works" in the history of TDR. (*A*) Wrong indication: TDR in a patient with isthmic type spondylolisthesis. (*B*) Wrong indication: TDR at L3-4 with a previously fractured L3 vertebral body. (*C*) Off-label use: TDR in degenerative lumbar scoliosis. (*D*) Off-label use: 4-level TDR combined with vertebroplasty in an osteoporotic patient. (*From* Harris WH. The first 50 years of total hip arthroplasty: lessons learned. Clin Orthop Relat Res 2009;467:28–31; with permission.)

event—the fall of the Berlin Wall on November 9, 1989. The first total disk implant (SB Charité I) was invented and first implanted at the Charité University Hospital of the Humboldt University in the former German Democratic Republic (East Germany). After the reunification of the two Germanys, Link (Waldemar Link GmbH & Co KG, Barkhausenweg 10,D-22,339 Hamburg, Germany), a well known West German implant manufacturer with long experience in total hip and knee manufacturing, took over the technology and developed the further generations of the SB Charité total disk implant, which then became the first total disk prosthesis on the market.

THE TOTALLY UNEXPECTED

Applying new technologies implies the risk for unexpected adverse events or complications. The pioneers of THR certainly did not expect to create a new iatrogenic disease, periprosthetic osteolysis.[41,43] Total disks that are not mobile after the implantation are one result that nobody expected. Suboptimal placement of the implant and

segmental hyperlordosis due to sagittal imbalance are most probably responsible for this so-called locked-in scenario.[44–47] It is not clear whether loss of range of motion over time, heterotopic ossifications, or spontaneous fusions, which can occur in a small percentage of patients, are really unexpected.[48] It seems that a segment with a prosthetic disk behaves like a normal segment when it comes to the natural course.

RESEARCH SOLUTIONS—SCIENCE AND RANDOMIZED CONTROLLED TRIALS

Scientific workup in medicine takes time. It took 93 years between the first publication of an instrumented lumbar fusion in May 1908 and the first randomized controlled trial (RCT), which showed scientific evidence for the use of fusion in low back pain.[1,12] In 2000, 46 years after the description of laminectomy for the treatment of lumbar degenerative spinal stenosis, the first RCT proved its effectiveness.[49] Fortunately, it took just 21 years between the first implantation of a total disk (in former East Berlin in 1984) and the publication of the first Level I, evidence-based data in 2005.[32,34] The investigators proved "noninferiority" of the Charité disc (DePuy Spine, Raynham, MA, USA) as compared with BAK-cage (Orthofix Inc., Lewisville, TX, USA) supported anterior fusion. Although the success rates were not very convincing, neither were those in the control group after a 2-year follow-up. These results were recently confirmed after a 5-year follow-up period.[33] Two years later, the first RCT was published for the Prodisc Prosthesis (Synthes Inc, Paoli, PA, USA). In a study with 2 years of follow-up, Zigler and colleagues[36] demonstrated evidence for superior results of the Prodisc as compared with 360° fusion.

The Maverick disc (Medtronic, Memphis, TN, USA) was the third implant that received US Food and Drug Administration (FDA) approval. It proved to have less serious device-related adverse events and the patients returned to work earlier compared with stand-alone anterior interbody fusion. This study was the only one that compared two identical approaches (anterior interbody fusion vs TDR). Due to patent violations, this implant is currently not distributed in the United States.

The fourth RCT investigated the FlexiCore Disc (Stryker Spine, Allendale, NJ, USA).[35] In a 2-year follow-up of 67 patients from two sites that were involved in an FDA investigational device exemption (IDE) trial, the results were more or less the same as in other trials proving similar and, by some parameters, superior results compared with fusion. At the time this article was written (December 2010), the IDE study is completed and submitted, but the current status or results are unknown.

Recently, results of a RCT comparing two total disks were presented.[50] The Kineflex Disc (SpinalMotion, Mountain View, CA, USA) was compared with the Charité disc (control group) in 457 patients from 21 sites. Both groups showed significant improvement of clinical parameters, such as the Visual Analog Scale (VAS) and Oswestry Disability Index (ODI) scores, with no significant difference between the groups.[50] This IDE study is also completed and currently reviewed by the FDA.

Although scientific evidence was generated within a relatively short period of time, health care providers and health insurances in some countries still have difficulties accepting TDR as a standard procedure. From a scientific point of view, such attitudes seem to be driven by irrational fears:

- TDR could wipe away fusion technology and could lead to a dramatic increase in surgical procedures for low back pain.
- TDR would lead to uncontrollable increase of unforeseen sequelae, complications, and adverse events.

- TDR would dramatically increase the treatment costs for low back pain patients without improving the clinical results.

In countries where TDR has become a routine procedure, such developments have not been confirmed.

Costs

One concern of health care providers and insurance companies are the costs that are associated with new technology. In 2007, Guyer and colleagues[37] published an economic model of one-level lumbar arthroplasty versus fusion. The investigators analyzed the costs of the implant, hospital stay, operating room time, and so forth, and compared TDR with different types of lumbar fusion procedures (eg, transforaminal lumbar interbody fusion [TLIF], 360° fusion, anterior lumbar interbody fusion [ALIF]) and were able to show that, although the implant costs were similar to the other procedures, TDR is the least expensive type of treatment. In 2008, Patel and colleagues[38] were able to demonstrate that TDR costs are similar to TLIF or ALIF without BMP, that they are lower compared with TLIF or ALIF with BMP, and that they are definitely less when compared with 360° fusion. These results were confirmed as referred to the hospital charges for one-level procedures by Levin and colleagues.[39]

In summary, strong evidence has been published in the scientific literature that supports the safety and efficacy of TDR. Several prospective studies with 2-year to 5-year follow-up, as well as long-term results from outside the United States, prove that TDR results are at least as good as different types of fusion in comparable patient cohorts.[25,28,33,51] TDR is also similar or less expensive compared with various types of lumbar fusion procedures.[37–40] Although these results have been elaborated with different types of implants (different implant materials, different interfaces, varying kinematic characteristics, etc), there have been no significant differences in the overall clinical outcomes. This suggests that the influence of these different features on the outcome remains unclear.

Influence of Disk Pathology

The first years of TDR were dominated by discussions about the indication for this new type of treatment. The first prospective study analyzed the influence of different indications on the outcome of TDR.[30] Patients suffering from monosegmental or bisegmental degenerative disk disease with low back pain showed significant improvements in VAS and ODI within the first 3-year follow-up. It turned out that there were no significant differences between patients with or without Modic type I changes.

Influence of Previous Surgery

This study did not detect a significant difference in the clinical outcome when comparing patients with disk degeneration with or without previous discectomy surgery. This was confirmed by other independent study groups.[52–55] However, other investigators reported a negative effect on postoperative outcomes.[24,51,56–58] However, the results from these studies are not comparable with each other owing to differences in selection criteria. Patients with marked epidural scar tissue formation in the spinal canal on preoperative gadolinium diethylenetriaminopentaacetic acid-magnetic resonance imaging, as well as patients with significant facet joint alterations from the previous operation and patients with sciatica, were routinely excluded.[30]

Influence of Age

Similar findings were observed concerning the influence of age on the clinical outcomes of TDR. Several investigators described contradictory results with better outcomes in patients younger or older than 45 years.[55] Other investigators could not prove an influence of age on outcome.[53,59] There is, however, a general consensus that TDR should not be implanted in patients with reduced bone mineral density. In randomized controlled FDA IDE studies, patients with osteoporosis, osteopenia, or any type of metabolic bone disease were excluded.[32,35,36] There is still an ongoing discussion about which patients should have a dual energy x-ray absorptiometry (DXA) scan preoperatively. In a prospective series, DXA scans were performed in all women older than 45 years of age, in all men older than 55 years of age, as well as in all patients in whom either radiographs or the medical history showed signs or risk factors of osteopenia or osteoporosis.[29,60]

As compared with hip or knee arthroplasty, which can be performed even in elderly patients, TDR can rarely be performed in this age group. Besides the reduced bone mineral density, most of the older patients have other contraindications against TDR, such as spinal stenosis, degenerative deformities (de novo-scoliosis, degenerative spondylolisthesis, etc), as well as symptomatic and advanced facet joint osteoarthritis. All of these factors lead to a more or less natural selection of a younger patient cohort.

Influence of Anatomic Segments and Number of Levels on Outcomes

Several investigators have described similar or even superior clinical results in patients with double level implantations compared with single level TDR.[61–64] Others have described inferior clinical outcomes in multilevel implantations.[24,53] In a prospective series, the highest satisfaction rates were observed in patients with TDR at the level L4-5 (90.9% subjective patient satisfaction rate), followed by L5-S1 (78.9%). The lowest satisfaction rates were observed following double-level implantations—L4-5-S1 (65%).[29] The conclusion from these published data is that obviously TDR leads to good results in monosegmental implantations and the results also seem to be acceptable for selected bisegmental cases.

Complications

A wide variation of complication rates has been published in the last 16 years. The overall complication rates range from less than 1% to 39.7%.[24,28,36,51,54,63,65,66] At least part of these numbers represent the learning curves of individual surgeons. Access and technique-related complications seem to be dominant in most of the papers. The intraoperative and perioperative complication rates in the FDA IDE studies that were performed with the most widely used implants, Prodisc and Charité disc, did not show significant differences between the investigational and the control group.[32,36] Thus, previously published TDR complications rates are well within the range of complication rates that have been described for ALIF techniques.[67,68]

Reoperations

To date, there has been considerable concern that TDR might lead to frequent reoperations because of implant extrusions, subsiding, and/or loosening of the implant. These concerns were not confirmed in the studies published until now. The average reoperation rates within the first 2-years following TDR with the Prodisc and Charité disc were 3.7% and 5.4%, respectively.[32,36] McAfee and colleagues[69] published a reoperation rate of 8.8% following TDR in a series of 589 patients who received a disk replacement with the Charité disc. In another study, the reoperation rate within the first 2 years was 8.1%.[29] These rates do not differ from the ones published after lumbar fusion. Conversely, previously published reoperation rates following lumbar fusion procedures range between 11.9% and 27.4% within the first 3 to15 years postoperative.[14,17–21,23] The vast majority of reoperations in

TDR were performed in the early postoperative period and were mainly attributed to faults in either implantation technique or inappropriate indication for TDR.

Sagittal Balance

A postoperative sagittal malalignment is one potential disadvantageous effect of lumbar fusion procedures which may furthermore predispose the segments for adjacent level degeneration.[16,70–72] Conversely, previous studies have reported a maintained physiologic sagittal alignment following total lumbar disk replacement procedures.[27,47,73,74] While an improved sagittal alignment is one advantage of TDR over lumbar fusion procedures, a tendency for increased index-level hyperlordosis.[46,47,75,76] In a CT study, Liu and colleagues[75] reported a significant decrease of the facet joint articulation overlap in the sagittal plane and an increase in the facet joint space following an increase in the lumbar disk space. The authors concluded that an inappropriate increase of the disk space height will result in facet joint subluxation. Rohlmann and colleagues[76] similarly reported increasing intersegmental lordosis with increasing implant heights. The authors concluded that great care should be taken in choosing the optimal height and correct position of the implant. Clinical data similarly revealed an increased segmental lordosis and symptoms from the facet joints in a considerable number of patients postoperatively.[29,46,60] As a direct result of these studies, the authors have modified their disk replacement strategy over the years by choosing implants with less lordosis (≤6°) and the lowest available implant height (10 mm) for the majority of all patients.

Facet Joint Osteoarthritis

A variety of biomechanical studies have demonstrated increased facet joint pressures, segmental instability at the index level, and altered load patterns with sudden, instead of gradual, load increase in the facet joints following TDR.[54,77–87] Radiological studies have demonstrated an increased segmental hyperlordosis with the potential of subluxation of the facet joints.[45–47,74–76] Leivseth and colleagues[88] highlighted the disparity between the prosthesis and the anatomic center of rotation in patients treated with ProDisc II, particularly at the lumbosacral junction. Similarly, Rousseau and colleagues[83,89] highlighted aberrant centers of rotation following TDR and published possible consequences on facet joint contact forces.

Shim and colleagues[90] reported a 32% to 36.4% rate of degeneration of the facet joints

following TDR with Charité III and ProDisc II. Park and colleagues[91] observed progression of facet joint degeneration (FJD) in 29.3% of TDR segments at a follow-up of 32.2 months from grade 1 to grade 2, predominantly in women and 2-level TDR. In accordance with the above-mentioned studies by Shim and colleagues[90] and Park and colleagues,[91] other data similarly reveal a progression rate of FJD in a considerable number of patients (n = 44/220 facet joints; 20%).[44] The severity of FJD was, however, less than expected. A significant difference in FJD rates between the lumbosacral junction and the level L4-5 (23% vs 3.3%) was demonstrated.[44]

In summary, the data suggest that it is more likely a particular cohort of patients with inferior biomechanical compatibility that will experience complaints from the facet and sacroiliac joints[29,44,60] and who may stand an increased risk of developing FJD at later postoperative stages. Future studies will have to investigate whether these progressive degenerative changes will predominantly be limited to this particular cohort of patients with unfavorable biomechanical compatibility or if the overall patient population will be affected, which may have consequences for the long-term clinical results of lumbar disk replacement procedures.

Adjacent Segment Degeneration

Huang and colleagues[92] reported a 23.8% incidence (n = 10/42 segments) of adjacent level disease (ALD) following TDR with ProDisc I after a mean follow-up of 8.7 years. However, access to MRI was not available in the study setting. In a retrospective MRI and CT scan study, Park and colleagues[91] published a 4.3% progression rate of ALD in a cohort of 32 patients after a mean follow-up of 32.2 months following TDR with ProDisc II. Conversely, Shim and colleagues[90] reported a 19.4% to 28.6% incidence of ALD in a retrospective MRI investigation of 57 patients after a mean follow-up of 38 to 41 months.

An MRI analysis revealed a low incidence of ALD observed at 10.2% (n = 11/108) of all adjacent levels after an average follow-up of 53.4 months (range 24.1–98.7 months).[44] The degenerative changes were mild and signs of ALD occurred late postoperatively after an average follow-up of 62.5 months. Finally, the occurrence of ALD did not negatively affect the clinical symptomatology. Therefore, these results are in congruence with findings that have previously been published by a variety of independent biomechanical and radiological studies that demonstrated an unloading effect of TDR on adjacent levels compared with fusion procedures.[85,93–95]

Prognostic Factors

Predictors of outcome have been investigated for a variety of pathologies and interventions.[96–106] However, early detection of unsatisfactory late results remains a challenging task. Zindrick and colleagues[55] reported that the existing evidence does not provide any definite conclusions concerning factors that may affect postoperative outcomes. Guyer and colleagues[107] found that the only factor significantly related to the clinical outcome was the length of time off work before surgery. Patients who were off work for shorter durations, or not at all, were more likely to be in the best-outcome group compared with patients who were off work for an extended time before surgery.

Other data demonstrated that baseline ODI and early postoperative outcome parameters (≤ 6 months) revealed a significant and strong association with the final results following TDR.[31] Although the majority of patients with an early highly satisfactory outcome maintained satisfactory results at later follow-up stages, any significant improvement considered as "highly satisfied" is unlikely in a group of patients who reported an early unsatisfactory outcome. The findings from these studies may be helpful in an attempt to weigh both the patient's and the spine surgeon's expectations against any possible realistic achievements.

Sporting Activities Following TDR

Despite its widespread use in predominantly young and active patients, no previous study has addressed possibilities, limitations, and potential risks regarding athletic performance following TDR. Mechanical concerns remain and the implant's resilience regarding its load-bearing capacity during sporting activities is unknown. A prospective study cohort investigated the ability of TDR candidates to resume athletic abilities postoperatively.[108] The results demonstrate that patients were able to perform a variety of different sporting activities up to the level of competitive sports, extreme sports, and professional athletics. Sporting activity was resumed early postoperatively, within the first 3 (38.5%) to 6 (30.7%) months with peak performance being reached after 5.2 months. Minor implant subsidence was observed in 30% of all patients during the first 3 months with no further implant migration. Therefore, it was not attributed to the sporting activities. No evidence of implant wear was seen in radiological follow-up evaluations. However, owing to the young age of the patients and significant load-increase during athletic activities, concerns about the future of the implant still need to be investigated with larger patient cohorts, longer follow-up evaluations, and modified examination techniques.

THE ROLE OF ALTERNATIVES

The last observation of William H. Harris was that a new technology triggers the development of alternatives. In THR it was the search for new and better implant materials, such as ceramics, cross-linked ultra-high-molecular-polyethylene (UHMWPE), or new interfaces such as metal-metal, ceramics-ceramics or metal-UHMWPE that led to a continuous improvement of the technique as well as the clinical results. Regarding the development of TDR, the race for improvement of current implant materials has already begun. Metal-on-metal weight-bearing, ceramic disks, or viscoelastic materials are in the development pipelines of medical device companies. On the other hand, TDR has triggered the search and development of other nonfusion technologies. Dynamic pedicle screw-based fixation systems, interspinous spacers, as well as facet joint replacement technologies are examples.[109–120] Whether these technologies will lead to better outcomes in patients suffering from degenerative changes of the lumbar spine, and whether these outcomes will be superior, or at least the same compared with current standard techniques, remains to be established.

SUMMARY

In the nonscientific, political discussions lead by insurance companies, regulation authorities, and health care providers in some countries, lumbar fusion is generally accepted as the treatment of disease choice for low back pain due to lumbar degenerative disk spine. It is sometimes even glorified as a gold standard, although there has only been low evidence for that from the scientific literature.[1,121] Numerous scientific studies published worldwide revealed marked evidence that the results of lumbar fusion are inferior or, at the best, not inferior to the results observed following lumbar TDR in comparable patient cohorts.[32,33,35,36] There is growing evidence that lumbar fusion is associated with higher direct and indirect costs,[37–40] as well as with higher complication rates as compared with TDR.[2,5,7,9,37–40,67] There is also growing evidence that early results of TDR can be maintained after 5 years.[25,28,31,33,51] Similarly, there is evidence that the reoperation rates of lumbar fusion are higher compared with TDR.[14,17–21,23,32,33,35,36,69] Last, but not least, there is no evidence that TDR has led to a total increase of surgical treatment for degenerative lumbar spine disorders, especially in the United States.

Any type of new treatment technology should be thoroughly evaluated for safety and efficacy. However, the spine-treatment community should apply the same kind of stringent criticism to what is currently considered the gold standard treatment option for low back pain due to lumbar degenerative disk disease. Well-known negative side effects that have incited criticism for disk replacement technologies seem to be widely accepted for lumbar fusion procedures: high rates of adjacent level degenerative changes, adjacent level facet joint changes, considerable rates of revision surgeries and reoperation rates, nonunion or pseudarthrosis, facet or sacroiliac joint complaints, implant displacements, cranial screw facet joint violations, compromise of neurologic structures, and numerous others have been published.[14–23,70,122–127]

For degenerative lumbar disk disease, multiple RCTs with long follow-up periods show that no significant differences can be detected between varying treatment groups beyond 10-years of follow-up, independent of the type of treatment that was chosen. This points to the fact that the long-term progression of any degenerative pathology cannot be altered, whereas surgical intervention can significantly influence the short-term and mid-term outcome. The experience published in numerous papers demonstrates distinct advantages of TDR over lumbar fusion procedures for a small cohort of predominantly young and active patients, particularly within the early postoperative period. These experiences include earlier postoperative mobilization (same or first postoperative day) without the need for external support or bracing, shorter hospital stay, high rate of patients returning to work and resuming their professional activities, early resumption of athletic activities up to a very high competitive level,[108] lower reoperation rates, and a lower rate of adjacent level degeneration than what has previously been published for fusion candidates.

In summary, there is no surgical procedure in spinal surgery for which there is more scientific evidence than for TDR. It is common practice in the vast majority of spine centers across Europe and the results prove that it is a reasonable technology driven by medical needs with a number of benefits for our patients. Any general restriction for the use of this technology is not substantiated by the current scientific literature and, therefore, it is politically driven in some health care systems. This restriction denies the patient a useful and, in many aspects, beneficial type of surgical treatment of low back pain.

REFERENCES

1. Fritzell P, Hagg O, Wessberg P, et al. 2001 Volvo Award Winner in Clinical Studies: Lumbar fusion versus nonsurgical treatment for chronic low back pain: a multicenter randomized controlled trial from the Swedish Lumbar Spine Study Group. Spine 2001;26:2521–32 [discussion: 2532–4].

2. Crock HV. Anterior lumbar interbody fusion: indications for its use and notes on surgical technique. Clin Orthop Relat Res 1982;(165):157–63.

3. Dai LY, Jiang LS. Single-level instrumented posterolateral fusion of lumbar spine with beta-tricalcium phosphate versus autograft: a prospective, randomized study with 3-year follow-up. Spine (Phila Pa 1976) 2008;33:1299–304.

4. DiPaola CP, Molinari RW. Posterior lumbar interbody fusion. J Am Acad Orthop Surg 2008;16:130–9.

5. Greenough CG, Taylor LJ, Fraser RD. Anterior lumbar fusion: results, assessment techniques and prognostic factors. Eur Spine J 1994;3:225–30.

6. Karikari IO, Isaacs RE. Minimally invasive transforaminal lumbar interbody fusion: a review of techniques and outcomes. Spine (Phila Pa 1976) 2010;35:S294–301.

7. Kozak JA, Heilman AE, O'Brien JP. Anterior lumbar fusion options. Technique and graft materials. Clin Orthop Relat Res 1994;(300):45–51.

8. Obenchain TG. Laparoscopic lumbar discectomy: case report. J Laparoendosc Surg 1991;1:145–9.

9. Spivak JM, Neuwirth MG, Giordano CP, et al. The perioperative course of combined anterior and posterior spinal fusion. Spine (Phila Pa 1976) 1994;19:520–5.

10. Stauffer RN, Coventry MB. Anterior interbody lumbar spine fusion. Analysis of Mayo Clinic series. J Bone Joint Surg Am 1972;54:756–68.

11. Zucherman JF, Zdeblick TA, Bailey SA, et al. Instrumented laparoscopic spinal fusion. Preliminary results. Spine (Phila Pa 1976) 1995;20:2029–34 [discussion: 2034–5].

12. Lange F. Operative Behandlung der Spondylitis. Münchner Medizinische Wochenschrift 1909;56 [in German].

13. Weinstein JN, Lurie JD, Olson PR, et al. United States' trends and regional variations in lumbar spine surgery: 1992–2003. Spine (Phila Pa 1976) 2006;31:2707–14.

14. Gillet P. The fate of the adjacent motion segments after lumbar fusion. J Spinal Disord Tech 2003;16:338–45.

15. Carreon LY, Puno RM, Dimar JR 2nd, et al. Perioperative complications of posterior lumbar decompression and arthrodesis in older adults. J Bone Joint Surg Am 2003;85:2089–92.

16. Park P, Garton HJ, Gala VC, et al. Adjacent segment disease after lumbar or lumbosacral fusion: review of the literature. Spine 2004;29:1938–44.

17. Ciol MA, Deyo RA, Kreuter W, et al. Characteristics in Medicare beneficiaries associated with reoperation after lumbar spine surgery. Spine (Phila Pa 1976) 1994;19:1329–34.

18. Ghiselli G, Wang JC, Bhatia NN, et al. Adjacent segment degeneration in the lumbar spine. J Bone Joint Surg Am 2004;86:1497–503.

19. Malter AD, McNeney B, Loeser JD, et al. 5-year reoperation rates after different types of lumbar spine surgery. Spine (Phila Pa 1976) 1998;23:814–20.

20. Martin BI, Mirza SK, Comstock BA, et al. Reoperation rates following lumbar spine surgery and the influence of spinal fusion procedures. Spine 2007;32:382–7.

21. Taylor VM, Deyo RA, Ciol M, et al. Surgical treatment of patients with back problems covered by workers compensation versus those with other sources of payment. Spine (Phila Pa 1976) 1996; 21:2255–9.

22. Carreon LY, Glassman SD, Howard J. Fusion and nonsurgical treatment for symptomatic lumbar degenerative disease: a systematic review of Oswestry Disability Index and MOS Short Form-36 outcomes. Spine J 2008;8:747–55.

23. Martin BI, Mirza SK, Comstock BA, et al. Are lumbar spine reoperation rates falling with greater use of fusion surgery and new surgical technology? Spine (Phila Pa 1976) 2007;32:2119–26.

24. Cinotti G, David T, Postacchini F. Results of disc prosthesis after a minimum follow-up period of 2 years. Spine 1996;21:995–1000.

25. David T. Long-term results of one-level lumbar arthroplasty: minimum 10-year follow-up of the CHARITE artificial disc in 106 patients. Spine 2007;32:661–6.

26. Delamarter RB, Fribourg DM, Kanim LE, et al. ProDisc artificial total lumbar disc replacement: introduction and early results from the United States clinical trial. Spine 2003;28:S167–75.

27. Le Huec J, Basso Y, Mathews H, et al. The effect of single-level, total disc arthroplasty on sagittal balance parameters: a prospective study. Eur Spine J 2005;14:480–6.

28. Lemaire JP, Carrier H, Ali el HS, et al. Clinical and radiological outcomes with the Charité artificial disc: a 10-year minimum follow-up. J Spinal Disord Tech 2005;18:353–9.

29. Siepe CJ, Mayer HM, Heinz-Leisenheimer M, et al. Total lumbar disc replacement: different results for different levels. Spine 2007;32:782–90.

30. Siepe CJ, Mayer HM, Wiechert K, et al. Clinical results of total lumbar disc replacement with ProDisc II: three-year results for different indications. Spine 2006;31:1923–32.

31. Siepe CJ, Tepass A, Hitzl W, et al. Dynamics of improvement following total lumbar disc replacement: is the outcome predictable? Spine (Phila Pa 1976) 2009;34:2579–86.

32. Blumenthal S, McAfee PC, Guyer RD, et al. A prospective, randomized, multicenter Food and Drug Administration investigational device exemptions study of lumbar total disc replacement with the CHARITE artificial disc versus lumbar fusion: part I: evaluation of clinical outcomes. Spine 2005;30:1565–75 [discussion: E387–91].

33. Guyer RD, McAfee PC, Banco RJ, et al. Prospective, randomized, multicenter Food and Drug Administration investigational device exemption study of lumbar total disc replacement with the CHARITE artificial disc versus lumbar fusion: five-year follow-up. Spine J 2009;9:374–86.

34. McAfee PC, Cunningham B, Holsapple G, et al. A prospective, randomized, multicenter Food and Drug Administration investigational device exemption study of lumbar total disc replacement with the CHARITE artificial disc versus lumbar fusion: part II: evaluation of radiographic outcomes and correlation of surgical technique accuracy with clinical outcomes. Spine 2005;30:1576–83 [discussion: E388–90].

35. Sasso RC, Foulk DM, Hahn M. Prospective, randomized trial of metal-on-metal artificial lumbar disc replacement: initial results for treatment of discogenic pain. Spine 2008;33:123–31.

36. Zigler J, Delamarter R, Spivak JM, et al. Results of the prospective, randomized, multicenter Food and Drug Administration investigational device exemption study of the ProDisc-L total disc replacement versus circumferential fusion for the treatment of 1-level degenerative disc disease. Spine 2007;32: 1155–62 [discussion: 1163].

37. Guyer RD, Tromanhauser SG, Regan JJ. An economic model of one-level lumbar arthroplasty versus fusion. Spine J 2007;7:558–62.

38. Patel VV, Estes S, Lindley EM, et al. Lumbar spinal fusion versus anterior lumbar disc replacement: the financial implications. J Spinal Disord Tech 2008; 21:473–6.

39. Levin DA, Bendo JA, Quirno M, et al. Comparative charge analysis of one- and two-level lumbar total disc arthroplasty versus circumferential lumbar fusion. Spine 2007;32:2905–9.

40. Kurtz SM, Lau E, Ianuzzi A, et al. National revision burden for lumbar total disc replacement in the United States: epidemiologic and economic perspectives. Spine (Phila Pa 1976) 2010;35: 690–6.

41. Harris WH. The first 50 years of total hip arthroplasty: lessons learned. Clin Orthop Relat Res 2009;467:28–31.

42. Buttner-Janz K, Schellnack K. [Intervertebral disk endoprosthesis–development and current status]. Beitr Orthop Traumatol 1990;37:137–47 [in German].

43. Dattani R. Femoral osteolysis following total hip replacement. Postgrad Med J 2007;83:312–6.

44. Siepe CJ, Zelenkov P, Sauri-Barraza JC, et al. The fate of facet joint and adjacent level disc degeneration following total lumbar disc replacement: a prospective clinical, x-ray, and magnetic resonance imaging investigation. Spine (Phila Pa 1976) 2010;35:1991–2003.

45. Kafer W, Clessienne CB, Daxle M, et al. Posterior component impingement after lumbar total disc replacement: a radiographic analysis of 66 ProDisc-L prostheses in 56 patients. Spine 2008;33:2444–9.

46. Siepe CJ, Hitzl W, Meschede P, et al. Interdependence between disc space height, range of motion and clinical outcome in total lumbar disc replacement. Spine 2009;34:904–16.

47. Cakir B, Richter M, Kafer W, et al. The impact of total lumbar disc replacement on segmental and total lumbar lordosis. Clin Biomech (Bristol, Avon) 2005;20:357–64.

48. Tortolani PJ, Cunningham BW, Eng M, et al. Prevalence of heterotopic ossification following total disc replacement. A prospective, randomized study of two hundred and seventy-six patients. J Bone Joint Surg Am 2007;89:82–8.

49. Amundsen T, Weber H, Nordal HJ, et al. Lumbar spinal stenosis: conservative or surgical management? a prospective 10-year study. Spine (Phila Pa 1976) 2000;25:1424–35 [discussion: 1435–6].

50. Guyer RD, Blumenthal S, Cappuccino A. 24-month follow-up of a prospective randomized comparison of two lumbar total disc replacements. 9th Annual Global Symposium of the Spine Arthroplasty Society (SAS) Congress. London, 2009.

51. Tropiano P, Huang RC, Girardi FP, et al. Lumbar total disc replacement. Seven to eleven-year follow-up. J Bone Joint Surg Am 2005;87:490–6.

52. Bertagnoli R, Yue JJ, Shah RV, et al. The treatment of disabling single-level lumbar discogenic low back pain with total disc arthroplasty utilizing the Prodisc prosthesis: a prospective study with 2-year minimum follow-up. Spine 2005;30:2230–6.

53. Chung SS, Lee CS, Kang CS. Lumbar total disc replacement using ProDisc II: a prospective study with a 2-year minimum follow-up. J Spinal Disord Tech 2006;19:411–5.

54. Lemaire JP, Skalli W, Lavaste F, et al. Intervertebral disc prosthesis. Results and prospects for the year 2000. Clin Orthop Relat Res 1997;(337):64–76.

55. Zindrick MR, Tzermiadianos MN, Voronov LI, et al. An evidence-based medicine approach in determining factors that may affect outcome in lumbar total disc replacement. Spine 2008;33:1262–9.

56. David T. Lumbar disc prosthesis: surgical technique, indications and clinical results in 22 patients with a minimum of 12 months follow-up. Eur Spine J 1993;1:254–9.

57. Le Huec JC, Basso Y, Aunoble S, et al. Influence of facet and posterior muscle degeneration on clinical results of lumbar total disc replacement: two-year follow-up. J Spinal Disord Tech 2005;18:219–23.

58. Zeegers WS, Bohnen LM, Laaper M, et al. Artificial disc replacement with the modular type SB Charite III: 2-year results in 50 prospectively studied patients. Eur Spine J 1999;8:210–7.

59. Bertagnoli R, Yue JJ, Nanieva R, et al. Lumbar total disc arthroplasty in patients older than 60 years of age: a prospective study of the ProDisc prosthesis with 2-year minimum follow-up period. J Neurosurg Spine 2006;4:85–90.

60. Siepe CJ, Korge A, Grochulla F, et al. Analysis of postoperative pain patterns following total lumbar disc replacement: results from fluoroscopically guided spine infiltrations. Eur Spine J 2008;17:44–56.

61. Delamarter RB, Bae HW, Kropf MA, et al. 1 versus 2 versus 3-level lumbar artificial disc replacement—a prospective report of clinical outcomes with the ProDisc-L device. Presented at the Annual Meeting of the International Society for the Study of the Lumbar Spine (ISSLS). Bergen, Norway, 2006.

62. Hannibal M, Thomas DJ, Low J, et al. ProDisc-L total disc replacement: a comparison of 1-level versus 2-level arthroplasty patients with a minimum 2-year follow-up. Spine 2007;32:2322–6.

63. Bertagnoli R, Kumar S. Indications for full prosthetic disc arthroplasty: a correlation of clinical outcome against a variety of indications. Eur Spine J 2002;11(Suppl 2):S131–6.

64. Bertagnoli R, Yue JJ, Shah RV, et al. The treatment of disabling multilevel lumbar discogenic low back pain with total disc arthroplasty utilizing the ProDisc prosthesis: a prospective study with 2-year minimum follow-up. Spine 2005;30:2192–9.

65. Griffith SL, Shelokov AP, Buttner-Janz K, et al. A multicenter retrospective study of the clinical results of the LINK SB Charité intervertebral prosthesis. The initial European experience. Spine 1994;19:1842–9.

66. Tropiano P, Huang RC, Girardi FP, et al. Lumbar disc replacement: preliminary results with ProDisc II after a minimum follow-up period of 1 year. J Spinal Disord Tech 2003;16:362–8.

67. Faciszewski T, Winter RB, Lonstein JE, et al. The surgical and medical perioperative complications of anterior spinal fusion surgery in the thoracic and lumbar spine in adults. A review of 1223 procedures. Spine (Phila Pa 1976) 1995;20:1592–9.

68. Polly DW Jr. Adapting innovative motion-preserving technology to spinal surgical practice: what should we expect to happen? Spine 2003;28:S104–9.

69. McAfee PC, Geisler FH, Saiedy SS, et al. Revisability of the CHARITE artificial disc replacement: analysis of 688 patients enrolled in the U.S. IDE study of the CHARITE Artificial Disc. Spine 2006;31:1217–26.

70. Umehara S, Zindrick MR, Patwardhan AG, et al. The biomechanical effect of postoperative hypolordosis in instrumented lumbar fusion on

instrumented and adjacent spinal segments. Spine 2000;25:1617–24.

71. Akamaru T, Kawahara N, Tim Yoon S, et al. Adjacent segment motion after a simulated lumbar fusion in different sagittal alignments: a biomechanical analysis. Spine 2003;28:1560–6.

72. Lazennec JY, Ramare S, Arafati N, et al. Sagittal alignment in lumbosacral fusion: relations between radiological parameters and pain. Eur Spine J 2000;9:47–55.

73. Chung SS, Lee CS, Kang CS, et al. The effect of lumbar total disc replacement on the spinopelvic alignment and range of motion of the lumbar spine. J Spinal Disord Tech 2006;19:307–11.

74. Tournier C, Aunoble S, Le Huec JC, et al. Total disc arthroplasty: consequences for sagittal balance and lumbar spine movement. Eur Spine J 2007; 16:411–21.

75. Liu J, Ebraheim NA, Haman SP, et al. Effect of the increase in the height of lumbar disc space on facet joint articulation area in sagittal plane. Spine 2006;31:E198–202.

76. Rohlmann A, Zander T, Bergmann G. Effect of total disc replacement with ProDisc on intersegmental rotation of the lumbar spine. Spine 2005;30:738–43.

77. Cunningham BW. Basic scientific considerations in total disc arthroplasty. Spine J 2004;4:219S–30S.

78. Cunningham BW, Gordon JD, Dmitriev AE, et al. Biomechanical evaluation of total disc replacement arthroplasty: an in vitro human cadaveric model. Spine 2003;28:S110–7.

79. Denoziere G, Ku DN. Biomechanical comparison between fusion of two vertebrae and implantation of an artificial intervertebral disc. J Biomech 2006;39:766–75.

80. Dooris AP, Goel VK, Grosland NM, et al. Load-sharing between anterior and posterior elements in a lumbar motion segment implanted with an artificial disc. Spine 2001;26:E122–9.

81. McAfee PC, Cunningham BW, Hayes V, et al. Biomechanical analysis of rotational motions after disc arthroplasty: implications for patients with adult deformities. Spine 2006;31:S152–60.

82. O'Leary P, Nicolakis M, Lorenz MA, et al. Response of Charité total disc replacement under physiologic loads: prosthesis component motion patterns. Spine J 2005;5:590–9.

83. Rousseau MA, Bradford DS, Bertagnoli R, et al. Disc arthroplasty design influences intervertebral kinematics and facet forces. Spine J 2006;6:258–66.

84. Rohlmann A, Mann A, Zander T, et al. Effect of an artificial disc on lumbar spine biomechanics: a probabilistic finite element study. Eur Spine J 2009;18:89–97.

85. Chen SH, Zhong ZC, Chen CS, et al. Biomechanical comparison between lumbar disc arthroplasty and fusion. Med Eng Phys 2009;31(2):244–53.

86. Rundell SA, Auerbach JD, Balderston RA, et al. Total disc replacement positioning affects facet contact forces and vertebral body strains. Spine 2008;33:2510–7.

87. Chung SK, Kim YE, Wang KC. Biomechanical effect of constraint in lumbar total disc replacement: a study with finite element analysis. Spine 2009;34:1281–6.

88. Leivseth G, Braaten S, Frobin W, et al. Mobility of lumbar segments instrumented with a ProDisc II prosthesis: a two-year follow-up study. Spine 2006;31:1726–33.

89. Rousseau MA, Bradford DS, Hadi TM, et al. The instant axis of rotation influences facet forces at L5/S1 during flexion/extension and lateral bending. Eur Spine J 2006;15:299–307.

90. Shim CS, Lee SH, Shin HD, et al. CHARITE versus ProDisc: a comparative study of a minimum 3-year follow-up. Spine 2007;32:1012–8.

91. Park CK, Ryu KS, Jee WH. Degenerative changes of discs and facet joints in lumbar total disc replacement using ProDisc II: minimum two-year follow-up. Spine 2008;33:1755–61.

92. Huang RC, Tropiano P, Marnay T, et al. Range of motion and adjacent level degeneration after lumbar total disc replacement. Spine J 2006;6:242–7.

93. Auerbach JD, Wills BP, McIntosh TC, et al. Evaluation of spinal kinematics following lumbar total disc replacement and circumferential fusion using in vivo fluoroscopy. Spine 2007;32:527–36.

94. Dmitriev AE, Gill NW, Kuklo TR, et al. The effect of multilevel lumbar disc arthroplasty on the operative- and adjacent-level kinematics and intradiscal pressures. An in vitro human cadaveric assessment. Spine J 2008;8(6):918–25.

95. Panjabi M, Malcolmson G, Teng E, et al. Hybrid testing of lumbar CHARITE discs versus fusions. Spine 2007;32:959–66 [discussion: 967].

96. Anderson PA, Schwaegler PF, Cizek D, et al. Work status as a predictor of surgical outcome of discogenic low back pain. Spine 2006;31:2510–5.

97. Du Bois M, Donceel P. A screening questionnaire to predict no return to work within 3 months for low back pain claimants. Eur Spine J 2008;17:380–5.

98. Enthoven P, Skargren E, Carstensen J, et al. Predictive factors for 1-year and 5-year outcome for disability in a working population of patients with low back pain treated in primary care. Pain 2006;122:137–44.

99. Hagg O, Fritzell P, Ekselius L, et al. Predictors of outcome in fusion surgery for chronic low back pain. A report from the Swedish Lumbar Spine Study. Eur Spine J 2003;12:22–33.

100. Hakkinen A, Ylinen J, Kautiainen H, et al. Does the outcome 2 months after lumbar disc surgery predict the outcome 12 months later? Disabil Rehabil 2003;25:968–72.

101. Junge A, Frohlich M, Ahrens S, et al. Predictors of bad and good outcome of lumbar spine surgery. A prospective clinical study with 2 years' follow up. Spine 1996;21:1056–64 [discussion: 1064–5].

102. Lawrence JT, London N, Bohlman HH, et al. Preoperative narcotic use as a predictor of clinical outcome: results following anterior cervical arthrodesis. Spine 2008;33:2074–8.

103. Mannion AF, Elfering A. Predictors of surgical outcome and their assessment. Eur Spine J 2006; 15(Suppl 1):S93–108.

104. Miettinen T, Leino E, Airaksinen O, et al. The possibility to use simple validated questionnaires to predict long-term health problems after whiplash injury. Spine 2004;29:E47–51.

105. Peolsson A, Vavruch L, Oberg B. Can the results 6 months after anterior cervical decompression and fusion identify patients who will have remaining deficit at long-term? Disabil Rehabil 2006;28: 117–24.

106. Saberi H, Isfahani AV. Higher preoperative Oswestry Disability Index is associated with better surgical outcome in upper lumbar disc herniations. Eur Spine J 2008;17:117–21.

107. Guyer RD, Siddiqui S, Zigler JE, et al. Lumbar spinal arthroplasty: analysis of one center's twenty best and twenty worst clinical outcomes. Spine (Phila Pa 1976) 2008;33:2566–9.

108. Siepe CJ, Wiechert K, Khattab MF, et al. Total lumbar disc replacement in athletes: clinical results, return to sport and athletic performance. Eur Spine J 2007;16:1001–13.

109. Cakir B, Carazzo C, Schmidt R, et al. Adjacent segment mobility after rigid and semirigid instrumentation of the lumbar spine. Spine (Phila Pa 1976) 2009;34:1287–91.

110. Grob D, Benini A, Junge A, et al. Clinical experience with the Dynesys semirigid fixation system for the lumbar spine: surgical and patient-oriented outcome in 50 cases after an average of 2 years. Spine 2005;30:324–31.

111. Putzier M, Schneider SV, Funk JF, et al. The surgical treatment of the lumbar disc prolapse: nucleotomy with additional transpedicular dynamic stabilization versus nucleotomy alone. Spine 2005;30:E109–14.

112. Stoll TM, Dubois G, Schwarzenbach O. The dynamic neutralization system for the spine: a multi-center study of a novel non-fusion system. Eur Spine J 2002;11(Suppl 2):S170–8.

113. Zucherman JF, Hsu KY, Hartjen CA, et al. A multicenter, prospective, randomized trial evaluating the X STOP interspinous process decompression system for the treatment of neurogenic intermittent claudication: two-year follow-up results. Spine (Phila Pa 1976) 2005;30: 1351–8.

114. Zucherman JF, Hsu KY, Hartjen CA, et al. A prospective randomized multi-center study for the treatment of lumbar spinal stenosis with the X STOP interspinous implant: 1-year results. Eur Spine J 2004;13:22–31.

115. Brussee P, Hauth J, Donk RD, et al. Self-rated evaluation of outcome of the implantation of interspinous process distraction (X-Stop) for neurogenic claudication. Eur Spine J 2008;17:200–3.

116. Kondrashov DG, Hannibal M, Hsu KY, et al. Interspinous process decompression with the X-STOP device for lumbar spinal stenosis: a 4-year follow-up study. J Spinal Disord Tech 2006;19:323–7.

117. Siddiqui M, Smith FW, Wardlaw D. One-year results of X Stop interspinous implant for the treatment of lumbar spinal stenosis. Spine (Phila Pa 1976) 2007;32:1345–8.

118. Mayer HM, Zentz F, Siepe C, et al. [Percutaneous interspinous distraction for the treatment of dynamic lumbar spinal stensois and low back pain]. Oper Orthop Traumatol 2010;22:495–511 [in German].

119. Siepe CJ, Heider F, Beisse R, et al. [Treatment of dynamic spinal canal stenosis with an interspinous spacer]. Oper Orthop Traumatol 2010;22:524–35 [in German].

120. Charles YP, Persohn S, Steib JP, et al. Influence of an auxiliary facet system on lumbar spine biomechanics. Spine (Phila Pa 1976) 2011;36(9):690–9.

121. Brox JI, Sorensen R, Friis A, et al. Randomized clinical trial of lumbar instrumented fusion and cognitive intervention and exercises in patients with chronic low back pain and disc degeneration. Spine (Phila Pa 1976) 2003;28:1913–21.

122. Goulet JA, Senunas LE, DeSilva GL, et al. Autogenous iliac crest bone graft. Complications and functional assessment. Clin Orthop Relat Res 1997;(339):76–81.

123. Kumar MN, Jacquot F, Hall H. Long-term follow-up of functional outcomes and radiographic changes at adjacent levels following lumbar spine fusion for degenerative disc disease. Eur Spine J 2001;10: 309–13.

124. Lee CK. Accelerated degeneration of the segment adjacent to a lumbar fusion. Spine 1988;13:375–7.

125. Shah RR, Mohammed S, Saifuddin A, et al. Radiologic evaluation of adjacent superior segment facet joint violation following transpedicular instrumentation of the lumbar spine. Spine 2003;28:272–5.

126. Cardoso MJ, Dmitriev AE, Helgeson M, et al. Does superior-segment facet violation or laminectomy destabilize the adjacent level in lumbar transpedicular fixation? An in vitro human cadaveric assessment. Spine 2008;33:2868–73.

127. Moshirfar A, Jenis LG, Spector LR, et al. Computed tomography evaluation of superior-segment facet-joint violation after pedicle instrumentation of the lumbar spine with a midline surgical approach. Spine 2006;31:2624–9.

Stem Cell Regeneration of the Intervertebral Disk

Daisuke Sakai, MD, PhD

KEYWORDS

- Intervertebral disk • Nucleus pulposus • Cell transplantation
- Stem cell • Regenerative medicine

The intervertebral disk (IVD) functions as an essential load absorber between all vertebrae by allowing bending, flexion, and torsion of the spine. IVD degeneration is a cell-mediated response to progressive structural failure and causes instability of the vertebral motion segments that are responsible for neural compressive manifestations and low back pain.[1] Prolonged segmental instability eventually leads to deformity of the spine and many clinical problems.[2] These manifestations have a high impact on society and the economy, including direct costs for medical treatment and insurance, lost productivity, and disability benefits. These direct and indirect costs are estimated at £12 billion per year in the United Kingdom and $50 billion in the United States.[1,2,3] Therefore, prevention and treatment of IVD degeneration should have significant effects on society and the economy.

CELLULAR MICROENVIRONMENT OF THE INTERVERTEBRAL DISK

The IVD comprises the central nucleus pulposus (NP), the surrounding annulus fibrosus (AF), and the vertebral end plate, which isolates the blood supply from penetrating the largest avascular organ in the human body.[4] Developmentally, the NP originates from the notochord, although in human and other animal species, such as the rat, chondrodystrophoid breed canines, and cattle, there is a marked change in cell and tissue morphology during the early stage of life.[5,6] In human adults, most NP cells resemble chondrocytes of other cartilaginous tissues. These cells are interspersed at low density (approximately 5000 cells/mm^3) and are sometimes arranged in clusters within the matrix.[7] In the surrounding AF, the cells are more typically fibroblastic with a density of approximately 9000 cells/mm^3 and display a fibrous matrix, comprising 15 to 25 lamellae of collagen fibers oriented alternately at approximately 60° to the vertical axis.[8] In-between the lamellae are the elastin and proteoglycan matrix, which reinforces the viscoelastic structure.[9] The vertebral end plate is characterized by a thin layer of chondrocytes and hyaline matrix, which resembles articular cartilage. A capillary network of blood vessels ending here, called the vascular buds, is found within the end plate and supplies approximately 80% of the nutrients needed to support the viability of IVD cells through diffusion. The microenvironment for these cells comprising the IVD is characterized by low oxygen tension and high lactic acid concentration and thus an acidic pH level, compared with the levels in the blood plasma.[10]

This work was supported in part by a Grant-in-Aid for Scientific Research and a Grant of The Science Frontier Program from the Ministry of Education, Culture, Sports, Science and Technology of Japan and a grant from AO Spine International.

The authors have nothing to disclose.

Department of Orthopaedic Surgery, Surgical Science and, Research Center for Regenerative Medicine, Tokai University School of Medicine, Shimokasuya 143, Isehara, Kanagawa 259-1193, Japan

E-mail address: daisakai@is.icc.u-tokai.ac.jp

STEM CELL APPLICATIONS IN INTERVERTEBRAL DISK RESEARCH

Decreased number and viability of the IVD cells, especially the NP cells, initiate disk degeneration, and maintaining the homeostasis and restoring the IVD tissue and function are important determinants of the cells' condition. Basic in vitro studies have shown that IVD cells have a low proliferative ability and that most cells in the adult human IVD are in a senescent state.[11] These facts have led researchers to focus on the idea of using stem cells to treat IVD degeneration.

Stem cells are characterized by the ability to self-renew and multipotent capabilities. The application of stem cells and stem cell research techniques in IVD research has been investigated from several directions. Use of new stem cell sources, such as induced pluripotent stem cells or embryonic stem cells, may provide new insight into the field of IVD research.

DEFINING ENDOGENOUS STEM CELL POPULATIONS IN THE ADULT INTERVERTEBRAL DISK

Recent stem cell research has reported the presence of a stem/progenitor cell system as the key to maintaining normal homeostasis and self-renewal in various organs. Decreased number and altered function of stem/progenitor cells cause dysfunction of the composing organ. Activation of the endogenous stem/progenitor cells is one approach for maintaining cellular homeostasis of the IVD. Risbud and colleagues[12] reported that cells isolated from degenerate human tissues express CD105, CD166, CD63, CD49a, CD90, CD73, p75 low-affinity nerve growth factor receptor, and CD133/1, proteins that are characteristic of marrow mesenchymal stem cells (MSCs) and that represent the differentiation ability toward osteogenesis, adipogenesis, and chondrogenesis. A study by Blanco and colleagues[13] compared the differentiation capabilities of MSCs induced from the bone marrow or the NP from the same 16 individuals and found that MSCs similar to bone marrow MSCs are present in the human NP, with the exception that NP MSCs show poor adipogenic differentiation. Feng and colleagues[14] reported that AF cells express several of the cell surface antigens sometimes associated with MSCs, including CD29, CD49e, CD51, CD73, CD90, CD105, CD166, CD184, and Stro-1, and two neuronal stem cell markers, nestin and neuron-specific enolase. Varying the stimulants added to the induction media determined whether AF cells differentiated into adipocytes, osteoblasts, chondrocytes, neurons, or endothelial cells.

These research data suggest that stimulation of endogenous stem cell populations may be effective for treating IVD degeneration or for providing cells for the allogeneic transplantation of somatic tissue-specific stem cells.

INDUCTION OF STEM CELLS FROM OTHER ORGANS OF THE BODY

Another scenario involves promoting the mobilization of stem cell populations from the stem cell pool, such as the bone marrow. In cerebral and cardiac infarctions, stem cells are recruited from the stem cell pool and mobilized by agents, such as stem cell growth factor or granulocyte colony-stimulating factor, to restore cells in the injured lesion.[15,16] This kind of system may not be applicable to IVD degeneration because there is no blood supply through which to mobilize the cells; however, there may be different pathways for stem cells to approach the IVD. Detailed research on this problem awaits investigation.

USING STEM CELLS AS FEEDER CELLS TO INTERVERTEBRAL DISK CELLS

Stem cells may serve as feeder cells to stimulate directly other cells in the environment by cell-to-cell contact or indirectly through the secretion of various factors. In a rabbit IVD cell culture, Yamamoto and colleagues[17] showed that direct cell-to-cell contact between NP cells and MSCs occurs across a membrane with 0.45-μm pores, which allowed only the processes to adhere to each other without more extensive contact between the cultured cells. The extent of cell adhesion was assessed by scanning electron microscopy, cell proliferation was evaluated by the WST-8 assay, and the syntheses of DNA and proteoglycans was evaluated by the uptake of ^{3}H and ^{35}S, respectively. The levels of various growth factors and the secretion of cytokines into the culture supernatant were measured using a cytokine protein array. The results were confirmed by electron microscopy and showed that MSCs and NP cells adhered to each other by extending processes across the membrane. The number of cells significantly increased in NP cells cocultured with MSCs and allowed cell-to-cell contact. In addition, the synthesis of DNA and proteoglycans increased significantly in the NP cells cocultured with MSCs when cell-to-cell contact was allowed. The analysis using the cytokine protein array revealed that the secretion of cytokines known to increase the activity of NP cells (transforming growth factor β1 [TGF-β1]), insulinlike growth factor 1, platelet-derived growth factor, and epidermal growth factor) was also significantly higher in the media collected from NP cells cocultured, allowing cell-to-cell contact. Compared with the conventional NP cell-activation method, the coculture system allowing intercellular adhesion with MSCs led to a marked increase in NP cell proliferation, DNA synthesis, and proteoglycan synthesis. A possible explanation is the increased secretion of various cytokines into the culture medium because of the direct contact with MSCs, which act as feeder cells.

In a preliminary study at the author's laboratory, NP cells activated by coculture that allows intercellular contact (**Fig. 1**) were implanted in an in vivo rabbit model of IVD degeneration.[18] The severity of degeneration was determined over time according to Nishimura's histologic classification. The severity of degeneration was compared between cells treated with the new and conventional methods of activation. The Nishimura grade 24 weeks after transplant was 0 in the normal control group without degeneration induction, 2.8 (the most severe degeneration) in the control group with no treatment, 2.2 in the group receiving NP cells activated by conventional coculture with AF cells, 1.8 in the group receiving NP cells activated by conventional coculture with MSCs, and 1.2 in the group receiving NP cells activated by coculture involving contact with MSCs, the smaller value reflected a significantly less degree of degeneration.

The positive results of this coculture system have been extended to preclinical studies using human cells. Watanabe and colleagues[19] showed that human NP cells obtained from surgery and cocultured with MSCs of the same patient demonstrate up-regulated cellular proliferation and matrix synthesis, as described in animal models.

Strassburg and colleagues[20] demonstrated in the same coculture system using degenerate and nondegenerate NP cells that cellular interactions between MSCs and degenerate NP cells may stimulate both MSC differentiation to an NP-like phenotype and the endogenous NP cell population to regain a nondegenerate phenotype, which consequently increases matrix synthesis for self-repair.

INDUCING STEM CELLS TOWARD THE INTERVERTEBRAL DISK CELL PHENOTYPE

Using the multipotent differentiation capacity of stem cells, the author attempted to induce MSC differentiation in a mixed coculture system with NP or AF cells in alginate beads (**Fig. 2**). IVD tissue was retrieved during surgery for a burst fracture in a 19-year-old man. Under a microscope, the tissue was separated approximately into the NP and inner and outer AF. The separated tissue was digested with 0.02% pronase (Sigma) and 0.0125% collagenase P (Roche) for 8 hours to obtain cells for primary culture. The NP, inner AF, and outer AF cells were cultured and passaged twice and labeled with PKH26 red fluorescent dye (Sigma). Human MSCs were obtained commercially (Cambrex) and genetically labeled with green fluorescent protein (GFP) by infection with a retrovirus vector. The NP, inner AF, or outer AF cells were cocultured with MSCs in alginate beads in a 50:50 ratio at a density of 30,000 cells/bead. The cells were cocultured for 3 weeks in DMEM + 10% fetal bovine serum, and the cells were recovered. The recovered cells were analyzed, and GFP-positive MSCs were separated by flow cytometry (BD FACSVantage). Characterization of the recovered MSCs by flow cytometry showed that, in forward scatter analysis, the size of MSCs changed markedly after the coculture. MSCs cocultured with NP cells showed significantly greater average cell size, whereas cells cocultured with inner or outer AF cells had a smaller average cell size. The internal complexity analyzed by side scatter showed that MSCs cocultured with NP cells became more complex and that MSCs cocultured with inner or

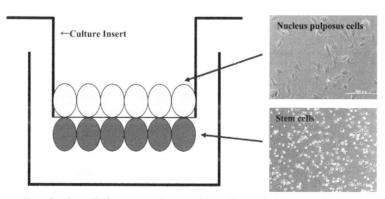

Fig. 1. Use of stem cells as feeder cells for up-regulation of NP cell metabolism. Coculture system allowing cell-to-cell contact.

Mixed 3D coculture system

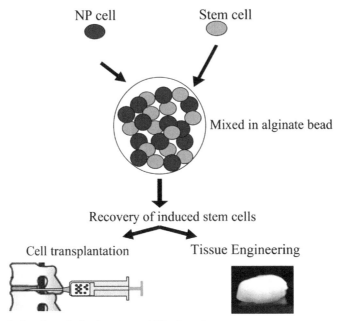

Fig. 2. Use of stem cells for direct induction toward NP phenotype.

outer AF cells became less complex. These characteristics reflected the NP or inner or outer AF cell phenotype of the cocultured opponent. MSCs cocultured with NP cells expressed type II collagen and keratin sulfate, whereas the expression of type I collagen was more intense in cells cocultured with outer AF cells compared with the MSCs before coculture. Gene expression analysis by reverse transcription–polymerase chain reaction (RT-PCR) also confirmed that coculture with different IVD cells in the same 3-D environment led to differentiation of MSCs toward the direction of the cocultured opponent. These experiments showed that the mixed coculture system in alginate is an effective tool for inducing differentiation to MSCs.

Korecki and colleagues[21] hypothesized that MSCs can be differentiated toward the NP cell phenotype if cultured with notochordal cell-conditioned medium. This medium was prepared from notochordal cells maintained in serum-free medium for 4 days. MSCs were cultured in the notochordal cell-conditioned medium, control, or chondrogenic medium. Significantly greater glycosaminoglycan accumulation was found in cell pellets treated with notochordal cell-conditioned medium compared with other media. The notochordal-conditioned medium treatment increased collagen III gene expression. There was a trend for increased expression of laminin-β1 and decreased expression of Sox9 and collagen II relative to the TGF-β group.

Chen and colleagues[22] cocultured synovium-derived stem cells and NP cells in a serum-free pellet system treated with varying doses of TGF-β. The coculture of synovium-derived stem cells and NP cells in a pellet system displayed similar differentiation properties to those of NP cells alone (high levels of collagen II, aggrecan, and Sox9; low level of collagen I; and no collagen X) when treated with high doses of TGF-β1. The coculture and NP cells alone shared a similar higher ratio of aggrecan to collagen II. Hypoxia-inducible factor 1α (HIF-1α) was also up-regulated in the cocultured pellets at day 7 and decreased by day 14 with the time of pellet tissue maturation. The rationale for these in vitro induction methods aims at providing the opportunity to study the cell differentiation pathways of IVD and stem cells and conditioning stem cells before transplantation into the degenerated disk.

TRANSPLANTATION OF STEM CELLS INTO THE INTERVERTEBRAL DISK

In 2003, Sakai and colleagues[23] first reported on transplantation of MSCs into a rabbit disk degeneration model. In the following study, the transplanted autologous MSCs were tagged with GFP, transplanted into a rabbit disk degeneration model, and followed for 48 weeks MRI and radiography.[24,25] Immunohistochemistry was performed to assess the expression of chondroitin sulfate; keratin sulfate; types I, II, and IV collagen; HIF-1α and HIF-1β and HIF-2α and HIF-2β; glucose transporter (GLUT)-1 and GLUT-3; and matrix metalloproteinase (MMP)-2. They also applied RT-PCR to quantify the expression levels of the genes for aggrecan, versican, types I and II collagen, interleukin (IL)-1β, IL-6, tumor necrosis factor (TNF)-α, MMP-9, and MMP-13. MRI and radiographic results confirmed the regenerative effects of the procedure. GFP-positive cells were detected in the nucleus throughout the study. The percentage of positive cells increased from 21% $\pm$ 6% at 2 weeks to 55% $\pm$ 8% at 48 weeks; this increase proved that the MSCs survived and proliferated. Immunohistochemistry showed positive staining of all proteoglycan epitopes and type II collagen in some of the GFP-positive cells. MSCs expressed HIF-1α, MMP-2, and GLUT-3, and this phenotypic activity was compatible with that of NP cells. RT-PCR showed significant restoration of aggrecan, versican, and type II collagen gene expression, and significant suppression of TNF-α and IL-1β genes in the transplantation group. These results show that MSCs transplanted into degenerating disks in vivo can survive, proliferate, and differentiate into cells that express the phenotype of NP cells but suppressed inflammatory genes.

Since the first report using the rabbit model in 2003, various animal studies have demonstrated the feasibility of transplantation of MSCs into the IVD and regenerative effects. Crevensten and colleagues[26] used a 15% hyaluronan gel as a carrier and injected fluorescently labeled MSCs into rat coccygeal disks. Although the number of retained MSCs decreased significantly during the first 2 weeks after injection, the initial cell number was restored after 4 weeks and cell viability and disk height were maintained. These results indicate that the injected cells started to proliferate within the rat disk. Zhang and colleagues[27] implanted allogeneic MSCs containing the marker gene LacZ from young rabbits into rabbit IVDs to determine the potential of this cell-based approach. The transplanted allogeneic MSCs survived and increased the proteoglycan content within the disk, an observation that supports the use of these cells as a potential treatment for IVD degeneration. Hiyama and colleagues[28] confirmed the effectiveness of transplantation of MSCs in large animal models, such as chondrodystrophoid breed canines given a nucleotomy, which have closer morphological features of the human IVD compared to other animals to humans. They also showed that transplanted MSCs expressed FasL after transplantation into the NP region, suggesting the preservation of immune privilege in the transplanted MSCs. These findings are to some

extent similar to the results of rabbit studies that used primarily notochordal NP cells.

Leung and colleagues[29] investigated allogeneic transplantation of MSCs and reported multiple advantages of such transplantation for treating disk disease. They reasoned that if the NP is an immune-privileged environment, then by presenting less antigen, MSCs should be able to escape alloantigen recognition. Moreover, xenogeneic transplantation of bone marrow MSCs has also been investigated in rats and porcine models and was proved effective.[30,31]

MSCs from other sources have also been studied. MSCs from adipose tissue have been reported as another potential cell source. Adipose tissue is considered an abundant, expendable, and easily accessible source of MSCs. The use of these cells may eliminate the need for in vitro expansion, which raises the possibility of a 1-step regenerative treatment method. Hoogendoorn and colleagues[32] reported that adipose-derived MSCs may be beneficial for cell therapy for IVD disease because they are isolated more easily than are bone marrow MSCs. Ganey and colleagues[33] studied the efficacy of autologous adipose tissue–derived stem cells in promoting disk regeneration in a canine disk injury model and found improved disk matrix production and overall disk morphology. Partial nucleotomy was performed at 3 lumbar levels, and the animals were allowed to recover for 6 weeks before receiving either adipose-derived stem cells in hyaluronic acid carrier, hyaluronic acid alone, or no treatment. The 3 experimental disks plus the 2 adjacent control disks were assessed for up to 12 months. The disks that received the adipose-derived cells more closely resembled the healthy controls, as evidenced by the matrix translucency, compartmentalization of the AF, and cell density within the NP. Matrix analysis of type II collagen and aggrecan demonstrated superior regenerative stimulation in the disks treated with adipose stem cells compared with the carrier-only group or no treatment group.

MSCs were recently transplanted into the human IVD to test their potential to regenerate the degenerated disk. Yoshikawa and colleagues[34] transplanted autologous bone marrow MSCs into IVDs showing vacuum phenomenon and instability in two patients going under decompression surgery for spinal stenosis. The MSCs were cultured in medium containing autogenous serum. During surgery, fenestration was performed on the stenosed spinal canal, and pieces of collagen sponge containing autologous MSCs were then grafted percutaneously to the degenerated IVD. Two years after surgery, radiography and CT showed improvements in the vacuum phenomenon in both patients. T2-weighted MRI showed high signal intensity in the IVDs with cell grafts, indicating high moisture content. Roentgenkymography showed less lumbar disk instability.

LIMITATIONS AND TASKS FOR THE FUTURE

It is no question that biologic therapies will take over many of the current therapeutics in the field of orthopaedic surgery. The forerunners are the growth factors and application of bone morphogenetic proteins (BMPs), and in clinical trials, have demonstrated excellent advantage in achieving bony fusion with spinal fusion surgeries compared to autologous bone graft. Recently, however, there have been many reports on serious side effects caused by the use of BMPs with spine surgery.[35] These include inflammatory reactions, adverse back and leg pain events, radiculitis, retrograde ejaculation, urinary retention, bone resorption, and implant displacement. This fact warns all health care providers the pitfall of uncontrolled and underestimated use of biologics.

Feasibility in clinical use of stem cells has historically investigated in hematology/oncology field and has spread to different organs and thus, may lead us to be optimistic of potential side effects, however, cautions need to be seriously warranted. Although many animal studies and recent clinical trials have used stem cells in the treatment of IVD degeneration (**Fig. 3**), careful attention is needed in its application. An experimental study by Vadala et al. has warned using the rabbit model that cell leakage after MSC injection to the IVD may cause osteophyte formation.[36] As they suggest, considerations on cell carriers or annulus-sealing techniques may need to be assessed or perhaps, post-surgical rehabilitation protocols shall be investigated to minimize the leakage. Unintended differentiation and tumorigenesis is another potential risk that stem cell therapy usually faces. More precise definition of IVD cells and their characteristics are needed to understand better how to control the induction pathways. The criteria for successful application need careful investigation in the context of stem cell transplantation into humans.

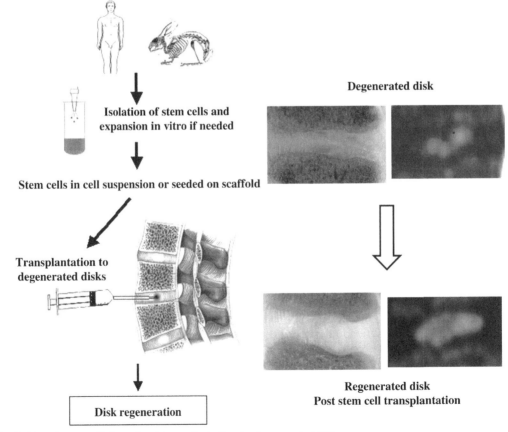

Fig. 3. Use of stem cells in a direct transplantation to degenerated IVD.

Much of the research on stem cell transplantation into the IVD focuses on regeneration of the NP rather than the AF or the vertebral end plate, probably because the NP is a cavity, which eases the application of stem cells. However, further understanding of methods to regenerate the AF and end plate is needed because end plate regeneration is important for securing the nutrition of the IVD microenvironment.

Despite all the limitations and risks, carefully designed clinical trials with appropriate informed consent are the only solution to find the answer and to define whether stem cell therapy will benefit patients with intervetrbral disk degeneration.

REFERENCES

1. Frymoyer JW, Cats-Baril WL. An overview of the incidence and costs of low back pain. Orthop Clin North Am 1991;22:263–71.

2. Deyo RA, Weinstein JN. Low back pain. N Engl J Med 2001;344:363–70.

3. Maniadakis N, Gray A. The economic burden of back pain in the UK. Pain 2000;84:95–103.

4. Buckwalter JA. Aging and degeneration of the human intervertebral disc. Spine 1995;20(11):1307–14.

5. Taylor JR, Twomey LT. The development of the human intervertebral disc. In: Ghosh P, editor. The biology of the intervertebral disc. Boca Raton (FL): CRC Press Inc.; 1988. p. 39–82.

6. Hunter CJ, Matyas JR, Duncan NA. Cytomorphology of notochordal and chondrocytic cells from the nucleus pulposus: a species comparison. J Anat 2004;205(5):357–62.

7. Maroudas A, Stockwell RA, Nachemson, et al. Factors involved in the nutrition of the human lumbar intervertebral disc: cellularity and diffusion of glucose in vitro. J Anat 1975;120(Pt 1):113–30.

8. Marchand F, Ahmed AM. Investigation of the laminate structure of lumbar disc anulus fibrosus. Spine 1990;15(5):402–10.

9. Yu J. Elastic tissues of the intervertebral disc. Biochem Soc Trans 2002;30(Pt 6):848–52.

10. Wuertz K, Godburn K, Neidlinger-Wilke, et al. Behavior of mesenchymal stem cells in the chemical microenvironment of the intervertebral disc. Spine 2008;33(17):1843–9.

11. Heathfield SK, Le Maitre CL, Hoyland JA. Caveolin-1 expression and stress-induced premature senescence in human intervertebral disc degeneration. Arthritis Res Ther 2008;10(4):R87.

12. Risbud MV, Guttapalli A, Tsai TT, et al. Evidence for skeletal progenitor cells in the degenerate human intervertebral disc. Spine 2007;32(23):2537–44.

13. Blanco JF, Graciani IF, Sanchez-Guijo FM, et al. Isolation and characterization of mesenchymal stromal cells from human degenerated nucleus pulposus: comparison with bone marrow mesenchymal stromal cells from the same subjects. Spine (Phila Pa 1976) 2010;35(26):2259–65.

14. Feng G, Yang X, Shang H, et al. Multipotential differentiation of human anulus fibrosus cells: an in vitro study. J Bone Joint Surg Am 2010;92(3):675–85.

15. Fujita J, Mori M, Kawada H, et al. Administration of granulocyte colony-stimulating factor after myocardial infarction enhances the recruitment of hematopoietic stem cell-derived myofibroblasts and contributes to cardiac repair. Stem Cells 2007;25(11):2750–9.

16. Kawada H, Takizawa S, Takanashi T, et al. Administration of hematopoietic cytokines in the subacute phase after cerebral infarction is effective for functional recovery facilitating proliferation of intrinsic neural stem/progenitor cells and transition of bone marrow-derived neuronal cells. Circulation 2006;113(5):701–10.

17. Yamamoto Y, Mochida J, Sakai D, et al. Upregulation of the viability of nucleus pulposus cells by bone-marrow-derived stromal cells: significance of direct cell-to-cell contact in co-culture system. Spine 2004;29:1508–14.

18. Nishimura K, Mochida J. Percutaneous reinsertion of the nucleus pulposus. An experimental study. Spine 1996;21:1556–63.

19. Watanabe T, Sakai D, Yamamoto Y, et al. Human nucleus pulposus cells significantly enhanced biological properties in a coculture system with direct cell-to-cell contact with autologous mesenchymal stem cells. J Orthop Res 2010;28(5):623–30.

20. Strassburg S, Richardson SM, Freemont AJ, et al. Co-culture induces mesenchymal stem cell differentiation and modulation of the degenerate human nucleus pulposus cell phenotype. Regen Med 2010;5(5):701–11.

21. Korecki CL, Taboas JM, Tuan RS, et al. Notochordal cell conditioned medium stimulates mesenchymal stem cell differentiation toward a young nucleus pulposus phenotype. Stem Cell Res Ther 2010;1(2):18.

22. Chen S, Emery SE, Pei M. Coculture of synovium-derived stem cells and nucleus pulposus cells in serum-free defined medium with supplementation of transforming growth factor-beta1: a potential application of tissue-specific stem cells in disc regeneration. Spine (Phila Pa 1976) 2009;34(12):1272–80.

23. Sakai D, Mochida J, Yamamoto Y, et al. Transplantation of mesenchymal stem cells embedded in atelocollagen gel to the intervertebral disc: a potential therapeutic model for disc degeneration. Biomaterials 2003;24:3531–41.

24. Sakai D, Mochida J, Iwashina T, et al. Differentiation of mesenchymal stem cells transplanted to

a rabbit degenerative disc model. Spine 2005;30:2379–87.

25. Sakai D, Mochida J, Iwashina T, et al. Regenerative effects of transplanting mesenchymal stem cells embedded in atelocollagen to the degenerated intervertebral disc. Biomaterials 2006;27:335–45.

26. Crevensten G, Walsh AJ, Ananthakrishnan D, et al. Intervertebral disc cell therapy for regeneration: mesenchymal stem cell implantation in rat intervertebral discs. Ann Biomed Eng 2004;32:430–4.

27. Zhang YG, Guo X, Xu P, et al. Bone mesenchymal stem cells transplanted into rabbit intervertebral discs can increase proteoglycans. Clin Orthop Relat Res 2005;430:219–26.

28. Hiyama A, Mochida J, Iwashina T, et al. Transplantation of mesenchymal stem cells in a canine disc degeneration model. J Orthop Res 2008;26:589–600.

29. Leung VY, Chan D, Cheung KM. Regeneration of intervertebral disc by mesenchymal stem cells: potentials, limitations, and future direction. Eur Spine J 2006;15:S406–13.

30. Wei A, Tao H, Chung SA, et al. The fate of transplanted xenogeneic bone marrow-derived stem cells in rat intervertebral discs. J Orthop Res 2009;3:374–9.

31. Henriksson HB, Svanvik T, Jonsson M, et al. Transplantation of human mesenchymal stems cells into intervertebral discs in a xenogeneic porcine model. Spine 2009;34(2):141–8.

32. Hoogendoorn RJ, Lu ZF, Kroeze RJ, et al. Adipose stem cells for intervertebral disc regeneration: current status and concepts for the future. J Cell Mol Med 2008;12(6A):2205–16.

33. Ganey T, Hutton WC, Moseley T, et al. Intervertebral disc repair using adipose tissue-derived stem and regenerative cells: experiments in a canine model. Spine 2009;34(21):2297–304.

34. Yoshikawa T, Ueda Y, Miyazaki K, et al. Disc regeneration therapy using marrow mesenchymal cell transplantation: a report of two case studies. Spine 2010;35(11):E475–80.

35. Carragee EJ, Hurwitz EL, Weiner BK. A critical review of recombinant human bone morphogenetic protein-2 trials in spinal surgery: emerging safety concerns and lessons learned. Spine J 2011;11:471–91.

36. Vadalà G, Sowa G, Hubert M, et al. Mesenchymal stem cells injection in degenerated intervertebral disc: cell leakage may induce osteophyte formation. J Tissue Eng Regen Med 2011. [Epub ahead of print].

Gene Therapy for Intervertebral Disk Degeneration

Barrett I. Woods, MD[a,b,]*, Nam Vo, PhD[a,b],
Gwendolyn Sowa, MD, PhD[a,c], James D. Kang, MD[a,b]

KEYWORDS

- Intervertebral disk degeneration • Treatment • Gene therapy

Intervertebral disk degeneration (IDD) is a common and potentially debilitating disease process that affects millions in the United States and worldwide. IDD has a variable presentation, from relatively benign to completely disabling, and can be associated with disk herniation, spinal stenosis, radiculopathy, myelopathy, instability, and low back pain. The socioeconomic impact of musculoskeletal disorders of the spine, such as IDD and low back pain, cannot be overstated because these conditions are the leading cause of disability in people 45 years and younger resulting in national economic losses of more than $90 billion annually.[1]

Despite the prevalence of IDD and its enormous socioeconomic impact, operative and nonoperative treatment options are suboptimal and associated with unpredictable outcomes. Current treatment options for IDD and the pathology associated with it include decompression, spinal fusion, diskectomy, electrothermal therapy, and arthroplasty, all addressing the clinical symptoms associated with this disease process (pain and mechanical instability) and not the underlying pathophysiology.[2–5] With advances in molecular as well as cellular biology researchers have begun to characterize the pathophysiologic pathways associated with disk degeneration and thus provided targets for potential biologic treatments to augment or reverse the course of IDD (see the articles by Leung and colleagues and Bae and colleagues elsewhere in this issue). This article briefly discusses the pathophysiology of disk degeneration, the premise behind gene therapy for the treatment of IDD, strategy for delivery, transfer of therapeutic genes to the disk, and safety concerns associated with its application.

PATHOPHYSIOLOGY OF INTERVERTEBRAL DISK DEGENERATION

The intervertebral disk is the largest avascular structure in the body and is composed of three morphologically distinct regions. The central nucleus pulposus is a gelatinous matrix rich in large aggregating proteoglycans, which imbibe water and may assist in the diffusion of nutrients from the periphery through maintenance of an osmotic gradient. The peripheral annulus fibrosis encases the nucleus pulposus and is a dense fibrotic tissue composed of concentric lamellae rich in type I collagen. The cartilaginous endplates are present at the cranial and caudal aspects of each disk and contain the peripheral vasculature, which nourishes the disk.

In concert these structures absorb and transmit mechanical stress to the vertebrae and surrounding musculoligamentous structures of

Disclosure: No conflicts of interest; the authors have nothing to disclose.
[a] The Ferguson Laboratory for Orthopaedic and Spine Research, University of Pittsburgh Medical Center, 200 Lothrop street, EBST 1641, Pittsburgh, PA 15213, USA
[b] Department of Orthopaedic Surgery, University of Pittsburgh Medical Center, Pittsburgh, PA, USA
[c] Department of Physical Medicine & Rehabilitation, University of Pittsburgh Medical Center, Pittsburgh, PA, USA
* Corresponding author. The Ferguson Laboratory for Orthopaedic and Spine Research, University of Pittsburgh Medical Center, 200 Lothrop street, EBST 1641, Pittsburgh, PA 15213.
E-mail address: woodbi@upmc.edu

Orthop Clin N Am 42 (2011) 563–574
doi:10.1016/j.ocl.2011.07.002

the spine. Maintenance of the morphologic distinctions between the nucleus pulposus and annulus fibrosis is essential for normal biomechanical function of the disk during loading (see the article by Inoue and Espinoza Orías elsewhere in this issue).[6]

The exact pathophysiology of degenerative disk disease has not yet been completely delineated; however, it is known to be influenced by the interaction between various genetic, biologic, and biomechanical factors.[7–10] In addition, the morphologic, biochemical, and radiographic changes, which occur with progressive degeneration of the intervertebral disk, have been well characterized. The hallmark of disk degeneration is the progressive loss of proteoglycans, which coincides with decreases in oxygen tension, free radical accumulation, decreased pH, and the increased activity of aberrant proteolytic enzymes.[11–13] With the loss of proteoglycans, the nucleus pulposus cannot maintain normal physiologic hydrostatic pressure, which results in the dehydration of the disk.[14] In addition, there is a progressive fibrosis of the nucleus pulposus as the ratio between type I and type II collagen increases.[15] As degeneration progresses, the nucleus pulposus and annulus fibrosis lose their morphologic distinction, which ultimately disrupts the finely balanced biomechanics of the disk and spine as a whole (**Fig. 1**).[14,16]

Several studies have indicated that the loss of proteoglycans within the disk is due to an imbalance between anabolism and catabolism within the disk, because proteolytic enzymes (matrix metalloproteinases and A disintegrin and metalloproteinase with thrombospondin) are up-regulated, whereas collagen and proteoglycan synthesis is diminished.[17–20] Over the past few years, key biologic factors that regulate disk extracellular matrix production, nutrition, cellular proliferation, signaling, and cell death have been identified.

The development of novel biologic treatments, such as gene therapy, have the potential to treat disk degeneration on a molecular level by correcting the biochemical imbalance within degenerating disks and thus potentially changing the natural history of this disease without the morbidity associated with surgery.

GENE THERAPY

The idea of gene therapy originated as a means to treat heritable genetic disorders by replacing defective genes with functional copies, thus curing the underlying disorder. The current concept of gene therapy has expanded to include the transfer of exogenous genes encoding therapeutic proteins into cells to treat disease. On transduction of this genetic material into the genome of the target cell, the host transcribes the transgene into mRNA, which is then translated by ribosome in the cytoplasm into the desired protein product. These protein products affect not only the metabolism of the host cell but also that of adjacent cells via a paracrine effect. The direct application of

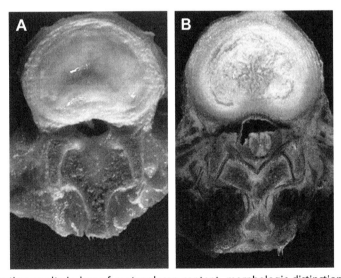

Fig. 1. Disk degeneration results in loss of proteoglycan content, morphologic distinction of the disk components, structural failure, and facet arthrosis. The loss of demarcation is clear in contrasting these two pictures as the type I/type II collagen ratio in the nucleus pulposus increases and becomes progressively more fibrotic. Loss of hydration causes decreased osmotic pressure, increased tensile forces, annulus fissures and loading of the posterior elements. (*A*) Healthy disk. (*B*) Disk degeneration in a 28 year old. (*From* Bullough PG. Orthopaedic pathology. 4th edition. Edinburgh; New York: Mosby; 2004; with permission.)

therapeutic exogenous proteins is inadequate because their short half-life within the cell precludes any long-term disease-modifying treatment. Gene therapy alters host cell DNA, thereby providing a mechanism for the sustained production of the desired therapeutic product.

The packaging of exogenous genes is a technically demanding and labor-intensive process. First, the enzyme reverse transcriptase is used to construct the complementary DNA (cDNA) of the gene of interest from mRNA. Next, the newly constructed cDNA is cloned in an expression plasmid under the control of an appropriate promoter, which drives the expression of the transgene. Finally, the completed expression plasmid (with the cDNA of the therapeutic gene) is integrated into a vector, which facilitates the entry of the exogenous gene into the host cell.

VECTORS

The success of gene therapy is dependent not only on sustained expression of the therapeutic gene but also efficient transfer of the genetic material to the host cell. With few exceptions, naked plasmid DNA alone is not an effective means of gene transfer. Therefore, the use of vectors is necessary to facilitate the transfer of genetic information to host cell. There are several types of vectors, most of which fall into one of two distinguishing classes: viral and nonviral.

Nonviral vectors include liposomes, gene guns, DNA-ligand complexes, and microbubble enhanced ultrasound. Liposomes are phospholipid vesicles that deliver the genetic material into the cell by fusing with the host's cellular membrane. DNA-ligand complexes and gene gun are other nonpathogenic vectors, which are inexpensive and easy to construct. Nishida and colleagues[21] illustrated that ultrasound transfection with microbubbles enhances the efficiency of plasmid DNA uptake into the nucleus pulposus of rats in vivo. The main issue with nonviral vectors is transient transgene expression due to low transfection efficiency into the host genome, thus making these vectors suboptimal for the treatment of chronic diseases in which the sustained production of the desire product is required for disease modification.

Viral vectors use the natural capability of viruses to infect host cells and thus transfer the viral genetic information into the host. Viral vectors are efficient at transducing the desired genetic material to the host cell, even into slowly dividing senescent cellular populations like those of the intervertebral disk. They are also associated with greater risks than nonviral vectors, however, such as cytotoxicity and immune-mediated response. Viral vectors used for gene therapy applications include adenovirus, adeno-associated virus (AAV), herpes simplex virus, lentivirus, retrovirus, and poxvirus. Each viral vector is associated with specific advantages and disadvantages. Therefore, proper selection of vector is critical to successful gene therapy. The most commonly used viral vectors for disk degeneration are adeno and AAV vectors.

Adenoviruses are double-stranded DNA viruses, which have the ability to infect many cell types. There are 47 known human serotypes, of which serotypes 2 and 5 are most commonly used for gene therapy applications. Adenovirus vectors are especially efficient at the transfer of genetic material to host cells, are relatively easy to construct at high titers, and can transduce nondividing quiescent cellular populations. These vectors are easily modifiable for gene therapy applications by the removal of the envelope E1 gene, which is essential for viral gene replication and expression.[22] In addition, the adenovirus genome does not integrate into that of the host cell and remains as an episome within the host cell's nucleus. Therefore, adenoviruses for gene therapy applications are thought to be associated with low rates of insertional mutagenesis during transduction in comparison with other vectors. The major limitation associated with the use of adenovirus vectors is the short duration of transgene expression in most tissues. This transient expression is attributed to the production of adenoviral antigens by the host cell, with the resulting immune response degrading the adenoviral episome within the nucleus, thus halting therapeutic protein production.[23,24] In addition, because the adenovirus is not integrated into the host cell's genome during cellular division, the episome is not replicated. Finally, wild-type adenoviral infections can cause upper respiratory and gastrointestinal illnesses. These issues, although concerning, likely have less clinical relevance due to the asvascular encapsulated nature of the disk. Currently, ways to minimize host adenoviral antigen production and viral protein expression are being investigated.

Unlike adenovirus, AAV is a parvovirus with a single-stranded DNA genome. AAV also has the ability to transfect multiple different cell types, much less efficiently, however, than the adenovirus. There are several distinct differences between adenovirus and AAV. First, the wild-type AAV is not associated with any human disease and thus there are fewer safety concerns with its application. The AAV vector integrates into a specific site on chromosome 19 without damaging the intrinsic genetic material present. Another beneficial feature is that

AAV has only two genes (Rep and Cap), which cannot self-replicate and require the presence of a helper virus. Therefore, in the absence of helper virus, there is no expression of intrinsic AAV gene products after transduction, limiting the cell-mediated immune response. The difficulty with using AAV vectors is that they can carry much less foreign (therapeutic) DNA than the adenovirus vector, and the purification of AAV is challenging because the helper virus must be isolated and removed. Despite these shortcomings, AAV has shown real promise as the conduit for successful gene therapy into musculoskeletal tissues. Currently improvements in vector immunogenicity as well as inducible and tissue-specific promoters are being developed. The selection of the appropriate vector is critical for successful gene therapy and depends on disease pathophysiology, therapeutic gene used, and strategy for delivery.

GENE DELIVERY STRATEGY

In addition to the selection of the appropriate gene and vector, another important consideration with gene therapy applications is the delivery strategy used. There are currently two basic strategies for the delivery of exogenous therapeutic genes into target cells. The in vivo strategy involves the direct transfer of the gene-vector complex to the targeted cellular population within the living host. The ex vivo strategy differs significantly because the targeted cells are isolated and removed from the living host. These cells are then cultured with transduction of the therapeutic gene occurring in vitro. The final step includes the reimplantation of the genetically altered cells back into the host (**Fig. 2**).

Theoretically, the ex vivo method may be a safer approach to gene therapy because the genetically altered cells are observed in vitro; therefore, the cells that show abnormal responses to the transfer of the therapeutic gene can be identified and isolated from the target cell population before reimplantation. There are several disadvantages, however, with the utlization of an ex vivo strategy for clinical gene therapy applications. First, there may be significant morbidity associated with the harvesting as well as the reimplanation of the targeted host cells. Second, often the in vivo environment from which the host cells are removed cannot be replicated in vitro. in vitro, the cells themselves maybe irreversibly altered, not making them suitable to reimplantion. This is of particular concern when considering gene therapy for IDD, because the harsh conditions the cells of the nucleus polposus experience (low oxygen tension, nutrients, and pH) cannot easily be replicated. Additionally in vitro cells are not subjected to biomechanical stimuli, which may be important to cellular signaling and cytokine production. Because of these reasons, most gene therapy applications for disk degeneration use an in vivo strategy for gene delivery.

MODULATION OF DISK CELL BIOLOGY

The foundation for the application of gene therapy to treat disk degeneration is rooted in the identification of exogenous proteins and cytokines, which have shown potential therapeutic benefits, albeit transient, when cultured with disk cells in vitro or directly into the disk in vivo.[25] As discussed

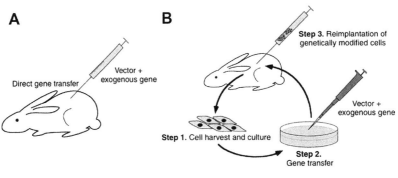

Fig. 2. (*A*) In vivo gene therapy involves the direct injection of vector-gene constructs into target tissues within the host. (*B*) In the ex vivo method target cells are harvested from the host, which are then transduced, expanded, and propagated in culture before reimplantation. (*From* Herkowitz HN, Rothman RH, Simeone FA. Rothman-Simeone, the spine. 5th edition. Philadelphia: Saunders Elsevier; 2006; with permission.)

previously, several studies suggest that the loss of proteoglycan associated with disk degeneration is due to an imbalance between catabolism and anabolism within the disk. Thus, the goal of gene therapy for the treatment of disk degeneration is to transfer genes, which corrects this imbalance, thereby slowing or reversing the loss of proteoglycans within the disk. Correction of the biochemical imbalances within the disk would likely facilitate the recovery and maintenance of normal disk morphology, thereby improving the biomechanical function of the disk and ultimately altering the natural course of this disease process. In addition, the intervertebral disk is a good target for gene therapy because it is encapsulated and avascular, thus acting as an immune-privileged organ allowing for sustained periods of transgene expression due to the lack of immune response to the therapeutic gene product or the intrinsic proteins produced by the vector.

Thompson and colleagues[26] were the first to demonstrate that in vitro proteoglycan synthesis within the disk could be up-regulated through the application of exogenous human transforming growth factor β1 (TGF-β1) in cultured canine disk tissue. There have been several subsequent studies that have identified other growth factors that have the ability to increase proteoglycan synthesis in intervertebral disk cells. Osada and colleagues[27] demonstrated increased proteoglycan synthesis in cultured bovine disk cells stimulated with exogenous insulin growth factor-1. Takegami and colleagues[28] illustrated a similar increase in proteoglycan synthesis in cultured rabbit nucleus pulposus cells exposed to exogenous osteogenic protein-1, in addition to the recovery of proteoglycan content lost in cells exposed to inflammatory cytokine interleukin (IL)-1. Li and colleagues[29] illustrated that exogenous of bone morphogenetic protein (BMP)-2 not only increased aggrecan expression but also stimulated osteogenic protein-1 expression, further boosting proteoglycan synthesis in cultured rat disk cells. Tim Yoon and colleagues[30] performed an in vitro study on rat intervertebral disk stimulated with BMP-2 and found that this growth factor not only increased cell proliferation and proteoglycan synthesis but also increased the mRNA of type II collagen, aggrecan, and Sox9 genes, which are all chondrocyte-specific genes (**Fig. 3**). In addition to the anabolic function of these growth factors, Gruber and colleagues[31] demonstrated that the exogenous application of IGF-I and platelet-derived growth factor significantly decreased the number of apoptotic disk cells in culture. Thus, these growth factors may have some utility in treating disk degeneration by

maintaining the disk cell population, phenotype, and proteoglycan content.

GENE THERAPY TO INTERVERTEBRAL DISKS

With the identification of potential therapeutic growth factors and cytokines, the idea of producing them endogenously using gene therapy arose. This idea was first expounded on by Wehling and colleagues[32] who performed an in vitro study using retroviral-mediated transfer of the bacterial enzyme β-galactosidase marker gene (LacZ) and the cDNA of the human IL-1 receptor antagonist to bovine endplate chondrocytes. Despite successfully transducing only approximately 1% of the cultured bovine cells, the transgene expression of IL-1 receptor antagonist was significantly increased over controls at 48 hours. From these data it was concluded that the ex vivo method of gene therapy may be a novel approach to the treatment of disk degeneration via the reimplantation of genetically altered disk cells. The first successful in vivo gene transfer was demonstrated by Nishida and colleagues,[33] who reported sustained transgene expression of adenoviral-mediated LacZ marker gene in skeletally mature New Zealand white rabbits. These rabbits showed no evidence of systemic illness, which was supported by the lack of cellular immune response histologically up to 3 months post-transduction, with evidence of transgene expression within the disk detected 1 year post-transduction (**Fig. 4**).[34] This study also demonstrated much more efficient transfer of genetic material than was previously reported, as in vitro transduction of LacZ in cultured rabbit cells was nearly 100% using the adenovirus vector.[33] In addition to these findings, Nishida and colleagues[33] found no change in the intradiscal expression of a genetic marker luciferase in rabbits immunized subcutaneously with the transgene-vector construct weeks before delivery into the disk. In other tissues, such as the testis and retina, their immune privilege characteristics have been attributed to the local expression of Fas ligand within their tissues, which induces apoptosis to invading Fas-positive T cells. Takada and colleagues[35] subsequently demonstrated the presence of Fas ligand in disk cells, specifically those of the nucleus pulposus, providing a mechanism to support the theory of the immune privilege status of the disk. These pivotal studies not only illustrated the potential of in vivo gene therapy for disk degeneration but also legitimized the claim that gene therapy into the intervertebral disk is feasible due to its immune-privileged nature.

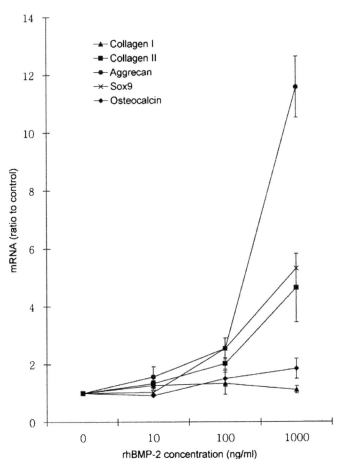

Fig. 3. Quantitation of mRNA levels using real-time polymerase chain reaction 7 days after application of recombinant human BMP (rhBMP)-2 to rat annulus cells in vitro. Normalization was performed with internal control (glyceraldehyde-3-phosphate dehydrogenase [GAPDH]) and a standard curve for each primer. Aggrecan, Sox9, and type II collagen were significantly increased at rhBMP-2 concentrations of 100 and 1000 ng/mL. Type I collagen levels did not change regardless of rhBMP-2 concentration. (*From* Tim Yoon S, Su Kim K, Li J, et al. The effect of bone morphogenetic protein-2 on rat intervertebral disk cells in vitro. Spine [Phila Pa 1976] 2003;28:1773–80; with permission.)

GENETIC TRANSFER OF THERAPEUTIC GENES

The next step in the evolution of gene therapy for the treatment of disk degeneration was to replace the marker gene (LacZ) with ones having therapeutic potential. Using an adenovirus vector, Nishida and colleagues[36] successfully transduced cDNA for TGF-β1 into the nucleus pulposus of lumbar rabbit disks. This study illustrated a 30-fold increase in synthesis of active TGF-β1 and a 5-fold increase in total production of this growth factor in disks injected with the adenovirus-gene complex (**Fig. 5**). In addition to the successful transduction of TGF-β1, proteoglycan synthesis increased 100% from baseline values. As in previous studies with vector-marker gene constructs, there was no evidence of a systemic of local immune response. Cells that received adenovirus TGF-β1 had increased synthesis of matrix components (proteoglycans and collagen) in comparison with those receiving the exogenous protein alone, which is likely due to the sustained expression produced by gene therapy. The transduced cells also exerted a paracrine effect on adjacent nontreated cells, because the viral load required to increase proteoglycan synthesis was much lower than that required to transduce the entire cell population of the disk. Assays for TGF-β1 and proteoglycan synthesis were also performed on disks transduced with a viral vector control gene construct (adeno-luciferase marker gene). There was no increase in TGF-β1 or proteoglycan synthesis detected in these disks indicating that the observed response in the treatment group was due to the presence of TGF-β1 and not a nonspecific response to the adenovirus vector.

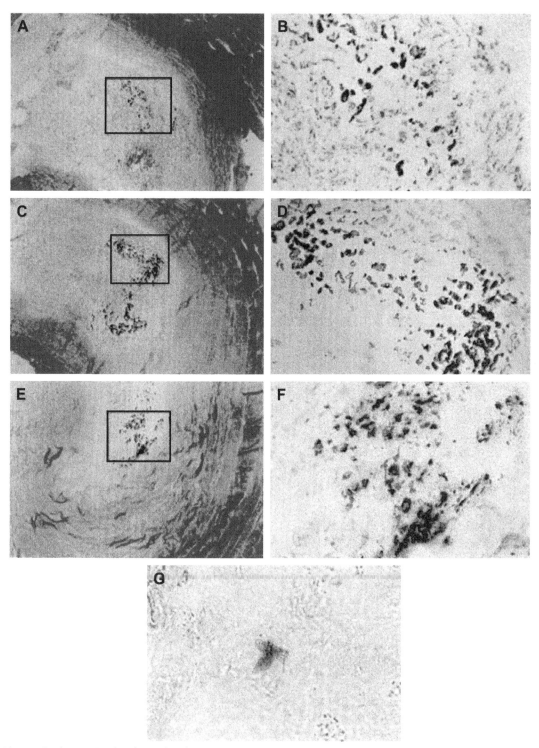

Fig. 4. Histology stained with X-Gal and eosin representing transgene expression of Ad-LacZ in rabbit lumbar intervertebral disks at 3 weeks (*A*, *B*), 6 weeks (*C*, *D*), 24 weeks (*E*, *F*), and 52 weeks (*G*) post-transduction. At 52 weeks, positive X-Gal staining was observed in the disks from 2 of the 3 rabbits; however, the intensity of the positive stain was significantly diminished from previous time periods (original magnifications ×40 [*A, C, E*], ×200 [*B, D, F*], and ×600 [*G*]). (*From* Nishida K, Kang JD, Gilbertson LG, et al. Modulation of the biologic activity of the rabbit intervertebral disk by gene therapy: an in vivo study of adenovirus-mediated transfer of the human transforming growth factor beta 1 encoding gene. Spine [Phila Pa 1976] 1999;24:2419–25; with permission.)

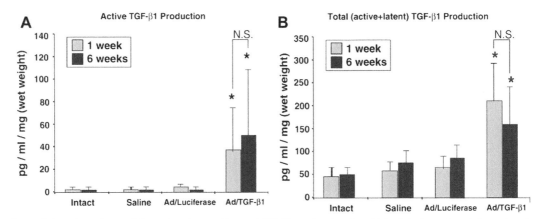

Fig. 5. (*A*) Active TGF-β1. (*B*) Total active and latent TGF-β1 production in rabbit disk tissue 1 and 6 weeks after in vivo transduction. Sustained transgene expression was present at 6 weeks, as there was no significant difference in active or total TGF-β1 production between the 1 and 6 week time points. Asterisks denotes a significant increase in TGF-β1 production in treatment group versus controls (*P*<.05). (*From* Nishida K, Kang JD, Gilbertson LG, et al. Modulation of the biologic activity of the rabbit intervertebral disk by gene therapy: an in vivo study of adenovirus-mediated transfer of the human transforming growth factor beta 1 encoding gene. Spine [Phila Pa 1976] 1999;24:2419–25; with permission.)

This study demonstrated that intervertebral disk cells not only could be transduced successfully with therapeutic genes but also were capable of producing enough growth factor to significantly modulate the biologic activity of the treated cell population. These results have been replicated in other studies using growth factors (BMP-2 and IGF-1) vector complexes that increase proteoglycan synthesis in a dose-dependant manner.[37,38] Tissue inhibitor of metalloproteinase 1 (TIMP-1), however, displayed the same ability when transduced into nucleus pulposus cells. TIMP-1 is an inhibitor of matrix metalloproteinases that breaks down the extracellular matrix components and is thus one of many regulators of the catabolic activity of the disk. Up-regulation of this anticatabolic cytokine was matrix protective by inhibiting the breakdown of existing proteoglycans within the disk. Wallach and colleagues[38] demonstrated increased proteoglycan synthesis in human disk cells cultured in 3-D pellets exposed to adenovirus TIMP-1 (**Fig. 6**). This finding provided credence to the hypothesis that the imbalance between catabolism and anabolism results in proteoglycan loss and that biologic modification could target increasing anabolism or decreasing catabolism in the disk.

Two other potentially disease-altering genes being investigated include LIM mineralization protein (LMP-1) and Sox9. LMP-1 is a regulatory protein that up-regulates the anabolic activity of BMPs in the disk. Yoon and colleagues[39] found significantly increased expression of BMP-2 and 7 mRNA after the in vitro transduction of

adenovirus LMP-1. This finding was correlated with an increase in proteoglycan synthesis both in vivo and in vitro after transduction of rat intervertebral disk cells. Sox9 is a transcription factor that has many responsibilities, including type II collagen expression, an essential component of the nucleus pulposus extracellular matrix. Human intervertebral disk cells treated with adenoviral vector Sox9 complex in vitro showed increase type II collagen production compared with controls.[40] As the pathophysiology of disk degeneration is better delineated, the use of certain specific therapeutic genes or a combination of those may be better suited for the biologic augmentation of diseased disk cells. Continued research is geared toward identifying more potentially therapeutic genes and improving the efficiency and safety of their delivery.

REGULATION OF PATHOLOGIC GENE EXPRESSION

RNA interference (RNAi) has emerged as another strategy for altering genetic information within diseased disk cells. RNAi reduces the overall production of a targeted gene product by the use of small interfering RNA (siRNA), which binds to the targeted mRNA in a sequence-specific manner, leading to either suppressed translation or enhanced degradation of the message. Thus, catabolic genes within the disk tissue can be targeted and silenced through siRNA-mediated destruction preventing translation of those genes. As with therapeutic exogenous genes, siRNA has

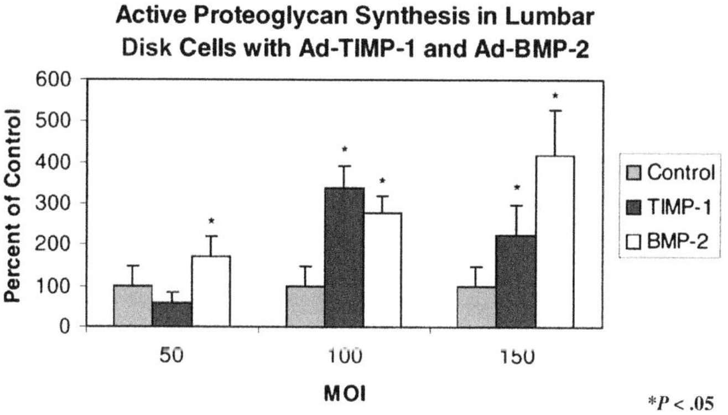

Active Proteoglycan Synthesis in Lumbar Disk Cells with Ad-TIMP-1 and Ad-BMP-2

Fig. 6. Measured proteoglycans in human lumbar disk cells cultured in 3-D pellet. Cells were transduced with Ad-TIMP-1 or Ad-BMP-2, and proteoglycans are expressed as percent measured in controls. An optimal response to Ad-TIMP-1 occurred at a multiplicity of infection (MOI) of 100 and resulted in a more than 300% increase in proteoglycan production from controls. Ad-BMP-2 application resulted in a dose-dependant increase in proteoglycan content. (*From* Wallach CJ, Sobajima S, Watanabe Y, et al. Gene transfer of the catabolic inhibitor TIMP-1 increases measured proteoglycans in cells from degenerated human intervertebral disks. Spine [Phila Pa 1976] 2003;28:2331–7; with permission.)

a short half-life. Kakutani and colleagues[41] demonstrated sustained down-regulation of specific targeted genes using DNA vector-siRNA complexes. In that study, expression of firefly luciferase was inhibited 94.7% in rat and 93.7% in human nucleus pulposus cells cultured in vitro that were treated with siRNA targeting this gene. This inhibitory effect was gone 3 weeks after initial treatment, however. RNAi may provide another mechanism to address the resultant imbalance between catabolism and anabolism in intervertebral disk cells; however, sustained down-regulation of specific target genes is required to treat chronic progressive disorders, such as IDD.

SAFETY CONSIDERATIONS

Due to the potential adverse effects associated with the use of viral vectors for gene therapy applications, current areas of investigation include strategies to reduced viral load required to produce significant therapeutic end product production, inducible on-off mechanisms, tissue-specific promoters, and AAV vector constructs. One strategy to amplify transgene expression while limiting viral load is to transduce combinations of anabolic genes on one viral vector. Experiments with various combinations of growth factors (TGF-β1, BMP-2, and IGF-1) show a synergistic effect amplifying the production of extracellular matrix components.[37] In this study,[37] human nucleus pulposus cells were isolated and cultured in vitro. On confluence, cells were subsequently transduced with one of the growth factors, a combination of two growth factors (TGF-β1 +

IGF-1, TGF-β1 + BMP-2, or IGF-1 + BMP-2), or all three growth factors using an adenovirus vector. Proteoglycan synthesis was significantly increased from control (180%–295%) when treated with one factor, and a synergistic effect was observed when cells were treated with a combination of two factors as increases in proteoglycan synthesis ranged from 322% to 398%. Cell cultures that received all three factors had a 471% increase in new proteoglycan synthesis. Future studies will determine if combinations of these anabolic growth factors in addition to anticatabolic factors, such as TIMP-1, have even greater effects on the biologic activity within the disk.

Another concern with the application of gene therapy is the inability to regulate transgene expression once successfully transduced into the host cell. Wallach and colleagues[42] demonstrated that accidental intradural injection of vector-therapeutic gene constructs (adenovirus encoding human [Ad]-TGF-β1) can result in severe histologic changes and paralysis in New Zealand white rabbits. Therefore, inducible systems to regulate transgene expression are being developed. Several inducible gene expression systems have been investigated, including systems using heat shock proteins, metallothionine, steroid regulatory promoters, tetracycline, and, most recently, the insect ecdysone receptor. Most of these inducible systems work by linking a ligand-activated promoter region to the potential therapeutic gene within the vector construct. There are two basic strategies for regulation, which depend on whether the exogenously applied ligand turns transgene expression "on" or "off." The Tet-On system is one in which transgene expression is activated by administration of a tetracycline derivative, and this inducible system has been incorporated into AAV vector constructs.[43] These Tet-On systems have demonstrated successful regulation of a marker gene in chondrocytes from New Zealand white rabbit knees.[44] Current research is investigating ways to increase efficiency of Tet-On systems and evaluate their control of therapeutic transgene expression in intervertebral disk cells. Additionally, regulation systems with tissue-specific promoters are being developed and would further optimize efficacy and minimize treatment side effects.

The use of less pathologic viral vector constructs, such as AAV, have also been investigated as alternatives to adenovirus vectors. The efficacy of AAV vector transduction in comparison with adenovirus was explored on nucleus pulposus cells in vitro and in vivo.[45] Despite approximately half the transgene expression seen with adenovirus in vitro and in vivo, there was sustained production of the luciferase marker at all time points up to 6 weeks. Additionally, the overall transduction achieved with AAV vector LacZ marker was high, setting the precedent for the use of AAV vector for gene therapy applications to treat disk degeneration. The use of AAV vector to transduce therapeutic anabolic and anticatabolic genes (BMP-2 and TIMP-1) is currently being investigated.

SUMMARY

IDD is a common and potentially debilitating disease process affecting millions of Americans and other populations each year. Current treatments address resultant symptoms and not the underlying pathophysiology of disease. This has spawned the development of biologic treatments, such as gene therapy, which attempt to correct the imbalance between catabolism and anabolism within degenerating disk cells. The identification of therapeutic genes and development of successful delivery systems have resulted in significant advances in this novel treatment. Continued investigation of the pathophysiology of disk degeneration, however, as well as safety mechanisms for the application of gene therapy are required for clinical translation.

ACKNOWLEDGMENTS

The Pittsburgh Foundation.

REFERENCES

1. Luo X, Pietrobon R, Sun SX, et al. Estimates and patterns of direct health care expenditures among individuals with back pain in the United States. Spine (Phila Pa 1976) 2004;29:79–86.
2. Buijs PC, Lambeek LC, Koppenrade V, et al. Can workers with chronic back pain shift from pain elimination to function restore at work? qualitative evaluation of an innovative work related multidisciplinary programme. J Back Musculoskelet Rehabil 2009; 22:65–73.
3. Bono CM, Lee CK. Critical analysis of trends in fusion for degenerative disc disease over the past 20 years: influence of technique on fusion rate and clinical outcome. Spine (Phila Pa 1976) 2004;29: 455–63 [discussion: Z5].
4. Hwang SL, Hwang YF, Lieu AS, et al. Outcome analyses of interbody titanium cage fusion used in the anterior discectomy for cervical degenerative disc disease. J Spinal Disord Tech 2005;18:326–31.
5. Karasek M, Bogduk N. Twelve-month follow-up of a controlled trial of intradiscal thermal anuloplasty for back pain due to internal disc disruption. Spine (Phila Pa 1976) 2000;25:2601–7.
6. Hubert MG, Vadala G, Sowa G, et al. Gene therapy for the treatment of degenerative disk disease. J Am Acad Orthop Surg 2008;16:312–9.
7. Kelsey JL, Githens PB, Walter SD, et al. An epidemiological study of acute prolapsed cervical intervertebral disc. J Bone Joint Surg Am 1984;66:907–14.
8. Noponen-Hietala N, Kyllonen E, Mannikko M, et al. Sequence variations in the collagen IX and XI genes are associated with degenerative lumbar spinal stenosis. Ann Rheum Dis 2003;62:1208–14.
9. Pluijm SM, van Essen HW, Bravenboer N, et al. Collagen type I alpha1 Sp1 polymorphism, osteoporosis, and intervertebral disc degeneration in older men and women. Ann Rheum Dis 2004;63:71–7.
10. Sambrook PN, MacGregor AJ, Spector TD. Genetic influences on cervical and lumbar disc degeneration: a magnetic resonance imaging study in twins. Arthritis Rheum 1999;42:366–72.
11. Colombini A, Lombardi G, Corsi MM, et al. Pathophysiology of the human intervertebral disc. Int J Biochem Cell Biol 2008;40:837–42.
12. Buckwalter JA. Aging and degeneration of the human intervertebral disc. Spine (Phila Pa 1976) 1995;20:1307–14.
13. Urban JP, Roberts S. Degeneration of the intervertebral disc. Arthritis Res Ther 2003;5:120–30.
14. Urban JP, McMullin JF. Swelling pressure of the inervertebral disc: influence of proteoglycan and collagen contents. Biorheology 1985;22:145–57.
15. Roberts S, Evans H, Trivedi J, et al. Histology and pathology of the human intervertebral disc. J Bone Joint Surg Am 2006;88(Suppl 2):10–4.

16. Butler D, Trafimow JH, Andersson GB, et al. Discs degenerate before facets. Spine (Phila Pa 1976) 1990;15:111–3.

17. Kang JD, Georgescu HI, McIntyre-Larkin L, et al. Herniated lumbar intervertebral discs spontaneously produce matrix metalloproteinases, nitric oxide, interleukin-6, and prostaglandin E2. Spine (Phila Pa 1976) 1996;21:271–7.

18. Kang JD, Stefanovic-Racic M, McIntyre LA, et al. Toward a biochemical understanding of human intervertebral disc degeneration and herniation. Contributions of nitric oxide, interleukins, prostaglandin E2, and matrix metalloproteinases. Spine (Phila Pa 1976) 1997;22:1065–73.

19. Le Maitre CL, Freemont AJ, Hoyland JA. Localization of degradative enzymes and their inhibitors in the degenerate human intervertebral disc. J Pathol 2004;204:47–54.

20. Le Maitre CL, Freemont AJ, Hoyland JA. The role of interleukin-1 in the pathogenesis of human intervertebral disc degeneration. Arthritis Res Ther 2005;7:R732–45.

21. Nishida K, Doita M, Takada T, et al. Sustained transgene expression in intervertebral disc cells in vivo mediated by microbubble-enhanced ultrasound gene therapy. Spine (Phila Pa 1976) 2006;31:1415–9.

22. Robbins PD, Ghivizzani SC. Viral vectors for gene therapy. Pharmacol Ther 1998;80:35–47.

23. Tripathy SK, Black HB, Goldwasser E, et al. Immune responses to transgene-encoded proteins limit the stability of gene expression after injection of replication-defective adenovirus vectors. Nat Med 1996;2:545–50.

24. Yang Y, Nunes FA, Berencsi K, et al. Cellular immunity to viral antigens limits E1-deleted adenoviruses for gene therapy. Proc Natl Acad Sci U S A 1994;91:4407–11.

25. Evans CH, Robbins PD. Possible orthopaedic applications of gene therapy. J Bone Joint Surg Am 1995;77:1103–14.

26. Thompson JP, Oegema TR Jr, Bradford DS. Stimulation of mature canine intervertebral disc by growth factors. Spine (Phila Pa 1976) 1991;16:253–60.

27. Osada R, Ohshima H, Ishihara H, et al. Autocrine/paracrine mechanism of insulin-like growth factor-1 secretion, and the effect of insulin-like growth factor-1 on proteoglycan synthesis in bovine intervertebral discs. J Orthop Res 1996;14:690–9.

28. Takegami K, Thonar EJ, An HS, et al. Osteogenic protein-1 enhances matrix replenishment by intervertebral disc cells previously exposed to interleukin-1. Spine (Phila Pa 1976) 2002;27:1318–25.

29. Li J, Yoon ST, Hutton WC. Effect of bone morphogenetic protein-2 (BMP-2) on matrix production, other BMPs, and BMP receptors in rat intervertebral disc cells. J Spinal Disord Tech 2004;17:423–8.

30. Tim Yoon S, Su Kim K, Li J, et al. The effect of bone morphogenetic protein-2 on rat intervertebral disc cells in vitro. Spine (Phila Pa 1976) 2003;28:1773–80.

31. Gruber HE, Norton HJ, Hanley EN Jr. Anti-apoptotic effects of IGF-1 and PDGF on human intervertebral disc cells in vitro. Spine (Phila Pa 1976) 2000;25:2153–7.

32. Wehling P, Schulitz KP, Robbins PD, et al. Transfer of genes to chondrocytic cells of the lumbar spine. Proposal for a treatment strategy of spinal disorders by local gene therapy. Spine (Phila Pa 1976) 1997;22:1092–7.

33. Nishida K, Kang JD, Suh JK, et al. Adenovirus-mediated gene transfer to nucleus pulposus cells. Implications for the treatment of intervertebral disc degeneration. Spine (Phila Pa 1976) 1998;23:2437–42 [discussion: 2443].

34. Sobajima S, Kim JS, Gilbertson LG, et al. Gene therapy for degenerative disc disease. Gene Ther 2004;11:390–401.

35. Takada T, Nishida K, Doita M, et al. Fas ligand exists on intervertebral disc cells: a potential molecular mechanism for immune privilege of the disc. Spine (Phila Pa 1976) 2002;27:1526–30.

36. Nishida K, Kang JD, Gilbertson LG, et al. Modulation of the biologic activity of the rabbit intervertebral disc by gene therapy: an in vivo study of adenovirus-mediated transfer of the human transforming growth factor beta 1 encoding gene. Spine (Phila Pa 1976) 1999;24:2419–25.

37. Moon SH, Nishida K, Gilbertson LG, et al. Biologic response of human intervertebral disc cells to gene therapy cocktail. Spine (Phila Pa 1976) 2008;33:1850–5.

38. Wallach CJ, Sobajima S, Watanabe Y, et al. Gene transfer of the catabolic inhibitor TIMP-1 increases measured proteoglycans in cells from degenerated human intervertebral discs. Spine (Phila Pa 1976) 2003;28:2331–7.

39. Yoon ST, Park JS, Kim KS, et al. ISSLS prize winner: LMP-1 upregulates intervertebral disc cell production of proteoglycans and BMPs in vitro and in vivo. Spine (Phila Pa 1976) 2004;29:2603–11.

40. Paul R, Haydon RC, Cheng H, et al. Potential use of Sox9 gene therapy for intervertebral degenerative disc disease. Spine (Phila Pa 1976) 2003;28:755–63.

41. Kakutani K, Nishida K, Uno K, et al. Prolonged down regulation of specific gene expression in nucleus pulposus cell mediated by RNA interference in vitro. J Orthop Res 2006;24:1271–8.

42. Wallach CJ, Kim JS, Sobajima S, et al. Safety assessment of intradiscal gene transfer: a pilot study. Spine J 2006;6:107–12.

43. Chtarto A, Bender HU, Hanemann CO, et al. Tetracycline-inducible transgene expression mediated by a single AAV vector. Gene Ther 2003;10: 84–94.

44. Ueblacker P, Wagner B, Kruger A, et al. Inducible nonviral gene expression in the treatment of osteochondral defects. Osteoarthr Cartil 2004;12: 711–9.

45. Lattermann C, Oxner WM, Xiao X, et al. The adeno associated viral vector as a strategy for intradiscal gene transfer in immune competent and pre-exposed rabbits. Spine (Phila Pa 1976) 2005;30:497–504.

Tissue Engineering for Intervertebral Disk Degeneration

Victor Y.L. Leung, PhD[a], Vivian Tam, PhD[a],
Danny Chan, PhD[b], Barbara P. Chan, PhD[c],
Kenneth M.C. Cheung, MBBS(UK), MD (HK),
FRCS, FHKCOS, FHKAM(Orth)[d],*

KEYWORDS

• Intervertebral disk • Degeneration • Tissue engineering

Disease conditions are often manifested with the disruption of tissue structure and function, which the body is incapable of repairing. Advancement in various disciplines, including cell biology, developmental genetics, materials science, and biomechanics, has brought the realization that tissue engineering could assist tissue repair or replacement (see articles elsewhere in this issue by Inoue and Espinoza Orias, Bae and colleagues, and Woods and colleagues). Unlike cartilage engineering, the engineering of the intervertebral disk (IVD) has many challenges owing to its complexity and presence of extraordinary stresses related to its architecture and function. The IVD plays a crucial role in articulation of the spinal column and contributes to various body postures and force coordination in daily activities. Along with its role in articulation, the IVD has a major function in providing cushioning effects to the spine against axial load. As a result of the intensive mechanical stress, the IVD suffers from degeneration in a similar fashion to articular cartilage in loaded appendicular joints. The causes of IVD degeneration are not clear, although they are thought to be multifactorial, with a large contribution from both genetic and environmental components,[1,2]

and may share common biologic components exhibited in osteoarthritis.[3] Current treatments predominantly aim not to correct the degeneration but alleviate symptoms, such as back pain and sciatica, which are often manifested by severe IVD degeneration or radiculopathy caused by prolapse of the degenerated disk (see article elsewhere in this issue by Karppinen and colleagues). Conventional modalities range from surgical means, such as spinal segment fusion, laminectomy, and total disk/nucleus replacement, to noninvasive physiotherapies, such as ultrasound electrotherapy and traction.

Current theory suggests that when the IVD is degenerated, the articular unit has compromised mechanical function and, subsequently, the motion segment becomes unstable under load. Consequently, this may result in significant pain and neurologic irritations that can cause a severe decrease in daily activities of an individual. Although intervertebral fusion, the gold standard for treating symptomatic disk degeneration, may stabilize the segment and relieve symptoms, juxta-level degeneration may occur due to the observed hypermobility of the IVD adjacent to the fused segment (see article elsewhere in this issue by

[a] Department of Orthopaedics & Traumatology, The University of Hong Kong, Sassoon Road, Hong Kong SAR, China
[b] Department of Biochemistry, The University of Hong Kong, Sassoon Road, Hong Kong SAR, China
[c] Tissue Engineering Laboratory, Department of Mechanical Engineering, The University of Hong Kong, Pokfulam Road, Hong Kong SAR, China
[d] Department of Orthopaedics and Traumatology, Division of Spine Surgery, Li Ka Shing Faculty of Medicine, The University of Hong Kong, Professorial Block, 5th Floor, 102 Pokfulam Road, Pokfulam, Hong Kong SAR, China
* Corresponding author. Department of Orthopaedics and Traumatology, The University of Hong Kong, Queen Mary Hospital, Professorial Block, 5th Floor, 102 Pokfulam Road, Pokfulam, Hong Kong SAR, China.
E-mail address: cheungmc@hku.hk

Orthop Clin N Am 42 (2011) 575–583
doi:10.1016/j.ocl.2011.07.003
0030-5898/11/$ – see front matter © 2011 Published by Elsevier Inc.

Lund and Oxland).[4] Rebuilding an IVD of native function that allows appropriate interplay with other motion segment components, including the facet joints and ligaments, could therefore be promising in the removal of symptoms while simultaneously re-establishing spine kinematics. A recent study of IVD allograft transplantation to treat cervical disk herniation in humans supports this notion.[5] Although total disk replacement may potentially resolve the issue in a similar manner, long-term results suggest that artificial disk replacements frequently result in spontaneous fusion and are considered expensive spacers for fusion (see article elsewhere in this issue by Mayer and Siepe).[6] Bioengineering of the IVD may, therefore, provide an alternative solution to address the issue.

Tissue engineering can be achieved at different levels of complexity, from cell programming and scaffold modeling to cell-scaffold composite construction and multiscale tissue fabrication. Advances in understanding of IVD properties and techniques in its engineering at each of the levels may have an impact on the success of building a functional motion segment for treating disk degeneration. This review provides an account of the progress and challenges of IVD engineering and proposes what is needed to move forward and toward bedside translation.

DISK CELL ENGINEERING

The IVD is composed of multiple subunits that integrate seamlessly to form sophisticated and complex mechanical function. It has 3 main structures: a gelatinous nucleus pulposus (NP) core wrapped around and confined by a fibrous lamella structure, the annular fibrosus (AF), and cartilaginous endplates (CEPs) of the vertebrae sandwiching the NP and AF (see article elsewhere in this issue by Grunhagen and colleagues). The 3 compartments are different in mechanical properties and are functionally dependent on each other. These compartments are made up of various matrix components, predominantly collagens and proteoglycans, and comprise different cells that are thought to play roles in maintaining the matrix integrity. From a developmental point of view, IVD formation involves the diversification of cells from a primitive anlage consisting of the notochord and its surrounding mesenchymal cells, a process that involves vigorous cell differentiation during the embryonic stage and continual postnatal remodeling of its microenvironment, including the extracellular matrices.[7–9]

The primary role of the IVD is to provide mechanical support and motion, which is largely attributed to the viscoelastic properties (the viscous and elastic behavior under deformation) of the IVD.[10]

IVD-like properties and function may possibly be obtained by simply using acellular scaffolds or devices. Materials with desirable viscoelastic properties pertaining to IVD are often biodegradable, however, and, therefore, their function may not be sustained in the long term. Cell-containing constructs are advantageous with cells enable to remodel the scaffold template, thereby maintaining or enhancing matrix integrity. More importantly, IVD transplantation studies have demonstrated the integration of disk allograft to recipient vertebrae by biologic remodeling at the endplates, including that of misaligned disks, which were also found to self-correct postsurgery.[5] Because the self-correction is considered to eventually contribute to motion segment kinematics and stability in the long term, cellular IVD constructs would theoretically outperform acellular prosthetic devices in function.

The loss of integrity and viscoelasticity of the NP is one of the earliest observable events in disk degeneration, suggesting that the engineering of the NP is crucial to the success of a functional IVD construct. Considerable effort has been invested in understanding the NP, in particular, delineating the NP cell phenotype so as to facilitate NP cell engineering for the creation of cellular IVD constructs. Two cell populations are thought to exist in the NP: small nonvacuolated cells with a chondrocyte-like phenotype, and large vacuolated cells, often referred to as notochordal cells.[11] The large vacuolated NP cells have been shown to originate from the notochord,[8] whereas controversy still surrounds the origin of the chondrocyte-like cells, particularly in human NP. Nevertheless, recent studies have provided some insights to the molecular identity of the latter type of cells based on microarray-based gene expression profiles of NP cells from adult human,[12] bovine,[13] and chondrodystrophoid dog.[14] These studies did not yield common genetic markers that are translatable among different species but rather indicated the presence of species-specific markers, for example *PAX1* and *FOXF1* in human, *A2m* and *Anxa4* in canine, and *Snap25* and *Krt8* in bovine. Expression profile studies of rodent NP cells,[15] which predominantly consist of large vacuolated notochordal cells, also suggested that markers may not be shared with human NP cells, and indicated that notochordal and chondrocyte-like NP cells may be distinct in phenotypes. This is supported by cell sorting studies in which the two populations were separately extracted from the same animal for comparative analyses.[13,16] Nevertheless, recent studies suggest that a cross talk may possibly exist between the two cell populations, complicating the search of the true NP cell identity.[17,18]

IVD and articular cartilage have different mechanical properties. The transplantation of chondrocyte-like cells or the use of such cells in the engineering of NP constructs may not produce a disk with ideal function. Alternatively, future IVD engineering will likely use stem cells and other progenitor cell types to differentiate into NP cells and generate them in large quantity. Unless the phenotype and the functional characteristics of the notochordal and chondrocyte-like NP cell types are clearly defined, the generation of authentic NP cells from stem/progenitor cells and hence bioengineering of NP with native mechanical properties may not be achieved. In vitro studies have suggested that stimulation by co-culturing with NP cells,[19–22] induction of chondrogenic transcription factor SOX9,[23,24] or stimulation by chondrogenic growth factor transforming growth factor β1 (TGF-β1)[24–26] are attractive strategies to drive differentiation of adult stem cells, such as mesenchymal stem cells (MSCs), into NP-like cells. Whether or not the differentiated cells have attained an authentic NP cell or chondrocyte-like phenotype, however, remains elusive. Engineering the NP with chondrocytes is not desirable because it is likely that the construct will become hyaline cartilage instead of NP tissue and hence possess inappropriate viscoelastic properties.

Annulus fibrosus cells are generally referred to as fibrochondrocytes. This phenotype is based on the ability of AF cells to produce collagen I and III, in addition to collagen II and aggrecan, which are produced to a lower extent.[27] Compared with NP cells, the molecular phenotype of AF cells and their changes in disk degeneration are less clear. Although NP and AF are morphologically different and supposedly have different cell phenotypes, recent transcription profiling studies indicated that AF cells express a large number of nonhousekeeping genes at similar level to that of NP cells.[12–14] Nevertheless, other potential markers are suggested to be differentially expressed at higher levels in the AF relative to the NP, for example, *VCAM1* in human.[12] Fibromodulin has been shown to be a specific marker of the AF in rodent[28]; however, its expression pattern in humans or large animal models is unclear. Alternatively, although the CEP is assumed to be analogous to hyaline cartilage and consists of chondrocytes, the molecular phenotype of CEP cells is also not clear, and there is a lack of evidence that demonstrates their similarities. Histologic findings have suggested that there is a difference in the glycosaminoglycan composition and collagen VI and X expression between CEPs and growth plate cartilage.[9,29] It is not clear whether or not the use of chondrocytes in bioengineering can fully fulfill the function of the CEP.

ENGINEERING THE DISK MICROENVIRONMENT

The bulk of the IVD is composed of extracellular matrix, which plays prominent roles in the regulation of the disk cell environment and providing anchorage to disk cells. The extracellular matrix of the IVD, like cartilage, is comprised of mostly collagens, which provide tensile strength of the disk,[30] and proteoglycans, which function to reduce the internal friction in the disk matrix and to distribute load.[31] They also account for the viscoelastic behavior of the IVD, contributing to the shock-absorbing property.[32] Based on the relationship between function and form, materials that can mimic the anatomic architecture and mechanical properties of native IVD (reviewed by Nerurkar and colleagues[10]) are of interest to disk bioengineers.

Like hyaline cartilage, aggrecan and collagen II are the two main extracellular matrix components of mature NP. Although the NP in mature human IVD is thought to be analogous to articular cartilage, the nature of the matrix and hence their mechanical properties are not exactly the same.[33] NP in young individuals has a high proteoglycan to collagen content, with a suggested glycosaminoglycan-to-hydroxyproline ratio of 27:1, in comparison with a 2:1 ratio in hyaline cartilage.[34] The high proteoglycan content in the NP matrix facilitates the retainment of water, which attributes to the high hydrostatic pressure exhibited in the NP. Hydrogel scaffolds have been commonly used with the intention of simulating the NP microenvironment and entrapment of the newly deposited proteoglycan to facilitate the establishment of hydrostatic pressure. The effectiveness of various hydrogel-based scaffolds, either made from natural hydrophilic biomolecules or synthetic polymers, for NP engineering or repair has been documented. To date, alginate is one of most commonly adopted hydrogel scaffolds for NP cell culturing[35,36] due to its ease of manipulation, biodegradability, and inert bioactivities. Hyaluronic acid (HA) has been used for the treatment of osteoarthritic knee joints via the direct application into the synovial cavity, and in vivo studies propose that HA[37–40] or HA-derived hydrogel[41–43] may facilitate NP function and promote motion segment mechanics. Because the NP plays an important role in withstanding the compressive load so as to maintain disk height and range of motion of spinal segment, however, pure hydrogel scaffolds, which lack confined compressive strength, may not be adequate for NP engineering. Collagen I microspheres[44,45] and calcium polyphosphate[46] may, alternatively, provide good tensile and compressive strength to support stem cells or NP cells in NP engineering. Recent studies have focused on the generation of collagen-incorporated[47–49] or polymer-linked[50,51] hydrogels. These hybrid scaffolds mimic the native microenvironment of the NP to reproduce its viscoelastic and load distribution behavior within the IVD. Although swelling is known to provide the main load-bearing mechanism in the NP, the extensive collagen network inside the disk has also been suggested as supporting a considerable portion of load because the collagen fibril meshwork contributes to the compressive modulus to the tissue.[52] Moreover, collagens have been shown to act as a reservoir of signaling ligands, such as TGF-β1 and bone morphogenetic protein 2 for collagen II,[53] and are able to transduce mechanical signals,[54,55] therefore serving as important regulators of cell function and homeostasis.

In addition to NP engineering, current research has attempted to use injectable scaffolds as carriers to deliver cells with the aim of salvaging disk degeneration or on its own, as fillers for NP replacement using a minimally invasive approach.[49] Studies have also developed injectable materials that have the ability to self-assemble into a higher-order network, resulting in a solution-to-gel transition. For example, atelo-collagen (pepsin-digested collagen) can self–cross-link to form a fibrous meshwork,[56,57] and chitosan[26,58] and synthetic peptides[59–61] have been reported to self-assemble into a nanofiber network. Other natural biomolecules, including hyaluronan and chitosan, when modified with cross-linkable moieties are capable of chain polymerization through photochemical reactions.[62] These materials, as injectable media, may deliver cells of interest by providing a transient framework that prevents leakage of implants and allows for the accumulation of the extracellular matrix deposited by the introduced cells.

Although intradiscal pressure exerted by the NP plays an important role in disk function, it critically depends on the integrity of the AF. In addition, the trans-AF delivery system remains the commonly used way to manipulate the NP in clinical and experimental settings. The construction of AF may facilitate the repair of prolapsed disks and supplement nucleus replacement. Annulus closure devices[63] may possibly provide an effective means to treat prolapsed disks; however, they may restrict segment motion and possibly modify the load distribution in the IVD. AF construction is understandably indispensable to IVD engineering,

but effective bioengineering of AF may not be implemented without proper understanding of its microstructure and mechanics.

The AF lamellae are mainly composed of collagen I fiber bundles and have anisotropic mechanical behavior.[64] These bundles are approximately concentric to the lamellae around the NP, where the direction of alignment in one lamella differs to the next by 30°.[65] This angle-ply architecture of lamellae is thought to be designed to resist shear resulting from complex physiologic stresses, such as a combination of axial loading and torsion.[66,67] Annulus fibers are interconnected via intralamellar crossbridges[68] and interlamellar bridges.[69,70] In vitro studies showed that excess circumferential constraint may have a negative impact on NP cell metabolic activities,[71] which suggests that tissue rigidity needs to be carefully controlled during AF construction. The rigidity of the AF largely depends on the mechanical properties of the materials used during fabrication. Various materials have been tested for AF tissue construction, including porous silk,[72,73] polymer nanofibers,[38,66,74,75] poly-lactide/Bioglass composite,[76] and alginate/chitosan composite.[77] These scaffolds provide a framework of desirable mechanical and bioinductive properties for future AF engineering. An alternative is collagen gel[78,79] or collagen-glycosaminoglycan composite,[80] although fabrication into a specific geometry (such as fibers or lamella) or characteristic topographic template may be limited. Because AF cells are normally aligned with the lamella fibers, it may be ideal that AF constructs can be engineered through simultaneous controlled placement of AF cells and orientation of the matrix they interact with, such as using scaffolds with specifically designed microgrooves.[81]

Collagen fiber structure determines the mechanical strength and elasticity of the annulus. Recent studies in AF engineering have shed light on some important aspects of its structural properties at the molecular level. Nerurkar and colleagues[67,82] showed that, through electrospun nanofiber fabrication, a bilamellar tissue model with AF-like angle-ply architecture can be generated. By mechanical testing and modeling, they demonstrated that the bonding between the angle-ply lamellae is crucial to the resistance of interlamellar matrix to local deformations and, therefore, functions to reinforce the overall tensile response of AF architecture. Moreover, an in vitro study indicated that fibronectin can play a pivotal role in facilitating AF cell attachment and alignment on nanofibers,[83] implying that a synergy between collagen and other noncollagen matrix components may be required to provide AF cells a niche to attain appropriate activities. Altogether, these findings indicate that the AF structure is not just a multilayered fibrous tissue but built with a sophisticated hierarchy of intralamellar and interlamellar supramolecular interactions.

The CEP is involved in attachment of both AF and NP fibers.[84] Using a triphasic model, Hamilton and colleagues[85] also suggested that the CEP is a critical interface for bone-disk integration by providing an adhesive force that is resilient to shear loading. In addition, they reported that CEPs may secrete factors to stimulate proteoglycan and inhibit tumor necrosis factor α production in NP cells, suggesting CEPs have a role in regulating NP homeostasis.[86] CEPs are thought to be similar to articular cartilage and can be artificially engineered by plating and incubating chondrocytes at a high density on the target interface where they secrete matrices to model the interface into a cartilage layer.[85,87]

TOWARD WHOLE DISK ENGINEERING

By the time a degenerated disk becomes clinically symptomatic and requires treatment, the AF and endplate, in addition to NP, are also structurally altered or functionally incompetent. At a severely degenerated stage, the motion segment is often largely compromised not only because of malfunction of the disk but also due to secondary arthritic changes, such as facet joint degeneration and osteophyte formation. Transplantation of whole IVD seems to be a rational approach to replace severely degenerated spinal motion segments. This has been demonstrated recently in large animal models and in humans, where the transplantation of disk allografts was able to alleviate symptoms caused by the degenerated segment, thus a feasible option for treating disk degeneration.[5,88] It is still not clear, however, if allografts may be routinely applied in practice due to the limited availability of nondegenerated disk tissue from healthy donors and legislative regulations in using human cadavers. Artificial disk installation may provide an alternative to overcome the issues. The application of artificial disk replacements, however, may need to overcome additional hurdles, such as recipient-graft integration and demand in surgical precision that could possibly be overcome using organic disk grafts due to their biologic remodeling capacity.[5]

Although de novo bottom-up assembly of whole IVD is considered a challenging task, various attempts have been made to construct disk tissue prototypes with multicompartmental features. Nesti and colleagues[38] studied a biphasic model composed of an outer fibrous shell fabricated by electrospun nanofibers and an inner filling made of HA. Under stimulation with TGF, MSCs preimplanted in the two compartments were able to differentiate, transforming the composite into AF-like and NP-like structures. Mizuno and colleagues[89] were able to produce an IVD-like tissue by generating a composite of AF cell-seeded synthetic polymer mesh wrapping around an NP cell-seeded alginate filling, which was subsequently implanted subcutaneously for in vivo modeling and resulted in a collagen/proteoglycan-rich construct of enhanced mechanical properties. Another study by Wan and colleagues[90] tested the fabrication of a dual-layer composite consisting of bone matrix gelatin in one phase and chondrocyte-seeded, concentrically oriented polymer in another to replicate the inner and outer AF. Hamilton and colleagues[85] constructed a triphasic model to recapitulate the bone-CEP-NP organization. With the fabrication technique that replicates the angle-ply fiber organization of AF, Nerurkar and colleagues[82] engineered a biochemically and mechanically functional AF-NP composite with MSCs. Collectively, these studies reveal the possibility of artificially engineering disks, which are similar anatomically and mechanically to the native disk and thus have laid a valuable foundation for building a fully functional multiscale disk composite for total disk replacement. Future efforts are anticipated to build a complete CEP-NP-AF architecture to simulate the higher-order complexity of native disk tissues. An osteochondral interface with proper zonal organization between vertebrae and CEPs may also need to be carefully engineered to obtain satisfactory structural and functional complexity, such as via a collagen microencapsulation-based multilayer co-culture method.[91]

HURDLES AND PERSPECTIVES

The function of the IVD relies on an integrated dynamic interaction between the NP, AF, and CEPs. Therefore, de novo engineering of IVD would ultimately entail comprehensive knowledge of the biology and engineering techniques. At this stage, although the mechanical properties and functions of the individual compartments (ie, NP, AF, and CEPs) have been fairly well studied, there is limited understanding of the interaction among the compartments, for instance, which components are present in the interface between the NP and inner AF and how AF/NP fibers are attached to the CEPs. This is analogous to the interface between tendon and bone but with more complex mechanical moduli due to interplay among the disk compartments.

Moreover, disk cell engineering seems to be one of the main hurdles in the progress of IVD bioengineering. This could be partly due to an incomplete understanding of their phenotypes and their modulation during disk development and homeostasis. Studies of animal and ex vivo culture models, such as transgenic mice and bioreactor systems, may provide clues, such as specific genes or signaling factors, necessary for the induction of progenitors or stem cells to become disk-related cell types and to stably maintain the phenotype/characteristics of the derived cells in vitro. Alternatively, a better modeling of IVD microarchitecture may be achieved through molecular imaging and nanotechnology for better scaffold design and fabrication.

The engineering of a complete IVD is the first step of many, but the true challenge lies in the production of a fully functional IVD. Within a decade, complete bioengineering of all disk compartments will probably be enabled. In the long term, however, there may be a limitation in the available fabrication technology that enables the assembly of the building blocks to establish overall disk biomechanics. Perhaps to overcome the issue, a disk anlage, a primitive construct composing of distinctly engineered compartments, might be fabricated, subsequently allowing the construct (the so-called precursor tissue analog[92]) to evolve to form a mature IVD through native morphogenetic activities of disk cells, mimicking tissue growth and remodeling during the postnatal maturation process of the IVD.[7,9] Such a strategy may be realized with future advances in disk cell engineering and bioreactor systems for whole IVD culturing with mechanical stimulation.[60,93,94] Perhaps with advancement in tissue engineering and total disk replacement devices, it may be possible to combine both disciplines to create hybrid constructs with strengths in bioactivity, mechanical function, and durability.

Tissue engineering for IVD is in its infant stage when compared with articular cartilage engineering. In view of increasing the variety and sophistication of modalities available in cell biology, biomechanics, and tissue engineering, however, the bioengineering of whole functional IVD, hence its clinical application, could eventuate in the not too distant future.

REFERENCES

1. Chan D, Song Y, Sham P, et al. Genetics of disc degeneration. Eur Spine J 2006;15(Suppl 15):317–25.
2. Adams MA, Roughley PJ. What is intervertebral disc degeneration, and what causes it? Spine 2006;31: 2151–61.
3. Loughlin J. Knee osteoarthritis, lumbar-disc degeneration and developmental dysplasia of the hip - an emerging genetic overlap. Arthritis Res Ther 2011; 13:108.
4. Samartzis D, Lubicky JP, Herman J, et al. Symptomatic cervical disc herniation in a pediatric Klippel-Feil patient: the risk of neural injury associated with extensive congenitally fused vertebrae and a hypermobile segment. Spine 2006;31:E335–8.
5. Ruan D, He Q, Ding Y, et al. Intervertebral disc transplantation in the treatment of degenerative spine disease: a preliminary study. Lancet 2007;369:993–9.
6. Putzier M, Funk JF, Schneider SV, et al. Charite total disc replacement–clinical and radiographical results after an average follow-up of 17 years. Eur Spine J 2006;15:183–95.
7. Dahia CL, Mahoney EJ, Durrani AA, et al. Postnatal growth, differentiation, and aging of the mouse intervertebral disc. Spine 2009;34:447–55.
8. Choi KS, Cohn MJ, Harfe BD. Identification of nucleus pulposus precursor cells and notochordal remnants in the mouse: implications for disc degeneration and chordoma formation. Dev Dyn 2008;237: 3953–8.
9. Leung VY, Chan WC, Hung SC, et al. Matrix remodeling during intervertebral disc growth and degeneration detected by multichromatic FAST staining. J Histochem Cytochem 2009;57:249–56.
10. Nerurkar NL, Elliott DM, Mauck RL. Mechanical design criteria for intervertebral disc tissue engineering. J Biomech 2010;43:1017–30.
11. Hunter CJ, Matyas JR, Duncan NA. The notochordal cell in the nucleus pulposus: a review in the context of tissue engineering. Tissue Eng 2003;9:667–77.
12. Minogue BM, Richardson SM, Zeef LA, et al. Characterization of the human nucleus pulposus cell phenotype and evaluation of novel marker gene expression to define adult stem cell differentiation. Arthritis Rheum 2010;62:3695–705.
13. Minogue BM, Richardson SM, Zeef LA, et al. Transcriptional profiling of bovine intervertebral disc cells: implications for identification of normal and degenerate human intervertebral disc cell phenotypes. Arthritis Res Ther 2010;12:R22.
14. Sakai D, Nakai T, Mochida J, et al. Differential phenotype of intervertebral disc cells: microarray and immunohistochemical analysis of canine nucleus pulposus and anulus fibrosus. Spine (Phila Pa 1976) 2009;34:1448–56.
15. Lee CR, Sakai D, Nakai T, et al. A phenotypic comparison of intervertebral disc and articular cartilage cells in the rat. Eur Spine J 2007;16:2174–85.
16. Chen J, Yan W, Setton LA. Molecular phenotypes of notochordal cells purified from immature nucleus pulposus. Eur Spine J 2006;15(Suppl 15):303–11.
17. Gilson A, Dreger M, Urban JP. Differential expression level of cytokeratin 8 in cells of the bovine

nucleus pulposus complicates the search for specific intervertebral disc cell markers. Arthritis Res Ther 2010;12:R24.

18. Kim JH, Deasy BM, Seo HY, et al. Differentiation of intervertebral notochordal cells through live automated cell imaging system in vitro. Spine 2009;34:2486–93.

19. Richardson SM, Walker RV, Parker S, et al. Intervertebral disc cell-mediated mesenchymal stem cell differentiation. Stem Cells 2006;24:707–16.

20. Strassburg S, Richardson SM, Freemont AJ, et al. Co-culture induces mesenchymal stem cell differentiation and modulation of the degenerate human nucleus pulposus cell phenotype. Regen Med 2010;5:701–11.

21. Korecki CL, Taboas JM, Tuan RS, et al. Notochordal cell conditioned medium stimulates mesenchymal stem cell differentiation toward a young nucleus pulposus phenotype. Stem Cell Res Ther 2010;1:18.

22. Wei A, Chung SA, Tao H, et al. Differentiation of rodent bone marrow mesenchymal stem cells into intervertebral disc-like cells following coculture with rat disc tissue. Tissue Eng Part A 2009;15:2581–95.

23. Yang Z, Huang CY, Candiotti KA, et al. Sox-9 facilitates differentiation of adipose tissue-derived stem cells into a chondrocyte-like phenotype in vitro. J Orthop Res 2011;29:1291–7.

24. Richardson SM, Curran JM, Chen R, et al. The differentiation of bone marrow mesenchymal stem cells into chondrocyte-like cells on poly-l-lactic acid (PLLA) scaffolds. Biomaterials 2006;27:4069–78.

25. Risbud MV, Albert TJ, Guttapalli A, et al. Differentiation of mesenchymal stem cells towards a nucleus pulposus-like phenotype in vitro: implications for cell-based transplantation therapy. Spine 2004;29:2627–32.

26. Roughley P, Hoemann C, DesRosiers E, et al. The potential of chitosan-based gels containing intervertebral disc cells for nucleus pulposus supplementation. Biomaterials 2006;27:388–96.

27. Hayes AJ, Benjamin M, Ralphs JR. Extracellular matrix in development of the intervertebral disc. Matrix Biol 2001;20:107–21.

28. Smits P, Lefebvre V. Sox5 and Sox6 are required for notochord extracellular matrix sheath formation, notochord cell survival and development of the nucleus pulposus of intervertebral discs. Development 2003;130:1135–48.

29. Melrose J, Smith S, Knox S, et al. Perlecan, the multi-domain HS-proteoglycan of basement membranes, is a prominent pericellular component of ovine hypertrophic vertebral growth plate and cartilaginous endplate chondrocytes. Histochem Cell Biol 2002;118:269–80.

30. Iatridis JC, Weidenbaum M, Setton LA, et al. Is the nucleus pulposus a solid or a fluid? Mechanical behaviors of the nucleus pulposus of the human intervertebral disc. Spine 1996;21:1174–84.

31. Boxberger JI, Orlansky AS, Sen S, et al. Reduced nucleus pulposus glycosaminoglycan content alters intervertebral disc dynamic viscoelastic mechanics. J Biomech 2009;42:1941–6.

32. Mow VC, Guo XE. Mechano-electrochemical properties of articular cartilage: their inhomogeneities and anisotropies. Annu Rev Biomed Eng 2002;4:175–209.

33. Adams MA, Dolan P, McNally DS. The internal mechanical functioning of intervertebral discs and articular cartilage, and its relevance to matrix biology. Matrix Biol 2009;28:384–9.

34. Mwale F, Roughley P, Antoniou J. Distinction between the extracellular matrix of the nucleus pulposus and hyaline cartilage: a requisite for tissue engineering of intervertebral disc. Eur Cell Mater 2004;8:58–63 [discussion: 63–4].

35. Maldonado BA, Oegema TR Jr. Initial characterization of the metabolism of intervertebral disc cells encapsulated in microspheres. J Orthop Res 1992;10:677–90.

36. Chiba K, Andersson GB, Masuda K, et al. Metabolism of the extracellular matrix formed by intervertebral disc cells cultured in alginate. Spine 1997;22:2885–93.

37. Pfeiffer M, Griss P, Franke P, et al. Degeneration model of the porcine lumbar motion segment: effects of various intradiscal procedures. Eur Spine J 1994;3:8–16.

38. Nesti LJ, Li WJ, Shanti RM, et al. Intervertebral disc tissue engineering using a novel hyaluronic acid-nanofibrous scaffold (HANFS) amalgam. Tissue Eng Part A 2008;14:1527–37.

39. Ganey T, Hutton WC, Moseley T, et al. Intervertebral disc repair using adipose tissue-derived stem and regenerative cells: experiments in a canine model. Spine 2009;34:2297–304.

40. Pfeiffer M, Boudriot U, Pfeiffer D, et al. Intradiscal application of hyaluronic acid in the non-human primate lumbar spine: radiological results. Eur Spine J 2003;12:76–83.

41. Cloyd JM, Malhotra NR, Weng L, et al. Material properties in unconfined compression of human nucleus pulposus, injectable hyaluronic acid-based hydrogels and tissue engineering scaffolds. Eur Spine J 2007;16:1892–8.

42. Revell PA, Damien E, Di Silvio L, et al. Tissue engineered intervertebral disc repair in the pig using injectable polymers. J Mater Sci Mater Med 2007;18:303–8.

43. Nakashima S, Matsuyama Y, Takahashi K, et al. Regeneration of intervertebral disc by the intradiscal application of cross-linked hyaluronate hydrogel and cross-linked chondroitin sulfate hydrogel in a rabbit model of intervertebral disc injury. Biomed Mater Eng 2009;19:421–9.

44. Li CH, Chik TK, Ngan AH, et al. Correlation between compositional and mechanical properties of human

mesenchymal stem cell-collagen microspheres during chondrogenic differentiation. Tissue Eng Part A 2011;17:777–88.

45. Chan BP, Hui TY, Yeung CW, et al. Self-assembled collagen-human mesenchymal stem cell microspheres for regenerative medicine. Biomaterials 2007;28:4652–66.

46. Seguin CA, Grynpas MD, Pilliar RM, et al. Tissue engineered nucleus pulposus tissue formed on a porous calcium polyphosphate substrate. Spine 2004;29:1299–306 [discussion: 1306–7].

47. Alini M, Li W, Markovic P, et al. The potential and limitations of a cell-seeded collagen/hyaluronan scaffold to engineer an intervertebral disc-like matrix. Spine 2003;28:446–54 [discussion: 453].

48. Calderon L, Collin E, Velasco-Bayon D, et al. Type II collagen-hyaluronan hydrogel—a step towards a scaffold for intervertebral disc tissue engineering. Eur Cell Mater 2010;20:134–48.

49. Collin EC, Grad S, Zeugolis DI, et al. An injectable vehicle for nucleus pulposus cell-based therapy. Biomaterials 2011;32:2862–70.

50. Abbushi A, Endres M, Cabraja M, et al. Regeneration of intervertebral disc tissue by resorbable cell-free polyglycolic acid-based implants in a rabbit model of disc degeneration. Spine 2008;33:1527–32.

51. Endres M, Abbushi A, Thomale UW, et al. Intervertebral disc regeneration after implantation of a cell-free bioresorbable implant in a rabbit disc degeneration model. Biomaterials 2010;31:5836–41.

52. Aladin DM, Cheung KM, Ngan AH, et al. Nanostructure of collagen fibrils in human nucleus pulposus and its correlation with macroscale tissue mechanics. J Orthop Res 2010;28:497–502.

53. Zhu Y, Oganesian A, Keene DR, et al. Type IIA procollagen containing the cysteine-rich amino propeptide is deposited in the extracellular matrix of prechondrogenic tissue and binds to TGF-beta1 and BMP-2. J Cell Biol 1999;144:1069–80.

54. Alexopoulos LG, Youn I, Bonaldo P, et al. Developmental and osteoarthritic changes in Col6a1-knockout mice: biomechanics of type VI collagen in the cartilage pericellular matrix. Arthritis Rheum 2009;60:771–9.

55. Guilak F, Alexopoulos LG, Upton ML, et al. The pericellular matrix as a transducer of biomechanical and biochemical signals in articular cartilage. Ann N Y Acad Sci 2006;1068:498–512.

56. Jakobsen RJ, Brown LL, Hutson TB, et al. Intermolecular interactions in collagen self-assembly as revealed by Fourier transform infrared spectroscopy. Science 1983;220:1288–90.

57. Sakai D, Mochida J, Yamamoto Y, et al. Transplantation of mesenchymal stem cells embedded in Atelocollagen gel to the intervertebral disc: a potential therapeutic model for disc degeneration. Biomaterials 2003;24:3531–41.

58. Chenite A, Chaput C, Wang D, et al. Novel injectable neutral solutions of chitosan form biodegradable gels in situ. Biomaterials 2000;21:2155–61.

59. Kisiday J, Jin M, Kurz B, et al. Self-assembling peptide hydrogel fosters chondrocyte extracellular matrix production and cell division: implications for cartilage tissue repair. Proc Natl Acad Sci U S A 2002;99:9996–10001.

60. Chan SC, Gantenbein-Ritter B, Leung VY, et al. Cryopreserved intervertebral disc with injected bone marrow-derived stromal cells: a feasibility study using organ culture. Spine J 2010;10:486–96.

61. Henriksson HB, Svanvik T, Jonsson M, et al. Transplantation of human mesenchymal stems cells into intervertebral discs in a xenogeneic porcine model. Spine (Phila Pa 1976) 2009;34:141–8.

62. Ifkovits JL, Burdick JA. Review: photopolymerizable and degradable biomaterials for tissue engineering applications. Tissue Eng 2007;13:2369–85.

63. Bron JL, van der Veen AJ, Helder MN, et al. Biomechanical and in vivo evaluation of experimental closure devices of the annulus fibrosus designed for a goat nucleus replacement model. Eur Spine J 2010;19:1347–55.

64. Elliott DM, Setton LA. Anisotropic and inhomogeneous tensile behavior of the human anulus fibrosus: experimental measurement and material model predictions. J Biomech Eng 2001;123:256–63.

65. Cassidy JJ, Hiltner A, Baer E. Hierarchical structure of the intervertebral disc. Connect Tissue Res 1989;23:75–88.

66. Nerurkar NL, Mauck RL, Elliott DM. ISSLS prize winner: integrating theoretical and experimental methods for functional tissue engineering of the annulus fibrosus. Spine 2008;33:2691–701.

67. Nerurkar NL, Baker BM, Sen S, et al. Nanofibrous biologic laminates replicate the form and function of the annulus fibrosus. Nat Mater 2009;8:986–92.

68. Pezowicz CA, Robertson PA, Broom ND. Intralamellar relationships within the collagenous architecture of the annulus fibrosus imaged in its fully hydrated state. J Anat 2005;207:299–312.

69. Schollum ML, Robertson PA, Broom ND. A microstructural investigation of intervertebral disc lamellar connectivity: detailed analysis of the translamellar bridges. J Anat 2009;214:805–16.

70. Schollum ML, Robertson PA, Broom ND. ISSLS prize winner: microstructure and mechanical disruption of the lumbar disc annulus: part I: a microscopic investigation of the translamellar bridging network. Spine 2008;33:2702–10.

71. Hamilton DJ, Pilliar RM, Waldman S, et al. Effect of circumferential constraint on nucleus pulposus tissue in vitro. Spine J 2010;10:174–83.

72. Chang G, Kim HJ, Vunjak-Novakovic G, et al. Enhancing annulus fibrosus tissue formation in

porous silk scaffolds. J Biomed Mater Res A 2010; 92:43–51.

73. Chang G, Kim HJ, Kaplan D, et al. Porous silk scaffolds can be used for tissue engineering annulus fibrosus. Eur Spine J 2007;16:1848–57.

74. Nerurkar NL, Elliott DM, Mauck RL. Mechanics of oriented electrospun nanofibrous scaffolds for annulus fibrosus tissue engineering. J Orthop Res 2007;25:1018–28.

75. Yang L, Kandel RA, Chang G, et al. Polar surface chemistry of nanofibrous polyurethane scaffold affects annulus fibrosus cell attachment and early matrix accumulation. J Biomed Mater Res A 2009;91:1089–99.

76. Wilda H, Gough JE. In vitro studies of annulus fibrosus disc cell attachment, differentiation and matrix production on PDLLA/45S5 Bioglass composite films. Biomaterials 2006;27:5220–9.

77. Shao X, Hunter CJ. Developing an alginate/chitosan hybrid fiber scaffold for annulus fibrosus cells. J Biomed Mater Res A 2007;82:701–10.

78. Bowles RD, Williams RM, Zipfel WR, et al. Self-assembly of aligned tissue-engineered annulus fibrosus and intervertebral disc composite via collagen gel contraction. Tissue Eng Part A 2010;16:1339–48.

79. Sato M, Asazuma T, Ishihara M, et al. An atelocollagen honeycomb-shaped scaffold with a membrane seal (ACHMS-scaffold) for the culture of annulus fibrosus cells from an intervertebral disc. J Biomed Mater Res A 2003;64:248–56.

80. Saad L, Spector M. Effects of collagen type on the behavior of adult canine annulus fibrosus cells in collagen-glycosaminoglycan scaffolds. J Biomed Mater Res A 2004;71:233–41.

81. Johnson WE, Wootton A, El Haj A, et al. Topographical guidance of intervertebral disc cell growth in vitro: towards the development of tissue repair strategies for the anulus fibrosus. Eur Spine J 2006;15(Suppl 3):S389–96.

82. Nerurkar NL, Sen S, Huang AH, et al. Engineered disc-like angle-ply structures for intervertebral disc replacement. Spine (Phila Pa 1976) 2010;35:867–73.

83. Attia M, Santerre JP, Kandel RA. The response of annulus fibrosus cell to fibronectin-coated nanofibrous

polyurethane-anionic dihydroxyoligomer scaffolds. Biomaterials 2011;32:450–60.

84. Wade KR, Robertson PA, Broom ND. A fresh look at the nucleus-endplate region: new evidence for significant structural integration. Eur Spine J 2011. [Epub ahead of print].

85. Hamilton DJ, Seguin CA, Wang J, et al. Formation of a nucleus pulposus-cartilage endplate construct in-vitro. Biomaterials 2006;27:397–405.

86. Arana CJ, Diamandis EP, Kandel RA. Cartilage tissue enhances proteoglycan retention by nucleus pulposus cells in vitro. Arthritis Rheum 2010;62:3395–403.

87. Waldman SD, Grynpas MD, Pilliar RM, et al. Characterization of cartilagenous tissue formed on calcium polyphosphate substrates in vitro. J Biomed Mater Res 2002;62:323–30.

88. Luk KD, Ruan DK, Lu DS, et al. Fresh frozen intervertebral disc allografting in a bipedal animal model. Spine 2003;28:864–9 [discussion: 870].

89. Mizuno H, Roy AK, Zaporojan V, et al. Biomechanical and biochemical characterization of composite tissue-engineered intervertebral discs. Biomaterials 2006;27:362–70.

90. Wan Y, Feng G, Shen FH, et al. Biphasic scaffold for annulus fibrosus tissue regeneration. Biomaterials 2008;29:643–52.

91. Cheng HW, Luk KD, Cheung KM, et al. In vitro generation of an osteochondral interface from mesenchymal stem cell-collagen microspheres. Biomaterials 2011;32:1526–35.

92. Nishimura I, Garrell RL, Hedrick M, et al. Precursor tissue analogs as a tissue-engineering strategy. Tissue Eng 2003;9(Suppl 1):S77–89.

93. Gantenbein B, Grunhagen T, Lee CR, et al. An in vitro organ culturing system for intervertebral disc explants with vertebral endplates: a feasibility study with ovine caudal discs. Spine 2006;31:2665–73.

94. Illien-Junger S, Gantenbein-Ritter B, Grad S, et al. The combined effects of limited nutrition and high-frequency loading on intervertebral discs with endplates. Spine 2010;35:1744–52.

Emerging Technologies for Molecular Therapy for Intervertebral Disk Degeneration

Won C. Bae, PhD[a], Koichi Masuda, MD[b],*

KEYWORDS

- Back pain ● Animal model ● Disk injection ● Growth factor
- Cytokine ● MRI

INTERVERTEBRAL DISK DEGENERATION AND HOMEOSTASIS OF THE EXTRACELLULAR MATRIX

Intervertebral disk (IVD) degeneration is one of the major causes of low back pain and lumbar disk herniation.[1] Biologically, the cells in the disk actively regulate the homeostasis of the IVD extracellular matrix (ECM) by maintaining a balance between anabolism and catabolism. The modulation of disk cell metabolism involves a variety of molecules (eg, cytokines, enzymes, enzyme inhibitors, and growth factors) that act in a paracrine and/or autocrine fashion. The degeneration of an IVD may result from the loss of steady state metabolism maintained in the normal disks, due to an imbalance between the anabolic and catabolic processes. The proteoglycan (PG) content of the ECM and the rate of PG synthesis decreased markedly with age and degeneration, similar to the case in articular cartilage.[2–10] The anabolic regulators include polypeptide growth factors, such as insulinlike growth factor 1 (IGF-1), transforming growth factor β (TGF-β), and the bone morphogenetic proteins (BMPs).[11,12] Catabolic regulators include many cytokines, notably interleukin 1 (IL-1)[13,14] and tumor necrosis factor (TNF)-α,[13–15] which influence the synthesis of matrix-degrading enzymes, such as the matrix metalloproteinases (MMPs).[16–21] Alterations in both anabolic and catabolic processes are thought to play key roles in the onset and progression of IVD degeneration; the biochemical processes that regulate these changes are important to understand for the development of effective treatments of disk degeneration.

CATABOLIC MEDIATORS AND ENZYMES IN DISK DEGENERATION

Under pathologic conditions, including IVD degeneration,[22] physical injury (eg, puncture or stab wounds),[16,23] and abnormal mechanical loading,[24,25] the IVD expresses cytokines and proteinases. Although macrophages that infiltrate herniated tissue or granulation tissue seem to be the major source of these cytokines,[26–28] recent studies indicate that IVD cells may also synthesize these molecules in an autocrine fashion.[29] In particular, increases in both protein and mRNA levels of IL-1α and its major regulator, TNF-α, have been observed in degenerated or herniated IVD tissues and both are spontaneously expressed by these tissues in culture.[30–37]

This work was supported in part by Grant No. K01AR059764 and Grant No. P01AR48152 from the National Institutes of Health.
Disclosures: Koichi Masuda, MD—research/institutional support: DePuy Spine, Inc, and Stryker Biotech.
[a] Department of Radiology, University of California San Diego, 408 Dickinson Street, San Diego, CA 92103-8226, USA
[b] Department of Orthopaedic Surgery, University of California San Diego, 9500 Gilman Drive, La Jolla, CA 92093-0863, USA
* Corresponding author.
E-mail address: koichimasuda@ucsd.edu

The catabolic processes induced by cytokines are mediated by various enzymes, such as the MMPs[14,32,38–40] or the aggrecanases.[41] IL-1 has been shown to stimulate matrix degradation as well as to inhibit the synthesis of ECM macromolecules[42–45] with minimum effect on cell proliferation.[42] IL-1 induced the production of collagenase,[46] cyclooxygenase-2 (COX-2[47]), prostaglandin E2,[14,48] nitric oxide,[45,46] MMP-1,[49] total[47] and active[44] MMP-3, MMP-13,[21,45] the aggrecanase A disintegrin and metalloproteinase with thrombospondin motifs (ADAMTS)-4),[22,45] IL-6,[47] and monocyte chemoattractant protein-1.[50,51] Recently, IL-1β was shown to increase the sensitivity of IVD cells to shear stress,[52] suggesting that this cytokine is involved in the acceleration of degradation processes in IVDs subjected to biomechanical stress. Although IL-1 affects both synthetic and degradative processes, at lower concentrations, IL-1 was much more effective in inhibiting the synthesis of aggrecan than in stimulating its degradation in articular cartilage.[53–55] An epidemiologic study has shown that IL-1 gene cluster polymorphisms significantly increased the risk of disk degeneration; this has shed more light on the possible involvement of IL-1 in IVD degeneration.[56]

The effects of the inhibition of catabolic cytokines have been evaluated in several studies. IL-1 receptor antagonist (IL-1ra), applied in vitro to degenerated[57] and herniated[58] human disk tissues, reduced the expression of MMP-3.[57,58] IL-1ra pretreatment of nucleus pulposus (NP) cells from moderately degenerate human disks reduced the expression of ADAMTS-4 and MMP-3 in subsequent treatment with IL-1.[59] In another human cell culture study, the addition of IL-1ra and soluble TNF receptor significantly up-regulated PG synthesis, suggesting that IL-1 and TNF suppress PG de novo synthesis.[60] IL-1ra and other agents may benefit from administration of slow-release agents, such as IL-1ra mixed with thermally responsive elastin-like polypeptide (ELP)[59] or with gelatin hydrogel.[61] In addition to IL-1, TNF-α has gained attention in association with disk herniation.[34,35,37,62] TNF-α inhibition, using a monoclonal antibody in herniated human disk explants, showed suppression of MMP-3 levels[58]; other anti-TNF agents are beginning to be applied to reduce pain in patients with sciatica[1,63,64] and discogenic pain.[65] Other anticytokine therapeutics include the p38 mitogen-activated protein kinase (MAPK) inhibitor, which hindered the catabolic effects of IL-1,[66] as well as nuclear factor κB decoy, which reduced pain in a rat lumbar disk herniation model.[67]

ANABOLIC EFFECTS OF CYTOKINES AND GROWTH FACTORS ON IVD CELLS

A variety of growth factors and cytokines (**Table 1**) can alter IVD homeostasis and stimulate ECM synthesis by shifting cellular metabolism to a more anabolic state.[68] The effects of TGF-β on PG synthesis[11,69] and cell proliferation[69] were described early in the literature. Similar effects of IGF-1 have also been reported.[12] IGF-1 and platelet-derived growth factor (PDGF) were also shown to reduce the percentage of apoptotic anulus fibrosus (AF) cells induced by serum depletion in culture.[70]

Osteogenic protein-1 (OP-1),[71] which is a member of the BMP family, up-regulates the PG metabolism of IVD cells. OP-1 strongly stimulated the production and formation of the ECM by rabbit IVD cells[71]; similar effects were found using human IVD cells.[72] OP-1 also replenished PGs and collagens after depletion of the ECM after exposure of IVD cells to IL-1[43] or chondroitinase ABC (C-ABC).[73]

Growth and differentiation factor-5 (GDF-5), originally found to be a factor responsible for skeletal alterations in brachypodism mice,[74] is another member of the BMP family that has anabolic effects on IVD cells. GDF-5 stimulated PG and collagen type II expression by mouse IVD cells.[75] Recombinant human GDF-5 (rhGDF-5) enhanced cell proliferation and matrix synthesis and accumulation by cells from bovine NP and, to lesser extent, AF cells.[76]

Because biologic molecules, prepared in an autologous fashion, avoid certain regulatory complications, they may be useful clinically. Autologous IL-1ra has been used, along with IGF-1 and PDGF proteins, to reduce apoptosis of disk cells and their production of IL-1 and IL-6.[77] Platelet-rich plasma (PRP) can be produced by centrifugal separation of a patient's own blood in the operating room; it contains multiple growth factors concentrated at high levels. In vitro, PRP stimulated cell proliferation and matrix synthesis, as shown using porcine disk cells.[78] PRP induced cell proliferation and differentiation and facilitated NP-like tissue formation by human disk cells.[79]

INTRADISCAL THERAPEUTICS: ANIMAL STUDIES

To study the ability of growth factors and other therapeutic agents to stimulate repair in vivo (**Table 2**), small animal models, in which the degree of degeneration can be controlled, are useful. Rabbit lumbar[76,80–83] and rat caudal disks[84–87] have been used extensively, although other animal models exist.[85,86] Both physical injury, such as stab wound[7,88] or controlled needle puncture,[89,90] and chemical degradation[83–87] approaches have been used.

The in vivo efficacy of OP-1 injection has been evaluated in several animal studies. In adolescent rabbits, an injection of recombinant human OP-1, but not the lactose vehicle, reversed the reduction in disk height and worsened the magnetic resonance imaging (MRI) grade caused by an anular needle puncture.[80] In another study with the same experimental design, the injection of OP-1 restored dynamic viscoelastic biomechanical properties, such as elastic and viscous moduli, of puncture-degenerated IVDs.[81] OP-1 treatment was also effective in restoring disks that have been chemically degraded. C-ABC has been used as an alternative to chymopapain for chemonucleolysis[91–98] as well as an animal model of disk degeneration in the rat tail[84–87] and goat[85,86] disk. When OP-1 or vehicle was injected into rabbit disks degraded with C-ABC for 4 weeks, the disk height initially decreased (approximately 34%), then recovered and gradually approached the level of the normal control.[82]

rhGDF-5 is another promising growth factor whose efficacy has been evaluated in animal models. The efficacy of injecting a single dose of GDF-5 has been reported in the mouse caudal disk with degeneration induced by static compression.[99] In that study, GDF-5 induced an increase in disk height and the expansion of the inner AF fibrochondrocytic population into the NP. In a needle-puncture model of disk degeneration (4 weeks) in adolescent (5–6 months old) rabbits, a single injection of rhGDF-5 restored disk height (**Fig. 1**A) and improved MRI and histologic grading scores within approximately 6 weeks.[76] There are concerns that aged or degenerated disks might have lower cellularity, especially in the number of notochordal cells often found in normal adolescent rabbit disks,[100,101] and might respond poorly to growth factor treatment. Despite this, a study using 2-year-old rabbits showed that rhGDF-5 effectively recovered disk height (see **Fig. 1**B) as well as MRI and histologic grades after a 12-week observation period.[102] Biomechanical analyses indicated that the viscous and elastic moduli of the IVDs in the rhGDF-5-injected disks were significantly higher than those in the phosphate-buffered saline (PBS)-injected disks. Additionally, rhGDF-5 has shown efficacy in rabbit disks that have been degraded using thrombin,[83] a serine proteinase that results in cleavage of PGs and decreased disk height.[103,104] In this study, disks of adolescent rabbits were injected with thrombin

(100 U/10 μL) and the rabbits were maintained for 4 weeks. A single injection of rhGDF-5 (10 μg/10 μL) or saline was then given, and endpoint measures (MRI and gene expression) were determined 12 weeks later. Quantitative MRI was used to evaluate T2 and T1rho[105,106] magnetic resonance properties. T2 (**Fig. 2**A, C) and T1rho (see **Fig. 2**B, D) MRI maps showed maintenance of NP morphology and MRI values in rhGDF-5–treated disks. Both T2 (**Fig. 3**A) and T1rho (see **Fig. 3**B) values of the NP were higher in the rhGDF-5 group, approaching those of unoperated controls. Treatment with rhGDF-5 also reduced the level of expression for ADAMTS-5 (**Fig. 4**A), ADAMTS-4 (see **Fig. 4**B), COX-2 (see **Fig. 4**C), and vascular endothelial growth factor (VEGF) (see **Fig. 4**D), molecules related to PG degradation, pain, and neovascularization seen in degenerated IVDs.[107]

PRP is another agent that has been evaluated in animal models. Using a nucleotomy rabbit model, the effects of allograft PRP with or without gelatin hydrogel microspheres (to provide slow release and mechanical support) and PBS-only injectates were evaluated.[108] The PRP with microspheres group had markedly suppressed degeneration, compared with the PBS-only and PRP-only groups. A recent study by the same group reported additional findings that microspheres alone without PRP did not have therapeutic value, and that the PRP with microsphere group benefited from increased disk height, water content, expression of PG core protein and collagen II, and fewer apoptotic cells in the NP.[61] Although the use of a sustained delivery system has been effective in nucleotomy models in a less severe anular puncture model, an injection of PRP alone was sufficient to induce restoration of disk height and T2 MRI values.[109] The use of fibrin glue alone had a positive effect in a porcine nucleotomy model, where the fibrin glue resulted in the suppression of IL-6 and TNF expression, while restoring mechanical properties and glycosaminoglycan (GAG) content.[110]

A recent study has developed and evaluated the efficacy of an inhibitor for ADAMTS-5 expression using small interference RNA (siRNA).[111] First, the ability of siRNA to reduce ADAMTS-5 expression was determined using rabbit NP cells in vitro. Adolescent rabbit disks, punctured in the anulus to induce degeneration, were injected with either ADAMTS-5 or control siRNA. After 8 weeks, the disks receiving ADAMTS-5 siRNA had markedly better MRI and histology results (**Fig. 5**). The control group exhibited complete loss of NP tissues (see **Fig. 5**A, C) that had been replaced by a fibrocartilaginous tissue (see

Table 1
The in vitro effects of therapeutic agents

Agent	Target	Dose	Effect	Author
TGF-β	Mature canine IVD	1 ng/mL	PG synthesis increased up to 5×; higher in NP than AF	Thompson et al,[11] 1991
IGF-1	Mature canine IVD	20 ng/mL	PG synthesis marginally increased in NP	Thompson et al,[11] 1991
TGF-β	Human anulus cells, 3-D culture	0.25–5 ng/mL	Cell proliferation and PG synthesis increased; reduced apoptosis with serum depletion	Gruber et al,[69] 1997
IGF-1	Young and old bovine NP cells	0–1000 ng/mL	Cell proliferation and matrix synthesis stimulated; more IGF-1 receptors	Osada et al,[12] 1996
OP-1	Young rabbit NP and AF cells; alginate beads	0, 100, 200 ng/mL	Increased PG and collagen production and content	Masuda et al,[71] 2003
BMP-2	Rat IVD cells monolayer	0–1000 ng/mL	Increased cell number, GAG, expression for collagen, aggrecan at higher doses	Yoon et al,[129] 2003
OP-1	Human NP and AF cells, alginate beads	0, 100, 200 ng/mL	Maintained cell density, increased PG synthesis and accumulation	Imai et al,[72] 2007
OP-1	Rabbit IVD cells; alginate beads: IL-1α pre-exposure	200 ng/mL	IL-1α decreased PG and collagen; reversed and exceeded with OP-1	Takegami et al,[43] 2002
OP-1	Rabbit IVD cells; alginate bead: C-ABC pre-exposure	200 ng/mL	OP-1 up-regulated PG synthesis; greater effect after C-ABC pre-Tx than control	Takegami et al,[73] 2005
BMP-2	Human IVD cells	300, 1500 ng/mL	Increased PG synthesis, expression of aggrecan, collagen types I and II; no bone formation	Kim et al,[130] 2003
rhBMP-2 & 12	Human IVD cells in monolayer	25–300 ng/mL	PG, collagen synthesis increased in NP cells; minimal effect on AF cells	Gilbertson et al,[131] 2008

GDF-5	Bovine IVD cells; alginate bead	100, 200 ng/mL	Increased DNA and PG content; at higher dose, PG and collagen synthesis increased	Chujo et al,[76] 2006
PRP	Porcine IVD cells; alginate bead	10% PRP	Mild increase in cell proliferation; marked increase in PG and collagen synthesis and PG accumulation	Akeda et al,[78] 2006
TGF-β1 and PRP	Human NP cells	1 ng/mL TGF-β1 in PRP	NP cell proliferation and aggregation; increase in mRNA of SOX-9, collagen type II, aggrecan	Chen et al,[79] 2006
Ad-TIMP-1, Ad-BMP-2	IVD cells from human degenerated IVD	50–150 MOI	2000 pg/mL production of TIMP w/100 MOI at day 4; PG synthesis increased with both Ad-TIMP-1 and Ad-BMP-2	Wallach et al,[132] 2003
Dexa-methasone	Human disk herniation tissue explants	0.01 mM	Decreased MMP-1 and -3 levels	Genevay et al,[58] 2009
IL-1ra	Human disk herniation tissue explants	100 ng/mL	Decreased MMP-3 levels	Genevay et al,[58] 2009
IL-1ra	Human normal and degenerated disk tissues in situ with IL-1β treatment	100 ng/mL	IL-1ra reduced cytokine levels (MMP-3, -7, -13) and matrix degradation in all tissue types	Le Maitre et al,[57] 2007
IL-1ra/ELP	Human IVD cells (grade 2–3); alginate beads: IL-1ra pre-Tx, then IL-1β insult	4–8000 pM	Reduced ADAMTS-4, MMP-3 transcription	Shamji et al,[59] 2007
p38 MAPK inhibitor (SB 202,190)	Rabbit NP cells pre-Tx with IL-1	1 μM	Decreased message for collagen, aggrecan, IGF-1; increased message for iNOS, COX-2, MMP-3, IL-6	Studer et al,[66] 2008
TNF inhibitor mAb	Human IVD herniation tissue explants	10 μg/mL	Decreased MMP-3 levels	Fujita et al,[39] 1993

Abbreviations: Ad-TIMP-1, adenoviral vector delivering cDNA of tissue inhibitor of MMP-1; Ad-BMP-2, adenoviral vector delivering cDNA of BMP-2; iNOS, inducible nitric oxide synthase; mAb, monoclonal antibody; MOI, multiplicity of infection; Tx, treatment.

Table 2
The in vivo effects of intradiscal injection treatments

Agent	Species	Site	Model	Dose per Disk	Effect	Author
IGF-1	Rat	Tail	Static compression	8 ng/8 µL	Clustering of inner anulus cells after single injection	Walsh et al,[99] 2004
GDF-5	Rat	Tail	Static compression	8 ng/8 µL	Clustering of cells, increase in disk height (single injection)	Walsh et al,[99] 2004
TFG-β	Rat	Tail	Static compression	1.6 ng/8 µL	Proliferation of cells (multiple injections)	Walsh et al,[99] 2004
bFGF	Rat	Tail	Static compression	8 ng/8 µL	No response	Walsh et al,[99] 2004
OP-1	Rabbit	Lumbar	None (normal)	2 µg/10 µL	Increased disk height and PG content in NP	An et al,[133] 2005
OP-1	Rabbit	Lumbar	C-ABC: Co-injection	100 µg/10 µL	Increased disk height and PG content in NP	Imai et al,[134] 2003
OP-1	Rabbit	Lumbar	Needle puncture: Tx 4 wk later	100 µg/10 µL	Increased disk height and PG content in NP and AF, improvement of MRI and histology grades	Masuda et al,[80] 2006
OP-1	Rabbit	Lumbar	Needle puncture	100 µg/10 µL	Increased disk height and viscoelastic properties	Miyamoto et al,[81] 2006
OP-1	Rabbit	Lumbar	C-ABC: Tx 4 wk later	100 µg/10 µL	Increased disk height, PG content in NP and AF	Imai et al,[82] 2007
GDF-5	Rabbit	Lumbar	Needle puncture: Tx 4 wk later	1, 100 ng/10 µL; 1, 100 µg/10 µL	Increased disk height, improvement of MRI and histology grades	Chujo et al,[76] 2006
GDF-5	Rabbit	Lumbar	Thrombin-degraded: Tx 4 wk later	10 µg/10 µL	Increased disk height, improved T1rho and T2 values; decreased ADAMTS-4, -5, COX-9 expression	Bae et al,[83] 2009
BMP-2	Rabbit	Lumbar	Anular stab (5 × 7 mm)	100 µg/100 µL	More degeneration, vascularity and fibroblast	Huang et al,[135] 2007
PRP	Rabbit	Lumbar	Nucleotomy, immediate Tx	PRP + GHM (20 µL) or PRP (5 µL) + PBS (15 µL)	PRP + GHM group had less degeneration and increased PG; PRP + PBS group showed no differences	Nagae et al,[108] 2007
PRP	Rabbit	Lumbar	Nucleotomy, immediate Tx	20 µL of PRP + GHM, PBS + GHM, PRP + PBS; puncture-only	PRP + GHM had greater disk height, water content, mRNA for PG core protein and collagen type II collagen; fewer apoptotic cells in NP	Sawamura et al,[61] 2009
BMP-17	Sheep	Lumbar	Anular stab (3 × 6 mm), immediate Tx	300 µg/70 µL	BMP-17 maintained disk height, MRI and histology scores, NP cell density; increased PG and collagen synthesis	Wei et al,[136] 2009
ADAMTS-5 siRNA	Rabbit	Lumbar	Needle puncture: Tx 4 wk later	10 µg/10 µL	Improved MRI and histology scores	Seki et al,[111] 2009

Abbreviations: bFGF, basic fibroblast growth factor; GHM, gelatin hydrogel microspheres; Tx, treatment.

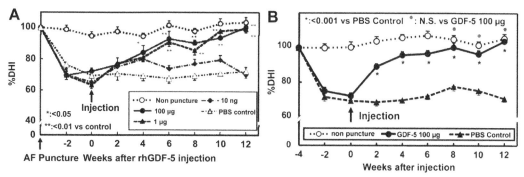

Fig. 1. Changes in the IVD height index (DHI) after anular puncture and rhGDF-5 injection. In a needle-puncture model of disk degeneration (4 weeks) in adolescent (5–6 month old) rabbits, a single injection of rhGDF-5 restored disk height (*A*). In a study using 2-year-old rabbits, disk height was also effectively recovered after a rhGDF-5 injection (*B*). (*Modified from* Chujo T, An HS, Akeda K, et al. Effects of growth differentiation factor-5 on the intervertebral disk—in vitro bovine study and in vivo rabbit disk degeneration model study. Spine [Phila Pa 1976] 2006;31[5]:2909; with permission; and Chujo T, An H, Takatori R, et al. In vivo effects of recombinant human growth and differentiation factor-5 on the repair of the mature rabbit intervertebral disk [abstract]. Spine J 2006;6[5]:23S–4S. [North American Spine Society, 21st Annual Meeting Proceeding, Seattle, WA]; with permission.)

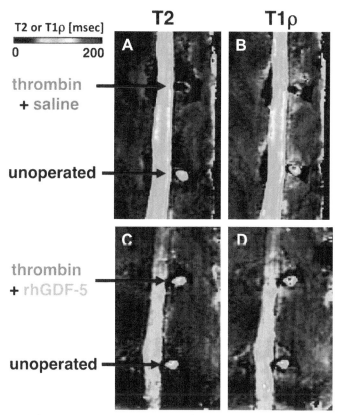

Fig. 2. Quantitative magnetic resonance parameter maps of thrombin-induced degraded rabbit lumbar spines after injection with the growth factor, rhGDF-5. Four weeks after thrombin injection (100 U/10 μL) into adolescent rabbit disks, a single injection of saline (10 μL) (*A, B*) or rhGDF-5 (10 μg/10 μL) (*C, D*) was given. T2 (*A, C*) and T1rho (*B, D*) MRI maps were obtained 12 weeks later. High magnetic resonance values in the nucleus pulposus regions are apparent in the samples treated with the growth factor (*C, D*). (*Modified from* Bae WC, Yoshikawa T, Kakutani K, et al. Effect of rhGDF-5 on the thrombin model of rabbit intervertebral disk degeneration: T1ρ quantification using 3T MRI [abstract]. Radiol Soc North Am 2009;95:SSE14–02; with permission.)

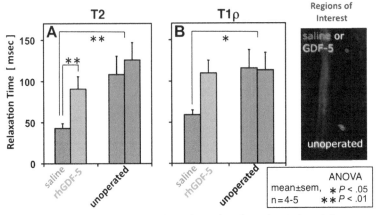

Fig. 3. Treatment with rhGDF-5 restored T2 and T1rho values after thrombin-induced degeneration in adolescent rabbit disks. Four weeks after thrombin injection (100 U/10 μL) into adolescent rabbit disks, a single injection of saline (10 μL) or rhGDF-5 (10 μg/10 μL) was given. T2 and T1rho MRI maps were obtained 12 weeks later. Regions of interest were selected to determine T2 and T1rho values in the NP. Both T2 (*A*) and T1rho (*B*) values of the NP were higher in the rhGDF-5–treated group, approaching those of the unoperated group. The saline group had significantly lower values compared with the unoperated control. (*Modified from* Bae WC, Yoshikawa T, Kakutani K, et al. Effect of rhGDF-5 on the thrombin model of rabbit intervertebral disk degeneration: T1ρ quantification using 3T MRI [abstract]. Radiol Soc North Am 2009;95:SSE14–02; with permission.)

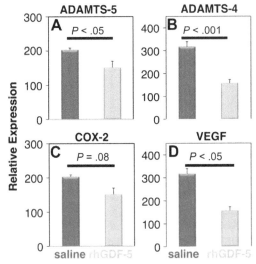

Fig. 4. Treatment with rhGDF-5 inhibits the expression of molecules related to disk degradation, pain, and neovascularization in thrombin-degenerated adolescent rabbit disks. Four weeks after thrombin injection (100 U/10 μL) into adolescent rabbit disks, a single injection of saline (10 μL) or rhGDF-5 (10 μg/10 μL) was given. Twelve weeks later, mRNA expression levels for ADAMTS-5 (*A*), ADAMTS-4 (*B*), COX-2 (*C*), and vascular endothelial growth factor (VEGF) (*D*), in saline-treated and rhGDF-5–treated disks showed a trend or significantly lower levels in the rhGDF-5–treated samples. (*Modified from* Masuda K, Pichika R, Kakutani K, et al. Intradiscal injection of recombinant human growth and differentiation factor-5 significantly suppressed the expression of cytokines, catabolic enzymes and pain markers in the rabbit anular puncture model [abstract]. Paper presented at the 35th Annual Meeting of the International Society of the Study of the Lumbar Spine. Miami (FL), May 4–8, 2009:47; with permission.)

Fig. 5E, G). In contrast, the ADAMTS siRNA group had maintained disk structure (see **Fig. 5**B, D), including a clearly distinguishable NP. Both MRI grade (**Fig. 6**A) and overall histology grade (see **Fig. 6**B) were significantly better for the ADAMTS siRNA group. The inhibition of degradative enzymes and catabolic cytokines provides a complimentary approach to treat degenerated disks at different levels of the modulation mechanism.

Several possible mechanisms governing the long-term effects of growth factor injection warrant further discussion. First, the residence time of an injected protein in the disk has not been solidly established. Some investigators have suggested a short half-life in the order of minutes,[112] whereas other investigators, using radiolabeling, have observed much greater times, likely more than 1 month (**Fig. 7**).[113] Both the structural integrity of the disk and injection location may affect the movement of injected materials in the disk. Second, it has been suggested that OP-1 binds to collagen molecules, which can explain its long-acting effects.[114] Finally, the duration of the anabolic effect resulting from a single exposure to a growth factor needs to be determined.

INJECTION THERAPEUTICS: EFFECT ON PAIN

In addition to the structural modifying effects of injection therapy seen in many preclinical animal studies, there is growing evidence that suggests its pain-relieving effects. In a rat model of pain in which degenerated disk tissue was applied to lumbar nerve roots, mechanical hyperalgesia was

Control siRNA   ADAMTS5 siRNA

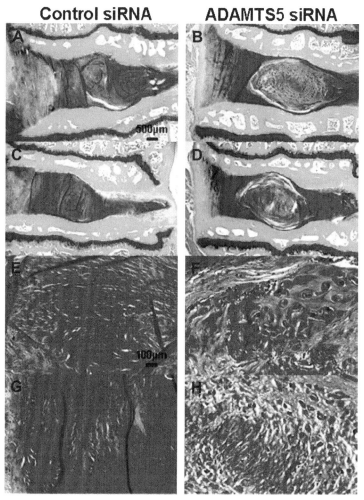

Fig. 5. Histology of anular puncture–induced degenerated adolescent rabbit disks injected with control siRNA or ADAMTS-5 siRNA. Representative safranin O–stained sections after injection of ADAMTS-5 siRNA or control siRNA in the rabbit anular puncture model of disk degeneration. Eight weeks after the siRNA injections, the control siRNA group displayed a complete loss of NP tissues that had been replaced by a fibrocartilaginous tissue (*A, C*). The severely degenerated disks that had received the control siRNA showed a loss of proteoglycans and the collapsed, wavy fibrocartilage lamellae typical of the AF, with associated fibrochondrocytes (*E, G*). In the ADAMTS-5 siRNA-injected disks, safranin O staining demonstrated the maintenance of IVD structure with a lightly stained matrix and large cells (*B, D*); the NP was rounded and bloated in appearance, and consisted of numerous large, vacuolated cells and smaller chondrocyte-like cells (*F, H*). A clear demarcation was seen between the NP and inner anulus in the ADAMTS-5 siRNA-injected disks (magnification ×20 [*A–D*] and ×100 [*E–H*]). Levels are L2/3 [*A, B, E,* and *F*] and L4/5 [*C, D, G,* and *H*]. (*Reproduced from* Seki S, Asanuma-Abe Y, Masuda K, et al. Effect of small interference RNA [siRNA] for ADAMTS5 on intervertebral disk degeneration in the rabbit anular needle-puncture model. Arthritis Res Ther 2009;11:R166; with permission.)

observed in the sham-injected and saline-injected groups but not in the OP-1–treated group.[115] The pain relief may have been due to the ability of OP-1 treatment to result in a reduction of immunohistologic staining for aggrecanase, MMP-13, substance P, TNF-α, and IL-1β.[116] These changes are consistent with the suppression by OP-1 treatment of the expression of IL-1β, TNF-α, IL-6, MMP-3, and aggrecanse-1 in IL-1 insulted human disk cells.[117] These results suggest that OP-1, in addition to being an anabolic mediator, is a catabolic regulator of the metabolism of IVD cells. OP-1 suppression of proinflammatory factors can also suppress a variety of pain markers, such as nerve growth factor, and can lead to pain reduction.

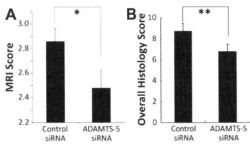

Fig. 6. MRI and histology grading scores of anular puncture–induced degenerated adolescent rabbit disks injected with control siRNA or ADAMTS-5 siRNA. (*A*) MRI assessment 8 weeks after siRNA injection, using a modified Thompson scale (1–4). The MRI grade in the ADAMTS-5 siRNA-treated disks show significantly better (*lower*) MRI grade compared with control siRNA-treated disks. (*B*) Histologic assessment for structure, cellularity, and matrix staining showed significantly better (*lower*) overall score (range 0–12) for ADAMTS-5 siRNA-treated samples. Mean ±SEM, n = 6. *$P<.05$, **$P<.01$; Mann-Whitney *U* test. (*Modified from* Seki S, Asanuma-Abe Y, Masuda K, et al. Effect of small interference RNA [siRNA] for ADAMTS5 on intervertebral disk degeneration in the rabbit anular needle-puncture model. Arthritis Res Ther 2009;11:R166; with permission.)

CONSIDERATIONS FOR INJECTABLE THERAPEUTICS AND THEIR LIMITATIONS

Although the clinical application of injectable therapeutics is being actively pursued, several limitations need to be considered. First, the target population of this therapeutic approach is mainly an aged population, which has fewer cells in the IVD than the normal population. IVD cell density is also lower in disks with advanced degeneration.[118] Because injection therapy seeks to influence existing cells in the disk, the appropriate stage of disk degeneration and age of the patients may need to be defined. For those with low cellularity, it may be possible to use a tissue-engineering approach. For example, a few functional cells recovered from herniated tissues or mesenchymal stem cells may be expanded for later use.[119–123]

In addition to cellular changes, nutritional supply and removal of metabolic wastes may be compromised by changes in the endplate, such as calcification seen in sclerosis. Hindrance of the nutritional pathway may render an injection therapy ineffective because the lack of nutrition may impair the synthesis of the disk matrix needed for repair. Similarly, when tissue-engineered cells are added to disks, they may not survive without a proper supply of nutrients to meet the demands of increased energy consumption. Thus, a noninvasive means to assess environmental conditions

(eg, changes in cartilage endplate) in the IVD is essential. Using a contrast-enhanced MRI method, the diffusion function of the endplate has been assessed indirectly in human subjects.[124,125] Recent advances in MRI, such as the ultrashort time-to-echo (UTE) technique,[125–127] allow for direct visualization (**Fig. 8**A) of regions of the cartilage endplate with high contrast, unlike conventional MRI sequences (see **Fig. 8**B). Abnormalities (see **Fig. 8**C) of the cartilage endplate in UTE MRI have been significantly associated with disk degeneration ($P<.01$, χ^2 test), as evaluated by Pfirrmann grading,[128] in approximately 30 cadaveric human lumbar spines. It would be useful to determine if the appearance of the cartilage endplate by MRI provides information on the time course of subsequent disk degeneration as well as the outcome of therapeutic treatments or the proper selection of patients.

Although much evidence of structural modifications in animal disk degeneration models has been demonstrated in this review, there are significant limitations to applying these results to human patients. Studies using large animals with disks of a size similar to those of the human that do not contain notochordal cells may be needed to answer the remaining issues of nutritional supply and cellular composition. The cost of studies using large animals and the ethical problems associated with these animals, however, are some of the issues that delay their use. In addition, pain measures have not been well established for large animals, making pain research difficult. Once a therapeutic agent is proved safe, however, a clinical trial on carefully selected patients (eg, those patients who would otherwise undergo spinal fusion) may be a good approach for testing therapeutic efficacy.

INJECTION THERAPEUTICS IN CLINICAL TRIALS

Several clinical trials involving intradiscal injection therapeutics are under way. These studies typically select patients exhibiting chronic moderate-to-severe discogenic pain, without involvement of nerve compression or facet joints, for which nonsurgical therapy has not been effective. Sponsored by Advanced Technologies and Regenerative Medicine and DePuy Spine, multicenter studies in the United States (ClinicalTrials.gov identifier: NCT01124006) and in Korea and Australia (NCT01158924 and NCT01182337) are currently (as of November 2010) recruiting patients to evaluate safety, tolerability, and effectiveness of single-injection of rhGDF-5 versus placebo, with

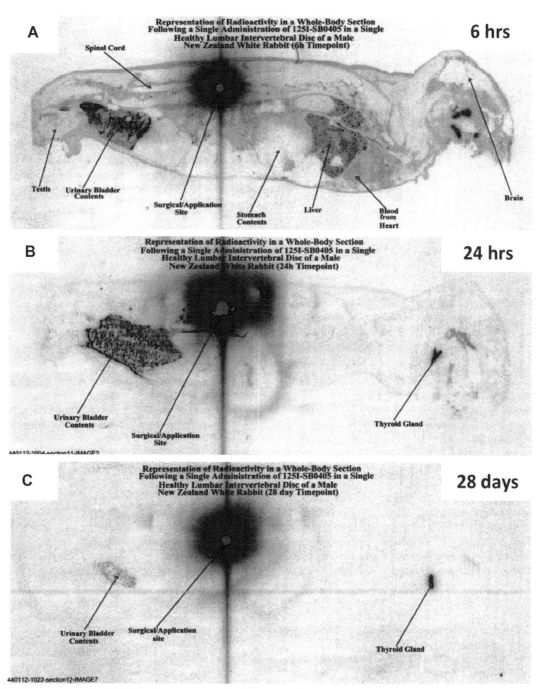

Fig. 7. Retention of radiolabeled BMP-7 in a rabbit disk. Normal rabbits that received a single intradiscal injection of ^{125}I-labeled BMP-7 (otherwise known as OP-1) were imaged using autoradiography (*A*) 6 hours, (*B*) 24 hours, or (*C*) 28 days after the injection. The signal from the radiolabeled BMP-7 is prominent even after 14 days. (*Modified from* Pierce A, Feng M, Masuda K, et al. Distribution, pharmacokinetics and excretion of 125-Iodine labeled BMP-7 [OP-1] following a single-dose administration in lumbar IVD or knee joint of NZW rabbits. Paper presented at the Sixth International Conference on Bone Morphogeneic Proteins. Cavtat (Croatia), October 11–15, 2006; with permission.)

outcome measures that include safety outcomes, pain, and MRI at 12 months.

Another study sponsored by Spinal Restoration (NCT01011816) will be evaluating the effects of injecting Biostat Fibrin Sealant on the time course of

pain reduction (visual analog scale) and function restoration (Roland-Morris Disability Questionnaire score) through 78 weeks, along with safety, on 260 patients. This study seeks to achieve a 30% decrease in pain and 30% improvement

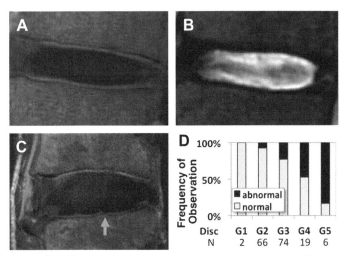

Fig. 8. Evaluation of region of cartilage endplate using UTE MRI. A normal lumbar disk imaged using UTE MRI (*A*) and conventional T2-weighted spin-echo MRI (*B*). Note the characteristic high-intensity lines (*A*) near the regions of cartilage endplate. The same regions appear dark in conventional MRI (*B*). Abnormalities, such as focal signal loss, have been observed (*arrow*) (*C*) and correlated with the grade of the adjacent disk (*D*). (*Modified from* Bae WC, Yoshikawa T, Znamirowski R, et al. Ultrashort time-to-echo MRI of human intervertebral disk endplate: association with disk degeneration. Proc Intl Soc Magn Reson Med 2010;18:534; with permission.)

in function. Once safety concerns are addressed in the current studies, it is hoped that later-stage studies with additional measures and a greater number of patients will reveal the mechanism of treatment as well as suitable patient selection.

SUMMARY

Abundant evidence for the efficacy of injectable therapeutics, including many growth factors, as treatment of IVD degeneration has been presented in studies using IVD cells in vitro as well as in preclinical in vivo animal studies. For animal studies, outcomes focused mainly on structural modification, and the effects of injection therapy on pain generation are not well known. Recent data obtained from small animal studies suggest that injection therapy can lead to modification of pain behaviors as well as changes in cytokine expression. Such results offer great potential for patients with chronic discogenic low back pain. Multiple clinical trials for injection therapy are now under way, and their results will be useful for establishing safety and efficacy injection treatments. In addition, for disks with advanced stages of degeneration, the prophylactic use of growth factor injection therapy, such as its application to disks adjacent to a fusion level, may be an alternative approach. Quantitative studies on the effects of a growth factor injection on pain reduction and on long-term cell survival using large animals are desirable. Diagnostic techniques to evaluate the disk environment, such as the MRI evaluation of

the cartilage endplate, may also become a desirable tool for patient selection. Furthermore, comprehensive studies looking at the muscles, facet joints, and vasculature that comprise the whole spinal structure are important to seek new innovative diagnostic and therapeutic approaches, encompassing surgical and conservative approaches.

REFERENCES

1. Karppinen J, Korhonen T, Malmivaara A, et al. Tumor necrosis factor-alpha monoclonal antibody, infliximab, used to manage severe sciatica. Spine (Phila Pa 1976) 2003;28:750.
2. Maeda S, Kokubun S. Changes with age in proteoglycan synthesis in cells cultured in vitro from the inner and outer rabbit annulus fibrosus. Responses to interleukin-1 and interleukin-1 receptor antagonist protein. Spine (Phila Pa 1976) 2000;25:166.
3. Antoniou J, Steffen T, Nelson F, et al. The human lumbar intervertebral disc: evidence for changes in the biosynthesis and denaturation of the extracellular matrix with growth, maturation, ageing, and degeneration. J Clin Invest 1996;98:996.
4. Buckwalter JA, Kuettner KE, Thonar EJ. Age-related changes in articular cartilage proteoglycans: electron microscopic studies. J Orthop Res 1985;3:251.
5. Buckwalter JA, Pedrini MA, Pedrini V, et al. Proteoglycans of human infant intervertebral disc. Electron microscopic and biochemical studies. J Bone Joint Surg Am 1985;67:284.

6. Cole TC, Ghosh P, Taylor TK. Variations of the proteoglycans of the canine intervertebral disc with ageing. Biochim Biophys Acta 1986;880:209.

7. Lipson SJ, Muir H. Experimental intervertebral disc degeneration: morphologic and proteoglycan changes over time. Arthritis Rheum 1981;24:12.

8. Melrose J, Ghosh P, Taylor TK, et al. A longitudinal study of the matrix changes induced in the intervertebral disc by surgical damage to the annulus fibrosus. J Orthop Res 1992;10:665.

9. Pearce RH, Grimmer BJ, Adams ME. Degeneration and the chemical composition of the human lumbar intervertebral disc. J Orthop Res 1987;5:198.

10. Nerlich AG, Schleicher ED, Boos N. 1997 Volvo Award winner in basic science studies. Immunohistologic markers for age-related changes of human lumbar intervertebral discs. Spine (Phila Pa 1976) 1997;22:2781.

11. Thompson JP, Oegema TJ, Bradford DS. Stimulation of mature canine intervertebral disc by growth factors. Spine (Phila Pa 1976) 1991;16:253.

12. Osada R, Ohshima H, Ishihara H, et al. Autocrine/paracrine mechanism of insulin-like growth factor-1 secretion, and the effect of insulin-like growth factor-1 on proteoglycan synthesis in bovine intervertebral discs. J Orthop Res 1996;14:690.

13. Ahn SH, Teng PN, Niyibizi C, et al. The effects of BMP-12 and BMP-2 on proteoglycan and collagen synthesis in nucleus pulposus cells from human degenerated discs. The 29th Annual Meeting of the International Society for the Study of the Lumbar Spine. Cleveland (OH), May 14–16, 2002, Proceedings: 49.

14. Takahashi H, Suguro T, Okazima Y, et al. Inflammatory cytokines in the herniated disc of the lumbar spine. Spine (Phila Pa 1976) 1996;21:218.

15. Miyamoto H, Saura R, Harada T, et al. The role of cyclooxygenase-2 and inflammatory cytokines in pain induction of herniated lumbar intervertebral disc. Kobe J Med Sci 2000;46:13.

16. Anderson DG, Izzo MW, Hall DJ, et al. Comparative gene expression profiling of normal and degenerative discs: analysis of a rabbit annular laceration model. Spine (Phila Pa 1976) 2002;27:1291.

17. Doita M, Kanatani T, Ozaki T, et al. Influence of macrophage infiltration of herniated disc tissue on the production of matrix metalloproteinases leading to disc resorption. Spine (Phila Pa 1976) 2001;26:1522.

18. Roberts S, Caterson B, Menage J, et al. Matrix metalloproteinases and aggrecanase: their role in disorders of the human intervertebral disc. Spine (Phila Pa 1976) 2000;25:3005.

19. Tsuru M, Nagata K, Ueno T, et al. Electron microscopic observation of established chondrocytes derived from human intervertebral disc hernia (KTN-1) and role of macrophages in spontaneous regression of degenerated tissues. Spine J 2001; 1:422.

20. Weiler C, Nerlich AG, Zipperer J, et al. 2002 SSE Award Competition in Basic Science: expression of major matrix metalloproteinases is associated with intervertebral disc degradation and resorption. Eur Spine J 2002;11:308.

21. Le Maitre CL, Freemont AJ, Hoyland JA. Localization of degradative enzymes and their inhibitors in the degenerate human intervertebral disc. J Pathol 2004;204:47.

22. Patel KP, Sandy JD, Akeda K, et al. Aggrecanases and aggrecanase-generated fragments in the human intervertebral disc at early and advanced stages of disc degeneration. Spine (Phila Pa 1976) 2007;32:2596.

23. Sobajima S, Shimer AL, Chadderdon RC, et al. Quantitative analysis of gene expression in a rabbit model of intervertebral disc degeneration by real-time polymerase chain reaction. Spine J 2005;5:14.

24. Yurube T, Nishida K, Suzuki T, et al. Matrix metalloproteinase (MMP)-3 gene up-regulation in a rat tail compression loading-induced disc degeneration model. J Orthop Res 2010;28:1026.

25. Iatridis JC, Godburn K, Wuertz K, et al. Region-dependent aggrecan degradation patterns in the rat intervertebral disc are affected by mechanical loading in vivo. Spine (Phila Pa 1976) 2011;36:203.

26. Doita M, Kanatani T, Harada T, et al. Immunohistologic study of the ruptured intervertebral disc of the lumbar spine. Spine 1996;21:235.

27. Gronblad M, Virri J, Tolonen J, et al. A controlled immunohistochemical study of inflammatory cells in disc herniation tissue. Spine (Phila Pa 1976) 1994;19:2744.

28. Baba H, Maezawa Y, Furusawa N, et al. Herniated cervical intervertebral discs: histological and immunohistochemical characteristics. Eur J Histochem 1997;41:261.

29. Rand N, Reichert F, Floman Y, et al. Murine nucleus pulposus-derived cells secrete interleukins-1-beta, -6, and -10 and granulocyte-macrophage colony-stimulating factor in cell culture. Spine (Phila Pa 1976) 1997;22:2598.

30. Ahn SH, Cho YW, Ahn MW, et al. mRNA expression of cytokines and chemokines in herniated lumbar intervertebral discs. Spine (Phila Pa 1976) 2002; 27:911.

31. Burke JG, Watson RW, Conhyea D, et al. Human nucleus pulposus can respond to a pro-inflammatory stimulus. Spine (Phila Pa 1976) 2003;28:2685.

32. Kang JD, Georgescu HI, McIntyre-Larkin L, et al. Herniated lumbar intervertebral discs spontaneously produce matrix metalloproteinases, nitric oxide, interleukin-6, and prostaglandin E2. Spine (Phila Pa 1976) 1996;21:271.

33. Weiler C, Nerlich AG, Bachmeier BE, et al. Expression and distribution of tumor necrosis factor alpha in human lumbar intervertebral discs: a study in surgical specimen and autopsy controls. Spine (Phila Pa 1976) 2005;30:44.

34. Igarashi T, Kikuchi S, Shubayev V, et al. 2000 Volvo Award winner in basic science studies: exogenous tumor necrosis factor-alpha mimics nucleus pulposus-induced neuropathology. Molecular, histologic, and behavioral comparisons in rats. Spine (Phila Pa 1976) 2000;25:2975.

35. Olmarker K, Larsson K. Tumor necrosis factor alpha and nucleus-pulposus-induced nerve root injury. Spine (Phila Pa 1976) 1998;23:2538.

36. Le Maitre CL, Freemont AJ, Hoyland JA. The role of interleukin-1 in the pathogenesis of human intervertebral disc degeneration. Arthritis Res Ther 2005;7: R732.

37. Le Maitre CL, Hoyland JA, Freemont AJ. Catabolic cytokine expression in degenerate and herniated human intervertebral discs: IL-1beta and TNFalpha expression profile. Arthritis Res Ther 2007;9:R77.

38. Liu J, Roughley PJ, Mort JS. Identification of human intervertebral disc stromelysin and its involvement in matrix degradation. J Orthop Res 1991;9:568.

39. Fujita K, Nakagawa T, Hirabayashi K, et al. Neutral proteinases in human intervertebral disc. Role in degeneration and probable origin. Spine (Phila Pa 1976) 1993;18:1766.

40. Kang JD, Georgescu HI, McIntyre-Larkin L, et al. Herniated cervical intervertebral discs spontaneously produce matrix metalloproteinases, nitric oxide, interleukin-6, and prostaglandin E2. Spine (Phila Pa 1976) 1995;20:2373.

41. Sztrolovics R, Alini M, Roughley PJ, et al. Aggrecan degradation in human intervertebral disc and articular cartilage. Biochem J 1997;326:235.

42. Shinmei M, Kikuchi T, Yamagishi M, et al. The role of interleukin-1 on proteoglycan metabolism of rabbit annulus fibrosus cells cultured in vitro. Spine (Phila Pa 1976) 1988;13:1284.

43. Takegami K, Thonar EJ, An HS, et al. Osteogenic protein-1 enhances matrix replenishment by intervertebral disc cells previously exposed to interleukin-1. Spine (Phila Pa 1976) 2002;27:1318.

44. Shen B, Melrose J, Ghosh P, et al. Induction of matrix metalloproteinase-2 and -3 activity in ovine nucleus pulposus cells grown in three-dimensional agarose gel culture by interleukin-1beta: a potential pathway of disc degeneration. Eur Spine J 2003;12:66.

45. Miyamoto K, Pichika R, An H, et al. Tumor Necrosis Factor-a exhibits potent effects on the metabolism of human intervertebral disc cells. Trans Orthop Res Soc 2005;30:188.

46. Sakuma M, Fujii N, Takahashi T, et al. Effect of chondroitinase ABC on matrix metalloproteinases and inflammatory mediators produced by intervertebral disc of rabbit in vitro. Spine (Phila Pa 1976) 2002;27:576.

47. Kang JD, Stefanovic-Racic M, McIntyre LA, et al. Toward a biochemical understanding of human intervertebral disc degeneration and herniation. Contributions of nitric oxide, interleukins, prostaglandin E2, and matrix metalloproteinases. Spine (Phila Pa 1976) 1997;22:1065.

48. Rannou F, Corvol MT, Hudry C, et al. Sensitivity of anulus fibrosus cells to interleukin 1 beta. Comparison with articular chondrocytes. Spine (Phila Pa 1976) 2000;25:17.

49. Akeda K, An H, Gemba T, et al. A new gene therapy approach: in vivo transfection of naked NFkB decoy oligonucleotide restored disc degeneration in the rabbit annular needle puncture model. Trans Orthop Res Soc 2005;30:45.

50. Yoshida M, Nakamura T, Kikuchi T, et al. Expression of monocyte chemoattractant protein-1 in primary cultures of rabbit intervertebral disc cells. J Orthop Res 2002;20:1298.

51. Jimbo K, Park JS, Yokosuka K, et al. Positive feedback loop of interleukin-1beta upregulating production of inflammatory mediators in human intervertebral disc cells in vitro. J Neurosurg Spine 2005;2:589.

52. Elfervig MK, Minchew JT, Francke E, et al. IL-1beta sensitizes intervertebral disc annulus cells to fluid-induced shear stress. J Cell Biochem 2001;82:290.

53. Arner EC, Pratta MA. Independent effects of interleukin-1 on proteoglycan breakdown, proteoglycan synthesis, and prostaglandin E2 release from cartilage in organ culture. Arthritis Rheum 1989;32:288.

54. Benton HP, Tyler JA. Inhibition of cartilage proteoglycan synthesis by interleukin I. Biochem Biophys Res Commun 1988;154:421.

55. Dingle JT, Horner A, Shield M. The sensitivity of synthesis of human cartilage matrix to inhibition by IL-1 suggests a mechanism for the development of osteoarthritis. Cell Biochem Funct 1991;9:99.

56. Solovieva S, Kouhia S, Leino-Arjas P, et al. Interleukin 1 polymorphisms and intervertebral disc degeneration. Epidemiology 2004;15:626.

57. Le Maitre CL, Hoyland JA, Freemont AJ. Interleukin-1 receptor antagonist delivered directly and by gene therapy inhibits matrix degradation in the intact degenerate human intervertebral disc: an in situ zymographic and gene therapy study. Arthritis Res Ther 2007;9:R83.

58. Genevay S, Finckh A, Mezin F, et al. Influence of cytokine inhibitors on concentration and activity of MMP-1 and MMP-3 in disc herniation. Arthritis Res Ther 2009;11:R169.

59. Shamji MF, Betre H, Kraus VB, et al. Development and characterization of a fusion protein between thermally responsive elastin-like polypeptide and

interleukin-1 receptor antagonist: Sustained release of a local antiinflammatory therapeutic. Arthritis Rheum 2007;56:3650.

60. Kakutani K, Kanaji A, Asanuma K, et al. Effect of IL-1 receptor antagonist and soluble TNF receptor on the anabolism of human intervertebral disc cells. Trans Orthop Res Soc 2008;33:442.

61. Sawamura K, Ikeda T, Nagae M, et al. Characterization of in vivo effects of platelet-rich plasma and biodegradable gelatin hydrogel microspheres on degenerated intervertebral discs. Tissue Eng Part A 2009;15:3719.

62. Yoshida M, Nakamura T, Sei A, et al. Intervertebral disc cells produce tumor necrosis factor alpha, interleukin-1beta, and monocyte chemoattractant protein-1 immediately after herniation: an experimental study using a new hernia model. Spine (Phila Pa 1976) 2005;30:55.

63. Genevay S, Stingelin S, Gabay C. Efficacy of etanercept in the treatment of acute, severe sciatica: a pilot study. Ann Rheum Dis 2004;63:1120.

64. Okoro T, Tafazal SI, Longworth S, et al. Tumor necrosis alpha-blocking agent (etanercept): a triple blind randomized controlled trial of its use in treatment of sciatica. J Spinal Disord Tech 2010;23:74.

65. Tobinick EL, Britschgi-Davoodifar S. Perispinal TNF-alpha inhibition for discogenic pain. Swiss Med Wkly 2003;133:170.

66. Studer RK, Gilbertson LG, Georgescu H, et al. p38 MAPK inhibition modulates rabbit nucleus pulposus cell response to IL-1. J Orthop Res 2008;26:991.

67. Suzuki M, Inoue G, Gemba T, et al. Nuclear factor-kappa B decoy suppresses nerve injury and improves mechanical allodynia and thermal hyperalgesia in a rat lumbar disc herniation model. Eur Spine J 2009;18:1001.

68. Masuda K, Oegema TR Jr, An HS. Growth factors and treatment of intervertebral disc degeneration. Spine (Phila Pa 1976) 2004;29:2757.

69. Gruber HE, Fisher EC Jr, Desai B, et al. Human intervertebral disc cells from the annulus: three-dimensional culture in agarose or alginate and responsiveness to TGF-beta1. Exp Cell Res 1997;235:13.

70. Gruber HE, Norton HJ, Hanley EN Jr. Anti-apoptotic effects of IGF-1 and PDGF on human intervertebral disc cells in vitro. Spine (Phila Pa 1976) 2000;25:2153.

71. Masuda K, Takegami K, An H, et al. Recombinant osteogenic protein-1 upregulates extracellular matrix metabolism by rabbit annulus fibrosus and nucleus pulposus cells cultured in alginate beads. J Orthop Res 2003;21:922.

72. Imai Y, Miyamoto K, An HS, et al. Recombinant human osteogenic protein-1 upregulates proteoglycan metabolism of human anulus fibrosus and nucleus pulposus cells. Spine (Phila Pa 1976) 2007;32:1303.

73. Takegami K, An HS, Kumano F, et al. Osteogenic protein-1 is most effective in stimulating nucleus pulposus and annulus fibrosus cells to repair their matrix after chondroitinase ABC-induced in vitro chemonucleolysis. Spine J 2005;5:231.

74. Storm EE, Huynh TV, Copeland NG, et al. Limb alterations in brachypodism mice due to mutations in a new member of the TGF beta-superfamily. Nature 1994;368:639.

75. Li X, Leo BM, Beck G, et al. Collagen and proteoglycan abnormalities in the GDF-5-deficient mice and molecular changes when treating disk cells with recombinant growth factor. Spine (Phila Pa 1976) 2004;29:2229.

76. Chujo T, An HS, Akeda K, et al. Effects of growth differentiation factor-5 on the intervertebral disc—in vitro bovine study and in vivo rabbit disc degeneration model study. Spine (Phila Pa 1976) 2006;31:2909.

77. Wehling P. Antiapoptotic and antidegenerative effect of an autologous IL-1ra/IGF-1/PDGF combination on human intervertebral disc cells in vivo. The 29th Annual Meeting of the International Society for the Study of the Lumbar Spine. Cleveland (OH), May 14–16, 2002, Proceedings: 49.

78. Akeda K, An HS, Pichika R, et al. Platelet-rich plasma (PRP) stimulates the extracellular matrix metabolism of porcine nucleus pulposus and anulus fibrosus cells cultured in alginate beads. Spine (Phila Pa 1976) 2006;31:959.

79. Chen WH, Lo WC, Lee JJ, et al. Tissue-engineered intervertebral disc and chondrogenesis using human nucleus pulposus regulated through TGF-beta1 in platelet-rich plasma. J Cell Physiol 2006;209:744.

80. Masuda K, Imai Y, Okuma M, et al. Osteogenic protein-1 injection into a degenerated disc induces the restoration of disc height and structural changes in the rabbit anular puncture model. Spine (Phila Pa 1976) 2006;31:742.

81. Miyamoto K, Masuda K, Kim JG, et al. Intradiscal injections of osteogenic protein-1 restore the viscoelastic properties of degenerated intervertebral discs. Spine J 2006;6:692.

82. Imai Y, Okuma M, An H, et al. Restoration of disc height loss by recombinant human osteogenic protein-1 injection into intervertebral discs undergoing degeneration induced by an intradiscal injection of chondroitinase ABC. Spine (Phila Pa 1976) 2007;32:1197.

83. Bae WC, Yoshikawa T, Kakutani K, et al. Effect of rhGDF-5 on the thrombin model of rabbit intervertebral disc degeneration: T1ρ quantification using 3T MRI. Radiol Soc North Am 2009;95:SSE14-02.

84. Norcross JP, Lester GE, Weinhold P, et al. An in vivo model of degenerative disc disease. J Orthop Res 2003;21:183.

85. Hoogendoorn RJ, Helder MN, Kroeze RJ, et al. Reproducible long-term disc degeneration in a large animal model. Spine (Phila Pa 1976) 2008;33:949.

86. Hoogendoorn RJ, Wuisman PI, Smit TH, et al. Experimental intervertebral disc degeneration induced by chondroitinase ABC in the goat. Spine (Phila Pa 1976) 2007;32:1816.

87. Boxberger JI, Auerbach JD, Sen S, et al. An in vivo model of reduced nucleus pulposus glycosaminoglycan content in the rat lumbar intervertebral disc. Spine (Phila Pa 1976) 2008;33:146.

88. Lipson SJ, Muir H. 1980 Volvo award in basic science. Proteoglycans in experimental intervertebral disc degeneration. Spine (Phila Pa 1976) 1981;6:194.

89. Masuda K, Aota Y, Muehleman C, et al. A novel rabbit model of mild, reproducible disc degeneration by an anulus needle puncture: correlation between the degree of disc injury and radiological and histological appearances of disc degeneration. Spine (Phila Pa 1976) 2005;30:5.

90. Sobajima S, Kompel JF, Kim JS, et al. A slowly progressive and reproducible animal model of intervertebral disc degeneration characterized by MRI, X-ray, and histology. Spine (Phila Pa 1976) 2005;30:15.

91. Eurell JA, Brown MD, Ramos M. The effects of chondroitinase ABC on the rabbit intervertebral disc. A roentgenographic and histologic study. Clin Orthop 1990;256:238.

92. Fry TR, Eurell JC, Johnson AL, et al. Radiographic and histologic effects of chondroitinase ABC on normal canine lumbar intervertebral disc. Spine (Phila Pa 1976) 1991;16:816.

93. Henderson N, Stanescu V, Cauchoix J. Nucleolysis of the rabbit intervertebral disc using chondroitinase ABC. Spine (Phila Pa 1976) 1991;16:203.

94. Kato F, Mimatsu K, Kawakami N, et al. Serial changes observed by magnetic resonance imaging in the intervertebral disc after chemonucleolysis. A consideration of the mechanism of chemonucleolysis. Spine (Phila Pa 1976) 1992;17:934.

95. Ando T, Kato F, Mimatsu K, et al. Effects of chondroitinase ABC on degenerative intervertebral discs. Clin Orthop 1995;318:214.

96. Sugimura T, Kato F, Mimatsu K, et al. Experimental chemonucleolysis with chondroitinase ABC in monkeys. Spine 1996;21:161.

97. Takahashi T, Kurihara H, Nakajima S, et al. Chemonucleolytic effects of chondroitinase ABC on normal rabbit intervertebral discs. Course of action up to 10 days postinjection and minimum effective dose. Spine (Phila Pa 1976) 1996;21:2405.

98. Yamada K, Tanabe S, Ueno H, et al. Investigation of the short-term effect of chemonucleolysis with chondroitinase ABC. J Vet Med Sci 2001;63:521.

99. Walsh AJ, Bradford DS, Lotz JC. In vivo growth factor treatment of degenerated intervertebral discs. Spine (Phila Pa 1976) 2004;29:156.

100. Kim KW, Lim TH, Kim JG, et al. The origin of chondrocytes in the nucleus pulposus and histologic findings associated with the transition of a notochordal nucleus pulposus to a fibrocartilaginous nucleus pulposus in intact rabbit intervertebral discs. Spine (Phila Pa 1976) 2003;28:982.

101. Scott NA, Harris PF, Bagnall KM. A morphological and histological study of the postnatal development of intervertebral discs in the lumbar spine of the rabbit. J Anat 1980;130:75.

102. Chujo T, An H, Takatori R, et al. In Vivo effects of recombinant human growth and differentiation factor-5 on the repair of the mature rabbit intervertebral disc. Spine J 2006;6:23S.

103. Asanuma K, Abe Y, Pichika R, et al. Direct cleavage by thrombin at the Arg375-Gly376 bond in the interglobular domain is involved in accelerated degradation of aggrecan by intervertebral disc cells. Trans Orthop Res Soc 2008;33:1420.

104. Asanuma K, Abe Y, Muehleman C, et al. A thrombin-injection model of disc degeneration in the rabbit. Trans Orthop Res Soc 2008;33:1394.

105. Duvvuri U, Reddy R, Patel SD, et al. T1rho-relaxation in articular cartilage: effects of enzymatic degradation. Magn Reson Med 1997;38:863.

106. Han ET, Busse RF, Li X. 3D segmented elliptic-centric spoiled gradient echo imaging for the in vivo quantification of cartilage T1rho. Int Soc Mag Res Med 2005;13:473.

107. Masuda K, Pichika R, Kakutani K, et al. Intradiscal injection of recombinant human growth and differentiation factor-5 significantly suppressed the expression of cytokines, catabolic enzymes and pain markers in the rabbit anular puncture model. The 35th Annual Meeting of the International Society of the Study of the Lumbar Spine. Miami (FL), May 4–8, 2009, Proceedings: 47.

108. Nagae M, Ikeda T, Mikami Y, et al. Intervertebral disc regeneration using platelet-rich plasma and biodegradable gelatin hydrogel microspheres. Tissue Eng 2007;13:147.

109. Obata K, Akeda K, Morimoto R, et al. Intradiscal injection of autologous platelet-rich plasma-serum induces the restoration of disc height in the rabbit anular needle puncture model. The 36th Annual Meeting of the International Society of the Study of the Lumbar Spine. Auckland (New Zealand), April 13–17, 2010, Proceedings: 12.

110. Buser Z, Kuelling F, Jane L, et al. Fibrin injection stimulates early disc healing in the porcine model. Spine J 2009;9:105S.

111. Seki S, Asanuma-Abe Y, Masuda K, et al. Effect of small interference RNA (siRNA) for ADAMTS5 on intervertebral disc degeneration in the rabbit anular

needle-puncture model. Arthritis Res Ther 2009;11: R166.

112. Larson JW 3rd, Levicoff EA, Gilbertson LG, et al. Biologic modification of animal models of intervertebral disc degeneration. J Bone Joint Surg Am 2006;88(Suppl 2):83.

113. Pierce A, Feng M, Masuda K, et al. Distribution, pharmacokinetics and excretion of 125-Iodine labeled BMP-7 (OP-1) following a single dose administration in lumbar IVD or knee joint of NZW rabbits. The Sixth International Conference on Bone Morphogenetic Proteins. Cavtat (Croatia), October 11–15, 2006.

114. Reddi AH. Morphogenetic messages are in the extracellular matrix: biotechnology from bench to bedside. Biochem Soc Trans 2000;28:345.

115. Kawakami M, Matsumoto T, Hashizume H, et al. Osteogenic protein-1 (osteogenic protein-1/bone morphogenetic protein-7) inhibits degeneration and pain-related behavior induced by chronically compressed nucleus pulposus in the rat. Spine (Phila Pa 1976) 2005;30:1933.

116. Chubinskaya S, Kawakami M, Rappoport L, et al. Anti-catabolic effect of OP-1 in chronically compressed intervertebral discs. J Orthop Res 2007; 25:517.

117. Pichika R, An H, Miyamoto K, et al. Suppressive effect of bone morphogenetic protein-7 on interleukin-1β mediated gene expression of cytokines and catabolic enzymes in human intervertebral disc cells. Ortho Res Soc Trans 2007;32:243.

118. Gruber HE, Hanley EN Jr. Analysis of aging and degeneration of the human intervertebral disc. Comparison of surgical specimens with normal controls. Spine (Phila Pa 1976) 1998;23:751.

119. Nishimura K, Mochida J. Percutaneous reinsertion of the nucleus pulposus. An experimental study. Spine (Phila Pa 1976) 1998;23:1531.

120. Okuma M, Mochida J, Nishimura K, et al. Reinsertion of stimulated nucleus pulposus cells retards intervertebral disc degeneration: an in vitro and in vivo experimental study. J Orthop Res 2000;18:988.

121. Anderson DG, Albert TJ, Fraser JK, et al. Cellular therapy for disc degeneration. Spine (Phila Pa 1976) 2005;30:S14.

122. Gruber HE, Johnson TL, Leslie K, et al. Autologous intervertebral disc cell implantation: a model using Psammomys obesus, the sand rat. Spine (Phila Pa 1976) 2002;27:1626.

123. Ganey T, Libera J, Moos V, et al. Disc chondrocyte transplantation in a canine model: a treatment for degenerated or damaged intervertebral disc. Spine (Phila Pa 1976) 2003;28:2609.

124. Rajasekaran S, Venkatadass K, Naresh Babu J, et al. Pharmacological enhancement of disc diffusion and differentiation of healthy, ageing and degenerated discs: results from in-vivo serial post-contrast MRI studies in 365 human lumbar discs. Eur Spine J 2008;17:626.

125. Rajasekaran S, Babu JN, Arun R, et al. ISSLS prize winner: a study of diffusion in human lumbar discs: a serial magnetic resonance imaging study documenting the influence of the endplate on diffusion in normal and degenerate discs. Spine (Phila Pa 1976) 2004;29:2654.

126. Bydder GM. New approaches to magnetic resonance imaging of intervertebral discs, tendons, ligaments, and menisci. Spine (Phila Pa 1976) 2002;27:1264.

127. Gatehouse PD, Bydder GM. Magnetic resonance imaging of short T2 components in tissue. Clin Radiol 2003;58:1.

128. Pfirrmann CW, Metzdorf A, Zanetti M, et al. Magnetic resonance classification of lumbar intervertebral disc degeneration. Spine (Phila Pa 1976) 2001;26: 1873.

129. Yoon TS, Su Kim K, Li J, et al. The effect of bone morphogenetic protein-2 on rat intervertebral disc cells in vitro. Spine (Phila Pa 1976) 2003;28:1773.

130. Kim DJ, Moon SH, Kim H, et al. Bone morphogenetic protein-2 facilitates expression of chondrogenic, not osteogenic, phenotype of human intervertebral disc cells. Spine (Phila Pa 1976) 2003;28:2679.

131. Gilbertson L, Ahn SH, Teng PN, et al. The effects of recombinant human bone morphogenetic protein-2, recombinant human bone morphogenetic protein-12, and adenoviral bone morphogenetic protein-12 on matrix synthesis in human annulus fibrosis and nucleus pulposus cells. Spine J 2008;8:449.

132. Wallach CJ, Sobajima S, Watanabe Y, et al. Gene transfer of the catabolic inhibitor TIMP-1 increases measured proteoglycans in cells from degenerated human intervertebral discs. Spine (Phila Pa 1976) 2003;28:2331.

133. An HS, Takegami K, Kamada H, et al. Intradiscal administration of osteogenic protein-1 increases intervertebral disc height and proteoglycan content in the nucleus pulposus in normal adolescent rabbits. Spine (Phila Pa 1976) 2005;30:25.

134. Imai Y, An H, Thonar E, et al. Co-injected recombinant human osteogenic protein-1 minimizes chondroitinase ABC-induced intervertebral disc degeneration: an in vivo study using a rabbit model. Trans Orthop Res Soc 2003;28:1143.

135. Huang KY, Yan JJ, Hsieh CC, et al. The in vivo biological effects of intradiscal recombinant human bone morphogenetic protein-2 on the injured intervertebral disc: an animal experiment. Spine (Phila Pa 1976) 2007;32:1174.

136. Wei A, Williams LA, Bhargav D, et al. BMP13 prevents the effects of annular injury in an ovine model. Int J Biol Sci 2009;5:388.

.

Index

Note: Page numbers of article titles are in **boldface** type.

A

Adjacent level disk disease, **529–541**
  causes of, 533–535
  incidence of, 529–533
  predisposing factors for, 529
Adjacent segment degeneration (ASD), **529–541**
  after lumbosacral fusion
    clinical studies on, 530–532
  causes of, 533–535
  as fusion disease, 537–538
  fusion technique and, 535–536
  incidence of, 529–533
  laminectomy and, 536
  protection from
    nonfusion technology in, 537
  risk factors for, 535–537
  sagittal balance and, 536–537
  TDR and, 548
Adjacent segment facet joint loads
  ASD due to, 534–535
Adjacent segment intervertebral motion
  ASD due to, 533–534
Adjacent segment Intradiskal pressure
  ASD due to, 534
Annulus fibrosus
  in IVD degeneration, 488
  IVD function and, 450–451
ASD. See Adjacent segment degeneration (ASD)

B

Back pain
  incidence of, 501
  low. See Low back pain
BAK-cage supported anterior fusion, 546
Behavioral therapy
  in chronic low back pain management, 519
Biologic therapies
  in IVD nutrition, 472–473
Blood supply
  to disk cells, 465–466

C

Cartilaginous endplate
  IVD function and, 452–453
  in supply of nutrients to disk cells, 466–467
Catabolic mediators
  in IVD degeneration, 585–586

Central sensitization
  in chronic low back pain, 517
Charité disk, 546
Contrast agents
  diffusion of
    in IVD degeneration, 505–506
Cytokine(s)
  anabolic effects on IVD cells, 586
  disk degeneration and, 453–454

D

Degenerative disk disease
  genetics in, 522–523
  maladaptive pain coping in, 522
  management of, **513–528**
  prognosis of, 522–523
Degenerative states
  ECM homeostasis and, 453–455
Disk cell engineering
  described, 576–577
Dual energy x-ray absorptiometry (DXA) scan
  prior to TDR, 547
DXA scan. See Dual energy x-ray absorptiometry (DXA) scan

E

ECM. See Extracellular matrix (ECM)
Environment
  disk cells interacting with, 455
Enzyme(s)
  in IVD degeneration, 585–586
Exercise therapy
  in chronic low back pain management, 519
Extracellular matrix (ECM)
  homeostasis of
    degenerative states and, 453–455
    IVD degeneration and, 585
  IVD function and, 450–453
Extracellular matrix (ECM) protein
  changes in
    in disk degeneration, 454–455

F

Facet joint osteoarthritis
  TDR and, 548
FlexiCore Disk, 546

Orthop Clin N Am 42 (2011) 603–606
doi:10.1016/S0030-5898(11)00087-3
0030-5898/11/$ – see front matter © 2011 Elsevier Inc. All rights reserved.

orthopedic.theclinics.com

G

Gene therapy
  for IVD degeneration, **563–574**
    described, 564–565
    disk cell biology modulation in, 566–567
    gene delivery strategy in, 566
    genetic transfer of therapeutic genes in,
      568–570
    pathologic gene expression regulation in,
      570–571
    safety considerations in, 571–572
    vectors in, 565–566
  to IVDs, 567
Genetics
  in chronic low back pain, 522–523
  in degenerative disk disease, 522–523
  human
    genome projects for, 481
    of lumbar disk degeneration, **479–486**. See also
      Lumbar disk degeneration, genetics of
Genome projects
  for human genetics, 481
Genotyping technologies, 481–482
Growth factors
  anabolic effects on IVD cells, 586

H

High-resolution magic angle spinning (HR-MAS)
  nuclear magnetic resonance (NMR) spectroscopy
  in IVD degeneration, 506–510
Homeostasis
  of ECM
    degenerative states and, 453–455
    IVD degeneration and, 585
HR-MAS NMR spectroscopy. See High-resolution
  magic angle spinning (HR-MAS) nuclear magnetic
  resonance (NMR) spectroscopy

I

Injection therapeutics
  in chronic low back pain management, 520–521
  for IVD degeneration, 592–596
    in clinical trials, 594–596
    considerations for, 594
    effects on pain, 592–593
    limitations of, 594
Intervertebral disk (IVD)
  biology of, **447–464**
  cellular microenvironment of, 555
  components of, 501–502
  degenerative components of
    material properties of, 487–488
  described, 448–449, 501
  development of, 449
  function of, 501

ECM and, 450–453
research on
  stem cell applications in, 556
solutes transport into
  direct visualization of, 468
stem cell regeneration of, **555–562**. See also
  Stem cell(s); Stem cell regeneration
stem cell transplantation into, 558–560
structural organization of, 449–450
structure of, **447–464**
Intervertebral disk (IVD) cells
  blood supply to, 465–466
  cytokines effects on
    anabolic effects of, 586
  disease states associated with, 455–457
  growth factors effects on
    anabolic effects of, 586
  interaction with environment, 455
  maintenance of, 455–457
  stem cells as feeder cells to, 556–557
  supply of nutrients to
    from blood vessels, 466
    cartilaginous endplate in, 466–467
    factors influencing rate of, 465–467
  viability and activity of
    extracellular nutrient-metabolite milieu in,
      468–472
    cell metabolism in regulation of, 469–470
    measured nutrient-metabolite
      concentrations in, 470
    modeling nutrient concentrations in,
      470–472
Intervertebral disk (IVD) degeneration
  biomechanics of, **487–499**
    degenerative changes in structural properties
      of motion segment, 488–490
    instability of lumbar spine and, 491–493
    instability of motion segment associated
      with, 490
  catabolic mediators and enzymes in, 585–586
  characteristics of, 502
  in chronic low back pain, 514–516
  components of
    material properties of, 487–488
  cytokines and, 453–454
  described, 502
  development of, 447–448
  diagnostic tools and imaging methods in, **501–511**
    diffusion of contrast agents, 505–506
    MRI diffusion measurements, 505
    MRI for biomechanical assessment, 506
    NMR spectroscopy, 506–510
    quantitative MRI, 504–505
  ECM protein changes in, 454–455
  gene therapy for, **563–574**. See also Gene
    therapy, for IVD degeneration
  homeostasis of ECM and, 585

intradiskal therapeutics for, 586–592
low back pain due to, 447
matrix metalloproteinase and, 453–454
molecular therapy for, **585–601**. *See also*
   Molecular therapy, for IVD degeneration
nutrient transport failure and, 467–468
pathophysiology of, 563–564
tissue engineering for, **575–583**. *See also* Tissue
   engineering, for IVD degeneration
Intervertebral disk (IVD) matrix
   diffusion through, 467
Intervertebral disk (IVD) nutrition, **465–477**
   biologic therapies in, 472–473
Intervertebral disk (IVD) phenotype
   inducing stem cells toward, 557–558
Intradiskal therapeutics
   for IVD degeneration, 586–592
IVD. *See* Intervertebral disk (IVD)

K

Kineflex Disk, 546

L

Laminectomy
   ASD related to, 536
Low back pain
   adverse effects of, 479
   chronic
      central sensitization in, 517
      disk degeneration in, 514–516
      genetics in, 522–523
      maladaptive pain coping in, 522
      management of, 517–522
         behavioral therapy in, 519
         exercise therapy in, 519
         initial clinical assessment in, 518
         injection therapy in, 520–521
         multidisciplinary rehabilitation in, 519–520
         pain medication in, 518–519
         surgical, 521–522
      prognosis of, 522–523
   consequences of, 447
   described, 513
   factors contributing to, 479
   IVD degeneration and, 447
   management of, 447
   prevalence of, 479
   types of, 513
Lumbar disk degeneration
   genetics of, **479–486**
      candidate gene studies in, 483
      current and future trends in, 483–484
         increasing sample size, 484
         marker selection and analysis, 483
         study design, 483–484

findings on, 483
genome projects for, 481
genotyping technologies, 481–482
human genome for studies of, 481
study strategies, 482–483
   linkage and association strategies, 482–483
phenotype of
   defining of, 480–481
Lumbar spine
   instability of
      IVD degeneration associated with, 491–493

M

Magnetic resonance imaging (MRI)
   for biomechanical assessment
      in IVD degeneration, 506
   quantitative
      in IVD degeneration, 504–505
Magnetic resonance imaging (MRI) diffusion
   measurements
      in IVD degeneration, 505
Magnetic resonance imaging (MRI) spectroscopy
   in IVD degeneration, 506–510
Matrix metalloproteinase
   disk degeneration and, 453–454
Maverick disk, 546
Molecular therapy
   for IVD degeneration, **585–601**
      emerging techniques
         injection therapeutics, 592–596. *See also*
            Injection therapeutics, for IVD
            degeneration
         intradiskal therapeutics, 586–592
      in vitro effects of, 588–589
      in vivo effects of, 590
Motion segment
   instability of
      IVD degeneration associated with, 490
   structural properties of
      degenerative changes in
         IVD degeneration associated with, 488–490
MRI. *See* Magnetic resonance imaging (MRI)

N

Nuclear magnetic resonance (NMR) spectroscopy
   in IVD degeneration, 506–510
Nucleus pulposus
   in IVD degeneration, 487–488
   IVD function and, 451–452
Nutrient(s)
   supply to disk cells
      factors influencing rate of, 465–467
      failure of
         disk degeneration associated with,
           467–468

Nutrition
    IVD, **465–477**. *See also* Intervertebral disk (IVD)
        nutrition

O

Osteoarthritis
    facet joint
        TDR and, 548

P

Pain
    back
        incidence of, 501
        low. *See* Low back pain
        injection therapeutics for IVD degeneration effects
            on, 592–593
Paracetamol
    in chronic low back pain management, 518–519
Prodisc Prosthesis, 546
Prosthetic total disk replacement, **543–554**.
    See also Total disk replacement (TDR)
Protein
    ECM
        changes in
            in disk degeneration, 454–455

Q

Quantitative MRI
    in IVD degeneration, 504–505

R

Rehabilitation
    multidisciplinary
        in chronic low back pain management,
            519–520

S

Sagittal balance
    TDR effects on, 548
Spectroscopy
    HR-MAS NMR
        in IVD degeneration, 506–510
    MRI
        in IVD degeneration, 506–510
    NMR
        in IVD degeneration, 506–510
Spinal fusion
    complication rates associated with, 543
    described, 543
Sporting activities

after TDR, 549
Stem cell(s)
    endogenous
        in adult IVD
            defining of, 556
        as feeder cells to IVD cells, 556–557
        inducing toward IVD phenotype, 557–558
        induction from other organs, 556
        in IVD research, 556
        transplantation into IVD, 558–560
Stem cell regeneration
    of IVD, **555–562**
        future of, 560–561
        limitations of, 560

T

TDR. *See* Total disk replacement (TDR)
THR. *See* Total hip replacement (THR)
Tissue engineering
    for IVD degeneration, **575–583**
        described, 575–577
        engineering disk microenvironment, 577–579
        perspectives on, 579–580
        problems related to, 579–580
        toward whole disk engineering, 579
Total disk replacement (TDR)
    age as factor in, 547
    alternatives to, 549
    anatomic segments effects on, 547
    ASD and, 548
    complications associated with, 545, 547
    costs related to, 546
    described, 543–544
    disk pathology effects on, 546–547
    DXA scan prior to, 547
    facet joint osteoarthritis and, 548
    previous surgery effects on, 547
    prognostic factors related to, 549
    prosthetic, **543–554**
        Pasteur's motto in, 544–545
        randomized controlled trials related to,
            545–549
        research solutions related to, 545–549
    reoperations after, 547–548
    sagittal balance and, 548
    sporting activities after, 549
Total hip replacement (THR)
    "skunk work" in, 544
Transplantation
    of stem cells
        into IVD, 558–560

United States Postal Service

Statement of Ownership, Management, and Circulation
(All Periodicals Publications Except Requestor Publications)

1. Publication Title	2. Publication Number	3. Filing Date
Orthopedic Clinics of North America	9 5 0 - 9 2 0	9/16/11

4. Issue Frequency	5. Number of Issues Published Annually	6. Annual Subscription Price
Jan, Apr, Jul, Oct	4	$269.00

7. Complete Mailing Address of Known Office of Publication (Not printer) (Street, city, county, state, and ZIP+4®)

Elsevier Inc.
360 Park Avenue South
New York, NY 10010-1710

Contact Person
Stephen Bushing

Telephone (Include area code)
215-239-3688

8. Complete Mailing Address of Headquarters or General Business Office of Publisher (Not printer)

Elsevier Inc., 360 Park Avenue South, New York, NY 10010-1710

9. Full Names and Complete Mailing Addresses of Publisher, Editor, and Managing Editor (Do not leave blank)

Publisher (Name and complete mailing address)

Kim Murphy, Elsevier, Inc., 1600 John F. Kennedy Blvd. Suite 1800, Philadelphia, PA 19103-2899

Editor (Name and complete mailing address)

David Parsons, Elsevier, Inc., 1600 John F. Kennedy Blvd. Suite 1800, Philadelphia, PA 19103-2899

Managing Editor (Name and complete mailing address)

Barbara Cohen-Kligerman, Elsevier, Inc., 1600 John F. Kennedy Blvd. Suite 1800, Philadelphia, PA 19103-2899

10. Owner (Do not leave blank. If the publication is owned by a corporation, give the name and address of the corporation immediately followed by the names and addresses of all stockholders owning or holding 1 percent or more of the total amount of stock. If not owned by a corporation, give the names and addresses of the individual owners. If owned by a partnership or other unincorporated firm, give its name and address as well as those of each individual owner. If the publication is published by a nonprofit organization, give its name and address.)

Full Name	Complete Mailing Address
Wholly owned subsidiary of	4520 East-West Highway
Reed/Elsevier, US holdings	Bethesda, MD 20814

11. Known Bondholders, Mortgagees, and Other Security Holders Owning or Holding 1 Percent or More of Total Amount of Bonds, Mortgages, or Other Securities. If none, check box. ☑ None

Full Name	Complete Mailing Address
N/A	

12. Tax Status (For completion by nonprofit organizations authorized to mail at nonprofit rates) (Check one)
The purpose, function, and nonprofit status of this organization and the exempt status for federal income tax purposes:
☐ Has Not Changed During Preceding 12 Months
☐ Has Changed During Preceding 12 Months (Publisher must submit explanation of change with this statement)

PS Form 3526, September 2007 (Page 1 of 3 (Instructions Page 3)) PSN 7530-01-000-9931 **PRIVACY NOTICE**: See our Privacy policy in www.usps.com

---

13. Publication Title			14. Issue Date for Circulation Data Below
Orthopedic Clinics of North America			July 2011

15. Extent and Nature of Circulation			Average No. Copies Each Issue During Preceding 12 Months	No. Copies of Single Issue Published Nearest to Filing Date
a. Total Number of Copies (Net press run)			1838	1600
b. Paid Circulation (By Mail and Outside the Mail)	(1)	Mailed Outside-County Paid Subscriptions Stated on PS Form 3541. (Include paid distribution above nominal rate, advertiser's proof copies, and exchange copies)	604	569
	(2)	Mailed In-County Paid Subscriptions Stated on PS Form 3541 (Include paid distribution above nominal rate, advertiser's proof copies, and exchange copies)		
	(3)	Paid Distribution Outside the Mails Including Sales Through Dealers and Carriers, Street Vendors, Counter Sales, and Other Paid Distribution Outside USPS®	517	552
	(4)	Paid Distribution by Other Classes Mailed Through the USPS (e.g. First-Class Mail®)		
c. Total Paid Distribution (Sum of 15b (1), (2), (3), and (4))		►	1118	1121
d. Free or Nominal Rate Distribution (By Mail and Outside the Mail)	(1)	Free or Nominal Rate Outside-County Copies Included on PS Form 3541	49	54
	(2)	Free or Nominal Rate In-County Copies Included on PS Form 3541		
	(3)	Free or Nominal Rate Copies Mailed at Other Classes Through the USPS (e.g. First-Class Mail)		
	(4)	Free or Nominal Rate Distribution Outside the Mail (Carriers or other means)	49	54
e. Total Free or Nominal Rate Distribution (Sum of 15d (1), (2), (3) and (4))		►	1164	1175
f. Total Distribution (Sum of 15c and 15e)		►	674	425
g. Copies not Distributed (See instructions to publishers #4 (page #3))			1818	1600
h. Total (Sum of 15f and g)		►		
i. Percent Paid (15c divided by 15f times 100)			96.05%	95.40%

16. Publication of Statement of Ownership

☐ If the publication is a general publication, publication of this statement is required. Will be printed in the October 2011 issue of this publication. ☐ Publication not required

17. Signature and Title of Editor, Publisher, Business Manager, or Owner

Stephen R. Bushing
Stephen R. Bushing - Inventory/Distribution Coordinator

Date September 16, 2011

I certify that all information furnished on this form is true and complete. I understand that anyone who furnishes false or misleading information on this form or who omits material or information requested on the form may be subject to criminal sanctions (including fines and imprisonment) and/or civil sanctions (including civil penalties).

PS Form 3526, September 2007 (Page 2 of 3)

Moving?

Make sure your subscription moves with you!

To notify us of your new address, find your **Clinics Account Number** (located on your mailing label above your name), and contact customer service at:

Email: journalscustomerservice-usa@elsevier.com

800-654-2452 (subscribers in the U.S. & Canada)
314-447-8871 (subscribers outside of the U.S. & Canada)

Fax number: 314-447-8029

Elsevier Health Sciences Division
Subscription Customer Service
3251 Riverport Lane
Maryland Heights, MO 63043

*To ensure uninterrupted delivery of your subscription, please notify us at least 4 weeks in advance of move.